Sjögren's Syndrome
A Clinical Handbook

Sjögren's Syndrome
A Clinical Handbook

Frederick B. Vivino, MD, MS, FACR

Chief
Division of Rheumatology
Penn Presbyterian Medical Center, Philadelphia
Pennsylvania
United States

Director
Penn Sjögren's Center, Philadelphia
Pennsylvania
United States

ELSEVIER

Elsevier
Radarweg 29, PO Box 211, 1000 AE Amsterdam, Netherlands
The Boulevard, Langford Lane, Kidlington, Oxford OX5 1GB, United Kingdom
50 Hampshire Street, 5th Floor, Cambridge, MA 02139, United States

Sjögren's Syndrome

Notices
Practitioners and researchers must always rely on their own experience and knowledge in evaluating and using any information, methods, compounds or experiments described herein. Because of rapid advances in the medical sciences, in particular, independent verification of diagnoses and drug dosages should be made. To the fullest extent of the law, no responsibility is assumed by Elsevier, authors, editors or contributors for any injury and/or damage to persons or property as a matter of products liability, negligence or otherwise, or from any use or operation of any methods, products, instructions, or ideas contained in the material herein.

ISBN: 978-0-323-67534-5

Publisher: Dolores Meloni
Acquisition Editor: Nancy Duffy
Editorial Project Manager: Samantha Allard
Production Project Manager: Sreejith Viswanathan
Cover Designer: Alan Studholme

Working together
to grow libraries in
developing countries

www.elsevier.com • www.bookaid.org

To Virginia and Jerome, my greatest sources of support; to Warren who got me interested in Sjögren's syndrome; and to my other colleagues who have taught me a lot.

Contents

CHAPTER 9   Sjögren's syndrome: peripheral and autonomic nervous system involvement................................ 153

David S. Younger, MD, MPH, MS

CHAPTER 10   Diagnosis and management of central nervous system Sjögren's syndrome................... 189

Pantelis P. Pavlakis, MD, PhD, Theresa Lawrence–Ford, MD, Shalini Mahajan, MD, Janet Lewis, MD, Arun Varadhachary, MD, Ianna Briggs, Elisabeth Goldberg, LMFT, Daniel J. Wallace, MD, FACP, MACR and Steven Mandel, MD

CHAPTER 11   Treatment of Sjögren's syndrome internal organ manifestations and constitutional symptoms 211

Rana Mongroo, MD, Bivin Varghese, MD and Steven Carsons, MD

Contributors

Richard F. Ambinder, MD, PhD
Professor of Oncology, Department of Oncology, Johns Hopkins University School of Medicine, Baltimore, MD, United States

Alan N. Baer, MD
Professor of Medicine, Division of Rheumatology, Department of Medicine, Johns Hopkins University School of Medicine, Baltimore, MD, United States

Matthew L. Basiaga, DO, MSCE
Senior Associate Consultant, Mayo Clinic, Rochester, MN, United States

Ianna Briggs
PLLC, Research Assistant, Neurology, Zuckerberg School of Medicine, New York City, NY, United States

Vatinee Y. Bunya, MD, MSCE
Assistant Professor, Cornea & External Disease, Ophthalmology, Scheie Eye Institute, Perelman School of Medicine at the University of Pennsylvania, Philadelphia, PA, United States

Steven Carsons, MD
Professor of Medicine, Chief, Division of Rheumatology, Allergy & Immunology, Department of Medicine, New York University Long Island School of Medicine, Mineola, NY, United States

Eliza F. Chakrabarty, MD, MPH
Arthritis & Clinical Immunology Program, Oklahoma Medical Research Foundation, Oklahoma City, OK, United States; Department of Medicine, College of Medicine, University of Oklahoma Health Sciences Center, Oklahoma City, OK, United States

Robert I. Fox, MD, PhD
Chief, Rheumatology Division, Scripps-XiMED Medical Center, La Jolla, CA, United States

Carla M. Fox, RN
Scripps-XiMED Medical Center, Clinic Administrator, La Jolla, CA, United States

Michael D. George, MD, MSCE
Assistant Professor of Medicine, Division of Rheumatology, University of Pennsylvania Perelman School of Medicine, Philadelphia, PA, United States

Elisabeth Goldberg, LMFT
PLLC, Research Assistant, Neurology, Zuckerberg School of Medicine, New York City, NY, United States

John A. Gonzales, MD
Francis I. Proctor Foundation and Department of Ophthalmology, University of California, San Francisco, CA, United States

Katherine M. Hammitt, MA
Vice President of Medical and Scientific Affairs, Sjögren's Foundation, Reston, VA, United States

Chadwick R. Johr, MD
Co-Director, Penn Sjögren's Center, Assistant Professor of Clinical Medicine, Rheumatology, Penn Presbyterian Medical Center, University of Pennsylvania Perelman School of Medicine, Philadelphia, PA, United States

Adriane Kilar, DMD
Massachusetts Institute of Technology, Cambridge, MA, United States

Theresa Lawrence–Ford, MD
Medical Director, CEO, Rheumatology, North Georgia Rheumatology Group, Gwinnett County, GA, United States

Yiu Tak Leung, MD, PhD
Assistant Professor, Department of Internal Medicine, Division of Rheumatology, Thomas Jefferson University Hospital, Philadelphia, PA, United States

Janet Lewis, MD
Associate Professor, Chief, Division of Rheumatology, University of Virginia, Charlottesville, VA, United States

Scott M. Lieberman, MD, PhD
Associate Professor of Pediatrics, Stead Family Children's Hospital and Carver College of Medicine, University of Iowa, Iowa City, IA, United States

Shalini Mahajan, MD
Assistant Professor, Department of Neurology, Cedars Sinai Medical Center Los Angeles, CA, United States

Steven Mandel, MD
Clinical Professor of Neurology, Donald and Barbara Zucker School of Medicine at Hofstra/Northwell, Lenox Hill Hospital, New York City, NY, United States

Mina Massaro-Giordano, MD
Assistant Professor, Cornea & External Disease, Ophthalmology, Scheie Eye Institute, Perelman School of Medicine at the University of Pennsylvania, Philadelphia, PA, United States

Rana Mongroo, MD
Fellow in Rheumatology, Division of Rheumatology, Allergy & Immunology, Department of Medicine, New York University Long Island School of Medicine, Mineola, NY, United States

Ghaith Noaiseh, MD
Associate Professor of Medicine, Division of Allergy, Clinical Immunology and Rheumatology, University of Kansas, Kansas City, KS, United States

Stephen E. Orlin, MD
Assistant Professor, Cornea & External Disease, Ophthalmology, Scheie Eye Institute, Perelman School of Medicine at the University of Pennsylvania, Philadelphia, PA, United States

Athena Papas, DMD, PhD
Distinguished Professor, Johansen Professor of Dental Research, Head of the Division Oral Medicine Department of Diagnostic Sciences, Tufts University School of Dental Medicine, Boston, MA, United States

Pantelis P. Pavlakis, MD, PhD
Assistant Attending, Department of Neurology, Hospital for Special Surgery, New York, NY, United States

Nora Sandorfi, MD
Associate of Medicine, Division of Rheumatology, University of Pennsylvania Perelman School of Medicine, Philadelphia, PA, United States

R. Hal Scofield, MD
Member, Arthritis & Clinical Immunology Program, Oklahoma Medical Research Foundation, Oklahoma City, OK, United States; Professor, Department of Medicine, College of Medicine, University of Oklahoma Health Sciences Center, Oklahoma City, OK, United States; Staff Physician, Associate Chief of Staff for Research, Medical Service, United States Department of Veterans Affairs Medical Center, Oklahoma City, OK, United States

Mabi L. Singh, DMD, MS
Associate Professor, Div. of Oral Medicine, Department of Diagnostic Sciences, Tufts University School of Dental Medicine, Boston, MA, United States

Sara M. Stern, MD
Assistant Professor of Pediatrics, University of Utah School of Medicine, Salt Lake City, UT, United States

Michael E. Sulewski, MD
Assistant Professor, Cornea & External Disease, Ophthalmology, Scheie Eye Institute, Perelman School of Medicine at the University of Pennsylvania, Philadelphia, PA, United States

Steven Taylor, MBA
CEO, Sjögren's Foundation, Reston, VA, United States

Arun Varadhachary, MD
Associate Professor of Neurology, Washington University School of Medicine in St. Louis, Saint Louis, MO, United States

Bivin Varghese, MD
Fellow in Rheumatology, Division of Rheumatology, Allergy & Immunology, Department of Medicine, New York University Long Island School of Medicine, Mineola, NY, United States

Frederick B. Vivino, MD, MS, FACR
Chief, Division of Rheumatology, Penn Presbyterian Medical Center, Director, Penn Sjögren's Syndrome Center, Professor of Clinical Medicine, University of Pennsylvania Perelman School of Medicine, Philadelphia, PA, United States

Daniel J. Wallace, MD, FACP, MACR
Associate Director, Rheumatology Fellowship Program, Board of Governors, Cedars-Sinai Medical Center, Professor of Medicine, David Geffen School of Medicine at UCLA, Los Angeles, CA, Unites States

David S. Younger, MD, MPH, MS
Department of Clinical Medicine, CUNY School of Medicine at City College, Graduate School of Public Health and Health Policy, City University of New York, New York, NY, United States

Preface

As medical history informs us, Sjögren's syndrome (SS) is now well over 100 years old but continues to pose significant diagnostic and therapeutic challenges for rheumatologists and other specialists. As the title implies *Sjögren's Syndrome: A Clinical Handbook* was written for clinicians. It was intended to be concise, easy to read, and to offer practical information on SS management.

A conscious effort was made to avoid exhaustive literature reviews and focus mainly on the most important clinical questions that every practitioner struggles with on a daily basis. The information herein is based on current clinical practice guidelines, other medical literature, and, whenever necessary, expert opinion. This book is formatted such that any reader can open any chapter, peruse the section headings, and immediately recognize the relevant content. This information will quickly inform rheumatologists, primary care physicians, ophthalmologists, optometrists, oral medicine specialists, dentists, neurologists, nurse practitioners, and other providers on current standards of care. In some instances the same topic is discussed and referenced in more than one chapter to provide more in-depth information.

In addition to the basic information every clinician should know, there are numerous novel highlights that are unique to this book. In the first chapter, we take a whirlwind tour of SS history dating back to the early case reports of the 1880s and are led to the present day to help us understand current problems and future directions. Chapter 2 provides an expanded differential diagnosis of the *sicca syndrome*, discusses the differences between classification and diagnostic criteria, and offers practical advice on SS diagnosis in the clinical setting. The third chapter contains numerous illustrations and an excellent discussion of oral pathophysiology that provides the necessary background for the proper diagnosis and treatment of various oral medicine problems. The chapter on ophthalmology (Chapter 4) provides a detailed review of published clinical practice guidelines for SS dry eyes, describes the risks of ocular surface surgery in SS, and discusses the problem of corneal neuropathies. Chapter 5 on childhood SS represents one of the most comprehensive and practical reviews on this subject that has been written thus far.

The middle part of this book focuses on the extraglandular manifestations that cause the most significant morbidity and mortality in SS. The sixth chapter contains a concise but thorough review of major constitutional symptoms/internal organ manifestations and numerous useful summary tables that provide a wealth of information at a glance. Chapter 7 provides a thorough, clinically oriented review of small and medium vessel vasculitis in SS, with further emphasis on vasculitis as a marker of disease severity and prognosis, especially when associated with cryoglobulinemia. Chapter 8 represents one of the most detailed and comprehensive reviews of lymphoproliferative disease in SS written to date, with special emphasis on lymphoma predictors and models as well as the pathophysiologic changes that characterize the transition from autoimmunity to malignancy.

The discussion of neurologic SS was purposely split into two parts. Chapter 9 provides an important, practical clinical overview of peripheral, cranial, and autonomic neuropathies in SS as well as a thoughtful discussion on the application and utility of various neurodiagnostic studies. In a similar fashion the 10th chapter tackles the ever challenging topic of central nervous system (CNS) SS and describes its relationship to other closely related CNS disorders including neuromyelitis optica and multiple sclerosis. Chapter 11 provides a state-of-the-art summary of treatment algorithms for the systemic and internal organ manifestations of SS, including a review of newly published clinical practice guidelines for the management of fatigue, musculoskeletal pain, and the use of biological therapy in this disease.

The last section of this clinical handbook covers several new and important topics that are rarely discussed in the SS literature. Chapter 12 presents a highly rigorous review of evidence-based complementary and alternative medicine, including recommendations on when it can be used for the treatment of SS. The 13th chapter provides much needed information on perioperative management strategies, including the dosing of immunosuppressive medications before and after surgery in order to prevent postoperative complications in the SS patient. Given the growing interest in using biological therapy and other immunosuppressive medications for SS, Chapter 14 on vaccines is very timely and gives practical advice on vaccine safety and efficacy based on the limited experience in SS and existing information for lupus and rheumatoid arthritis. Finally, we end with a very interesting chapter that discusses the value of social support in patients with chronic illness. Chapter 15 makes a very convincing argument that almost every SS patient would benefit from joining the national support group, the Sjögren's Foundation, Inc.

It is my sincere belief that the use of *Sjögren's Syndrome: A Clinical Handbook* will take the mystery out of SS diagnosis and management by providing clinicians with timely, practical information that can be utilized in daily practice. In my clinical experience, when informed practitioners work together as part of a multidisciplinary team for SS, we can not only improve outcomes in individual patients but also, more importantly, raise the overall standards of care. Hopefully, this book will move us closer toward that goal.

Frederick B. Vivino, MD, MS
Director, Penn Sjögren's Syndrome Center
Chief, Division of Rheumatology
Penn Presbyterian Medical Center
Professor of Clinical Medicine
University of Pennsylvania Perelman School of Medicine
Frederick.Vivino@pennmedicine.upenn.edu

Sjögren's syndrome: past, present, and future

Robert I. Fox, MD, PhD[1], Carla M. Fox, RN[2]

[1]*Chief, Rheumatology Division, Scripps-XiMED Medical Center, La Jolla, CA, United States;*
[2]*Scripps-XiMED Medical Center, Clinic Administrator, La Jolla, CA, United States*

Perspective

Sjögren's syndrome (SS) is a chronic autoimmune, rheumatic disorder most commonly characterized by dryness of eyes and mouth due to lymphocytic infiltration of the lacrimal and salivary glandular tissues. The condition has "benign" features that include dryness as well as vague myalgias, fatigue, and cognitive changes. These features are still poorly understood and treated. The benign symptoms represent the impact of the inflammatory process on the immune, neural, hormonal, and vascular signals necessary for normal secretory function or cognitive processes. In addition, SS patients have specific extraglandular manifestations affecting the renal, pulmonary, neural (both central and peripheral), hematopoietic, lymphatic, cardiac, and gastrointestinal systems.[1] Although there are clear overlaps with systemic lupus erythematosus (SLE), rheumatoid arthritis (RA), and scleroderma, there are also clear differences (serologic, clinical, pathogenic) that distinguish these disorders.

It is worth noting that in a multicenter study from excellent academic centers, the majority of patients with dry eyes due to SS were initially misclassified as having either SLE or RA based largely on the finding of a positive result in antinuclear antibody (ANA) or rheumatoid factor analysis.[2] This initial mislabeling of SS as another diagnosis deprives patients of adequate follow-up for their particular ocular and oral complications, as well as of the proper attention to the particular extraglandular manifestations that SS patients develop. It also hinders the enrollment in clinical trials of SS patients with significant extraglandular manifestations who may benefit from biological therapies but may still be sitting in pulmonary, renal, or hematology clinics undiagnosed or misdiagnosed.

Key points
- *"Benign" features such as fatigue, myalgias, cognitive dysfunction, and dryness are poorly understood.*
- *A variety of extraglandular manifestations occur that overlap with SLE, RA, and scleroderma.*

Sjögren's Syndrome. https://doi.org/10.1016/B978-0-323-67534-5.00001-6

SS has a worldwide distribution, and interestingly, the genomic associations differ in distinct ethnic groups, even though the histologic features of the tissue biopsies and epitopes recognized by autoantibodies show great similarities.[3–5] Comparison of genetic and nongenetic factors in these different groups may help find the common pathways important in clinical symptoms.

There are also important geographic differences that are associated with differences in clinical manifestations among various SS populations. For example, studies have shown that pulmonary arterial hypertension (PAH) in Chinese and Korean cohorts is more prevalent in SS and SLE patients than in those with scleroderma. However, we have many Chinese and Korean SS patients in the United States, and our registries do not reflect this shift in PAH incidence.[6] This type of comparison may lead the way to identify environmental factors that trigger PAH in people of different genetic backgrounds.

Key points
- *SS is frequently misdiagnosed as SLE or RA.*
- *Genomic associations differ in different ethnic groups.*
- *Geographic differences are associated with differences in disease manifestations.*

Brief review of the past—as "we only stand on the shoulders of past giants"

Early history

The traditional paragraph on the "history" of SS starts with Mikulicz, in 1892, describing a neck mass in a man with lymphocytic infiltrates and myoepithelial islands.[7] The term *Mikulicz syndrome* was used to describe the affected patients until the 1920s when it was subsequently discarded, as it failed to distinguish SS from other lymphocytic infiltrative processes such as tuberculosis and lymphoma.[8] Ironically, the recent recognition of the *IgG4 syndrome* (which occurs predominantly in men of this age and parallels Mikulicz's description) suggests that the original view of SS and Mikulicz syndrome as "identical disorders" was indeed incorrect.[9]

In retrospect, one of the earliest and most convincing descriptions of SS was given by a British physician, W. B. Hadden, who presented a case to his colleagues at the Clinical Society of London on March 9, 1888 (Fig. 1.1).[10] Dr. Hadden described a 65-year-old woman who was admitted to the hospital with a 7-month history of progressive dry mouth associated with dysphagia and the need to constantly drink fluids. As Dr. Hadden related, 2 months earlier "she had the occasion to cry but no tears would come." On examination, the patient was well appearing and her vital signs were normal. The only notable finding was the mouth; he recounted that "nearly all her teeth are wanting" and "the tongue was red, devoid of epithelium, and cracked in all directions like a crocodile's skin."

TRANSACTIONS

OF

THE CLINICAL SOCIETY

OF

LONDON.

VOLUME THE TWENTY-FIRST.

LONDON:
LONGMANS, GREEN, AND CO.
1888.

XXXVI.—*On "Dry Mouth," or Suppression of the Salivary and Buccal Secretions. By W. B. HADDEN, M.D. Read March 9, 1888.*

THE patient was a widow, æt. 65, who came under my care at St. Thomas's Hospital on December 1, 1887.

There was nothing of importance to note in the family history. With the exception of an attack of shingles nine years previously, and an attack of facial erysipelas six years later, she had been healthy until the onset of the present illness.

She stated that about seven months before she came under my notice her mouth gradually began to get dry, and that the dryness had steadily increased. To relieve the discomfort caused by the want of natural moisture she had to be constantly sipping fluid. She complained, too, that the act of swallowing was difficult and often painful. There was no history of the prolonged use of belladonna.

FIGURE 1.1

Dr. Hadden's case of dry mouth.

The patient spent 2 weeks in the hospital for observation and other diagnostic measures of the day. Finally, at the conclusion of the observation period, the decision was made to treat her with a medicinal remedy (tincture of jaborandi) administered both orally and subcutaneously. The patient responded and continued this therapy as an outpatient. Interestingly, the active ingredient in tincture of jaborandi, pilocarpine, was FDA-approved in tablet form some 110 years later as the first prescription drug for SS known as Salagen®.

In 1933, an ophthalmologist named HENRIK SJÖGREN (Fig. 1.2) described a constellation of ocular and oral dryness and arthritis in a large group of patients as part of his ophthalmology doctoral thesis in Scandinavia.[11] The present author had the honor to meet an elderly Dr. Sjögren in 1986 (at the time of the first International Symposium on Sjögren's Syndrome in Denmark)[12] shortly before his death at the age of 87 years from the complications of a stroke.

As an incentive to young researchers, it is important to note that Dr. Sjögren recounted how his thesis was given a poor grade and he was banished from academia to a remote region of Scandinavia to practice ophthalmology. He sustained himself during this "exile" and retained his "sanity" only by playing the piano until his early work was "rediscovered." This rediscovery occurred after translation of his thesis into English 10 years later, followed by a series of articles in the 1950s, beginning with a widely read *New England Journal* Clinical Pathology Conference by Drs. Morgan and Bloch.[13] Of importance, the basic clinical and pathologic features that we recognize today were clearly described in a study of 62 patients by Bloch et al. in 1956.[14] In 1957, Dr. Sjögren received well-deserved recognition, becoming an associate professor, docent, at the University of Gothenburg, and in 1965, the Swedish government honored him with the title of professor.

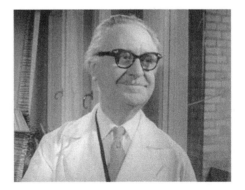

FIGURE 1.2

Dr. Sjögren at home during the twilight of his career.

The pioneers

In the United States, the next major steps in SS were presented in a large series of papers by Norman Talal et al. mainly during the 1960s and 1970s.[15–22] Equally important, Talal trained an entire generation of postdoctoral fellows, initially at the National Institutes of Health and later in San Francisco where he worked closely with outstanding members of the dental school, such as Greenspan and Daniels.[23–25] These former "postdoctoral fellows" and collaborators have formed the nucleus of SS research centers across the world, including teams in Japan led by Sugai and Miyasaka[26] and Saito and Tsubota.[27]

Talal also provided the scientific backing to the patient organization the Sjögren's Syndrome Foundation, Inc. (SSF) that allowed the clinical recognition and validation of SS as a disease with significant morbidity and the reception and input of SS patients into their unmet needs. Of course, other groups in the United States were entering the field such as Provost[28] and Tan and Reichlin (whose contributions are described later), whose postdoctoral fellows would also establish a central network of SS care and research.

Meanwhile in Europe, outstanding groups of researchers were forming study groups and research clinical centers of excellence for SS, including the groups led by Jonsson,[29] Manthorpe and Oxholm,[30,31] Konttinen,[32] Bombardieri and Vitali,[33] and Tzioufas, Mavragani, and Moutsopoulos.[34] The establishment of registries by Ramos-Casals and others[35] expanded our knowledge of disease manifestations, and the work by Mariette and colleagues led to renewed interest in clinical trials and outcome measures.[36]

In India, vibrant research sprang up in major cities under the direction of Sharma[37] and Agrawal and Pandya.[38] In China, centers of excellence were established by Chen[39] and Dong and Zhang[40] and were expanded by Guo.[41] As a tribute to these leaders, each of these centers has remained a leading center of SS clinical practice and research.

Although many other pioneers have not been listed here, the point is that a vibrant community of SS clinical and research excellence had been "seeded" by these researchers and was now ready to flourish with new approaches and new vitality.

Key points
- *Mikulicz's disease is now considered a manifestation of the IgG4 syndrome.*
- *Sjögren was not the first physician to describe SS but the first to provide a comprehensive description in a large group of patients.*
- *During the 1960s and 1970s, Talal and trainees created a legacy of interest in SS that spread to encompass almost the entire globe.*

Looking backward at the SS-A and SS-B autoantigens

The examination of autoantibodies and cloning of autoantigens relevant to SS was first performed by Tan in San Diego[42,43] and Reichlin (in Buffalo and later Oklahoma)[44,45] mostly during the 1980s. His team used a technique called immunodiffusion with serum from patients who had the initials "Ro" or "La." Although Dr. Reichlin was the first to find the association between "Ro" and "La" antibodies and the particular HLA-DR (human leukocyte antigen) genes in both SLE and SS patients, the work of Tan and the more powerful national autoantibody reference center at The Scripps Research Institute (TSRI) in San Diego led to our current use of the nomenclature "Sjögren's syndrome-associated antigen"(SS-A). The antibody recognizes an antigen that is actually composed of two different proteins of size 60 kDa and 52 kDa and RNA. (Full disclosure requires that I identify that Eng Tan was my Chairman upon my arrival at Scripps.) Dr. Tan and his team used these autoantibodies to "clone" the relevant cellular antigen using a technique called phage display library.

Key points
- *Reichlin and colleagues first noted the association between anti-Ro/La and certain HLA-DR genes.*
- *Tan and coworkers cloned the Ro antigen and coined the term anti-SS−A.*

Two interesting findings emerged quickly. First, the human autoantibodies were often directed at the active or binding site of the host protein. This is described later in which the antibody would bind at the same site where a virus might "find a home" and may have provided a way for the cell to protect itself.

Also, the particular autoantigens invariably possessed an unusual amino acid sequence such that they could resist the normal proteolytic digestion that comes with cell death (necrosis or apoptosis). In cellular terms, this meant that they lacked "caspase enzyme digestion sites" and could remain stably on the dying cell's surface in an "apoptotic" bleb. This resilience of the autoantigen and its ability to bind to the chaperone molecule (which contained single- and double-stranded RNA sequences) made it an ideal molecule to start a vicious cycle of autoimmunity in a person with the correct genetic predisposition (i.e., HLA-DR sequence).

A great deal of attention in the diagnostic criteria and pathogenesis is paid to the antibodies to the SS-A antigen, so it is worthy of a brief note to outline the history of this important cellular protein and its normal role. In 1983, striking similarities were noted between an adenovirus-associated RNA (VAI and VAII) and two small Epstein-Barr virus−encoded RNAs transcribed by RNA polymerase III. All these viral RNAs were "noncoding" but were found to coprecipitate with the anti-La protein[46] from SLE sera.[47] The Ro and La antigens were believed to bind to a tRNA-like structure that belonged to a family called hYRNA and serve as molecular chaperones.

Similar to the Victorian chaperone, a molecular chaperone escorted the relevant RNA to the correct and intended location within the cell, while protecting it from "degrading" circumstances. These chaperones also play a role in the control of transcription of DNA by interaction with chromatin and other initiation factors.

In patients who are genetically predisposed to a series of genes that regulate antibody production (particularly HLA-DR antigens and interferon regulatory genes), antibodies to SS-A may be present in "asymptomatic" individuals many years before any clinically detectable SS.[48] However, other genetic as well as environmental factors are also important for clinical disease expression.[48] For example, in an early study of identical twins by Reichlin, only three out of seven SS-A-positive twins both developed autoimmunity (i.e., concordance), whereas the remaining four remained normal during a 15-year follow-up (discordant for SLE or SS).[49] Similarly, a majority of SS-A-positive women who had fetuses with SS-A-related neonatal heart block did not develop SS[50] during many years of follow-up. Given the other hormonal factors and the microenvironment of the salivary or lacrimal glands (which are rich in growth factors and neural stimulatory signals), a self-perpetuating cycle of inflammation requires additional stimuli to develop and paralyze glandular function. Furthermore, these results instruct us that the finding of antibodies to SS-A in clinical screening does not always equate to a diagnosis of SS.

Key points
- *Anti-SS-A/SS-B recognize antigens that act as molecular chaperones for RNA and play a role in DNA transcription.*
- *Genetic, hormonal, and environmental factors play a role in the etiopathogenesis of SS.*
- *Not every anti-SS—A-positive patient will develop SS.*

Questions for the present
Classification and diagnosis

In the "present" section of this introductory chapter, an important advance to emphasize is the recent improvements in the classification criteria for SS[51] that are necessary for basic research, clinical trials by industry, and designation of endpoints by FDA regulators. These criteria and the guidelines for diagnostic testing suggested by both the European League Against Rheumatism (EULAR) and the American College of Rheumatology (ACR) are the subjects of Chapter 2 in this book. Despite these achievements, however, it is recognized that further modifications of these criteria will be required in the future, and subsets of patients with SS will likely need to be defined by genetic markers, other biomarkers, or other modalities such as ultrasonography.

In recent years, recruitment for clinical trials has led to increased awareness of SS among both physicians and patients. The aforementioned guidelines were developed to facilitate the identification of uniform groups of patients for research trials but by default are frequently used as diagnostic criteria by clinicians as well. However, in practice, rheumatologists rarely get minor salivary gland biopsies,[2] and both university and community pathologists rarely interpret them according to uniform guidelines.[52] This has led to an excessive reliance on the antibody to SS-A as a diagnostic test and a lack of understanding of the variables surrounding both false-positive and false-negative antibody test results. We know that a large subset of

SS patients (about one in three) will be seronegative and that failure to perform a biopsy in this group will miss diagnoses. Conversely, based on population studies, "false-"positive antibodies to the SS-A antigen also exist, and many of these individuals will not develop SS.

Additionally, other autoantibodies are described in SS that have diagnostic or prognostic value but are not routinely tested. For example, patients with antibodies that recognize the centromere-c antigen (anti-centromere antibodies) may exhibit some features of limited scleroderma in addition to SS, including an increased prevalence of Raynaud's phenomenon, and these antibodies may occur in up to 13% of SS patients.[53]

Key points
- *New classification criteria have advanced the research agenda.*
- *Additional biomarkers and/or new imaging studies are needed to move SS research to the next level.*
- *Excessive reliance on the results of serologic testing may lead to erroneous or missed diagnoses in SS.*

Clinical trials

The present is also dominated by numerous "failed" clinical trials. But it is not really fair to say the results represent true failure. In the recent studies of biological therapies, for example, we have gathered subjects with "benign" and "extraglandular" manifestations into a single group hoping to find differences after treatment in single or composite endpoints, with the goal of obtaining eventual FDA approval. The majority of SS patients enrolled in these studies do not have extraglandular disease, and the cohort is dominated by patients with "benign" symptoms. In a world of "personalized" medicine, we must evaluate particular manifestations and their response to therapy. By analogy, treatments for diabetic neuropathy approved by the FDA do not require that the underlying problem of diabetes or its multiple symptoms be eliminated. Of note, all the medications approved for SS to date have been studied with the focus on SS as a "single organ" disease.

Etiology and pathogenesis

Although the essential clinical features of SS (including its spectrum of autoantibodies and pathologic conditions) were outlined by Bloch et al. in 1956, we still really do not understand the underlying cause of SS. Its epidemiologic pattern suggests that both genetic and nongenetic factors (e.g., environmental or epigenetic modifications) play a role. Additionally, as SS is largely a disease of women, hormonal factors and Toll receptors (located on the X chromosome) must be important. The bimodal age of expression suggests the importance of hormonal changes that act either directly or indirectly on the normal processes of failed "tolerance" that characterize autoimmune diseases.

A common misconception is that the dryness of SS results entirely from destruction of the glands. Although parenchymal loss from apoptosis of glandular epithelial cells plays a role, histologic studies by researchers such as Roland Jonsson and Konttinen et al.[54–56] showed that even in patients with little or no saliva production, the majority of ductal/acinar structures as well as their innervation remain detectable. Apparently, the inflammatory microenvironment of cytokines and metalloproteinases prevents the orientation and functional activity of the residual secretory glands.[57,58] Thus glandular function depends on the temporal integration of neural and vascular signals in a precise pattern that can lead to secretory function.[58]

In ophthalmology, the importance of a "functional circuit" that links the unmyelinated afferents that go to the lacrimal nucleus in cranial nerve V, and then, subsequently, to the various parts of the cerebral cortex, is a relatively new concept described by Stern et al.[59,60] The components of the tear film and its stability were elaborated by Pflugfelder[61] and Dartt[57,62] who emphasized the additional role of the meibomian glands. The recognition that we must look at the entire "functional unit" as a goal for the future is really setting the "holy grail" for the next decade of dry eye research and may be applicable to other aspects of the disease. This approach should help us better understand the interface of the immune system, neural system, and hypothalamic axis.

Clinical challenges

There is a diminutive sound to the term "benign symptoms" in SS, as patients still struggle with dry eyes and dry mouth (Chapters 3 and 4) and both these symptoms can significantly compromise quality of life (Chapter 15). Dry eye symptoms continue to be the most common cause of patient distress in SS, and some studies suggest dry/painful eyes are now the most common cause for visits to ophthalmologists in the United States and United Kingdom.[63,64] The cost of medical evaluations and the myriad of over-the-counter "moisturizing" eye drops filling multiple pharmacy shelves reflect the scope of this problem and account for well over $175 billion in healthcare costs.[64] Medical economic analysis has recognized that being unable to fully participate at the workplace (a term called lack of "presentness") has a real cost over 5 times the cost of absenteeism.[65]

We live in an era where people increasingly work on computers (screen activity drops blink rate by 80%[66] and exacerbates dry eyes) in highly air-conditioned (low humidity) environments and deal with increasing stress related to economic factors, thus, further decreasing the secretory function by the adrenergic antagonism of cholinergic inputs. Therefore we should not be surprised by the "silent epidemic" that pervades ophthalmology clinics, where ocular discomfort remains among the most common reasons for patient referrals. To treat such volumes, rheumatologists and other providers are being educated to help SS patients deal with eye discomfort (Chapter 4) and are learning new terms such as "tear film instability" and "meibomian gland dysfunction." These conditions must be treated before other ocular lubricants or inflammatory drops can fully work. This is especially important because many rheumatologists will eventually assume the role of a primary care provider for SS patients and not every ophthalmologist or optometrist in the community is interested in dry eyes.

Similarly, dry mouth and its various health consequences continue to impact patients' overall condition. This problem negatively impacts the patient's nutrition (as they turn to "soft foods" high in sugar content), as well as socialization, and may lead to chronic anxiety, isolation, depression, and despair. The SS patient, in frustration, often turns to the Internet (which has become a citadel of misinformation) and sometimes succumbs to SS blogs and misleading "official SS"-appearing websites merchandizing "cures" and worthless products. Systemic therapies for dryness are currently available but limited by cholinergic side effects. Over-the-counter remedies are costly, time-consuming, and only provide transient relief at best. Clearly, better treatments are needed.

Patients may also complain to their rheumatologists of burning mouth and a "flare" of other symptoms in certain clinical situations. This scenario often occurs after treatment of a sinus infection or other infection by the primary care physician with antibiotics. This predisposes to the overgrowth of *Candida* species in the oral cavity and triggers mouth burning, increased oral discomfort, and decreased oral intake due to acute or chronic erythematous candidiasis. Stomatopyrosis and glossodynia make eating unpleasant and further compromise the patient's nutritional status and quality of life. It therefore behooves each and every provider to recognize the signs and symptoms of erythematous candidiasis, which frequently occurs as a complication of SS but can be easily managed (Chapter 3).

Another one of the most devastating and costly oral complications of SS is accelerated caries. SS patients have more caries, tooth extractions, and higher dental expenses over their lifetime than healthy controls.[67,68] Surprisingly, many SS patients, at the time of initial evaluation, receive little attention to this problem even by dental professionals. However, prevention of oral caries needs to become a full-time preoccupation for patients and a major priority for the dentist or oral medicine specialist, rheumatologist, and other members of the care team. The SSF has now published clinical practice guidelines for caries prophylaxis, thus emphasizing the importance of this problem and providing a treatment algorithm to follow.[69] Further research to more precisely define the risk factors for caries is needed.

Consideration of current research in SS will reveal that the "present" is largely dominated by studies on genomics, transcriptomics, and mechanisms of disease. The discoveries that may come from this work will undoubtedly provide the foundation for more targeted therapies in the future, the advent of personalized medicine in SS, and, perhaps, even a cure.

Key points
- *SS patients who have dry mouth often have intact salivary glands, suggesting other mechanisms for dryness besides tissue loss from apoptosis.*
- *Dry eyes and dry mouth are not trivial and can significantly impair quality of life.*
- *SS patients continue to have many unmet needs.*

Looking forward to to the future
Early diagnosis

In terms of future directions, better education of primary care physicians and other specialists on the proper use and interpretation of serologic tests would have an immediate impact on diagnostic accuracy. Given the fact that anti-SS—A positivity is frequently detected in ANA-negative SS patients, proper screening for SS would be best performed using a panel (ANA, anti-SS—A/SS—B). Additionally, if a strong clinical suspicion for SS exists, patients who are seronegative should be routinely referred for a lip biopsy to avoid missing the diagnosis. Finally, as the correlation between the severity of ocular and oral symptoms and the results of objective tests for dry eyes and dry mouth is often poor,[70,71] the clinician must always remember to pursue the entire diagnostic workup for SS in the appropriate clinical situation even in the absence of sicca symptoms. This is especially important when considering SS as a diagnosis in patients who present with extraglandular manifestations (e.g., peripheral or central nervous system SS) (Chapters 9 and 10) because, at the time of initial evaluation, sicca symptoms in this group are frequently minimal or nil. Thus for now, until a new diagnostic test with greater sensitivity and specificity is discovered, every patient deserves a comprehensive, systematic, multidisciplinary evaluation for SS in order to ensure a timely diagnosis.

Precision medicine and unmet needs

In the era of precision medicine, it is time to use a personalized medicine approach for SS and recognize that a variety of therapies such as the use of rituximab and abatacept and other treatments have indeed proven efficacious for extraglandular manifestations in certain SS patients.[72] The "one-size-fits-all approach" to treat SS has hindered care and should be abandoned.

Future advances in pharmacogenomics, epigenetics, cytokine research, or the discovery of other novel biomarkers will allow us to match specific therapies to specific patients and will lead to more cost-effective utilization of resources and, hopefully, greater availability of these treatments to SS patients down the road. Developments in this field should be greatly accelerated by the use of "artificial intelligence." Additionally, more clinical practice guidelines from the SSF and other organizations should be available to guide our therapeutic strategies.

A personalized medicine approach will also help us better focus our attention on the many unmet needs of this population. More aggressive treatment of "benign" and highly prevalent manifestations such as dry eyes, dry mouth, fatigue, and cognitive changes will not only significantly improve patient quality of life but also lower medical and dental costs related to common long-term complications.

The classification and treatment of neurologic signs and symptoms (both central and peripheral) as well as lymphoproliferative manifestations (Chapter 8) also remain significant challenges. To meet these needs, we will need to gain a better understanding of the interface of the various immune, endocrine, and neurologic factors that contribute to the pathogenesis of SS.

The full realization of precision medicine will be further accelerated by progress in genetic studies and, with the use of artificial intelligence, also enable future risk profiling for life-threatening complications (see Chapters 6−10). For example, the discovery of an association between mutations of the A20/TNFAIP3 gene and the development of mucosa-associated lymphoid tissue marginal zone B-cell lymphomas[73] in SS will undoubtedly stimulate more research in this area and may lead, in the future, to the first screening tests for lymphomas in SS.

Clinical trials

Advances in SS research using DNA and RNA sequencing[74] have already revealed fascinating cytokine and chemokine mechanisms that are associated with extraglandular manifestations and have led to an expanded panel of therapeutic targets in SS. We must therefore strengthen our partnership with the pharmaceutical industry and continue our concerted efforts to develop novel therapeutics for SS, including biological therapies that can halt the progression of the disease and/or prevent lymphoproliferation and its life-threatening manifestations.

Although past clinical trials of immunotherapies for SS have yielded disappointing results so far, we can learn from past mistakes. To achieve better outcomes, we need to enroll greater numbers of patients who not only meet the new classification criteria but also have extraglandular manifestations, as this group will most likely show short-term benefit from biologics. We must rethink entry criteria and avoid long washout periods from other treatments that leave patients vulnerable to disease progression and flares. Although a longer enrollment period would be required, in the long run, it may be more fruitful to study organ-specific (e.g., arthritis, interstitial lung disease) endpoints rather than composite endpoints. Quality-of-life endpoints should also be incorporated in all future trials, as these may prove to be the most efficacious way to demonstrate the value of a novel therapy.

Patients with "benign" symptoms are quite common and therefore easy to enroll in studies as a separate group. However, we need better efforts at screening for comorbidities such as depression or fibromyalgia that could influence trial results whenever endpoints such fatigue, pain, or cognitive dysfunction are studied. A multidisciplinary approach to the development of specific treatments for specific symptoms will drive this process. Longitudinal evaluation of patients with "benign disease" is also needed to determine the disease course and whether the parameters we study are valid endpoints. Although many challenges lie ahead, once the first therapeutic agent is FDA approved the floodgates will open.

Interdisciplinary care and future directions

Until a cure for SS is discovered, improved interdisciplinary cooperation between ophthalmology, rheumatology, oral medicine, neurology, and other specialties should be pursued in order to establish a multispecialty network for improved care. When considering the complexity of problems that these patients face, it would also seem logical to ask the rheumatologist to assist the family doctor in the role as primary care provider. Further reimbursement from healthcare insurers for cognitive services and coordination of care would help this model to flourish.

In moving forward, we also need to consider new paradigms of pathogenesis. Perhaps, we should view the immune system as the body's "sixth sense," as it sends lymphocytes out to the periphery to sense viral infections or apoptotic debris. We know that lymphocytes possess a full repertoire of neural actions, and an important part of the immune function may be to report back to the brain about the "situation in the remote provinces." Furthermore, as the patterns of cortical distribution of visual and oral signals have now been validated and biologically mapped, further study of the central nervous system may provide additional insight for a better understanding of key patient problems.

Through the millennium of Darwinian evolution, the importance of vision and taste has selected the neural and vascular innervation of the eye and mouth. Exploring this relationship may help solve many SS mysteries.

This intriguing book engages the expertise of multiple authors from various disciplines to define the most significant clinical problems in SS, and provides practical up-to-date advice to guide healthcare providers on disease management. More importantly, it extends the dialogue among multiple medical subspecialists, basic researchers, pathologists, and oral medicine specialists, all of whom contribute to the care of these patients. It also provides a basic vocabulary as we move into a most exciting next decade where we expect to see significant advances in our knowledge of the pathogenesis, epidemiology, and treatment of SS using a multidisciplinary research approach.

Key points
- *Multidisciplinary care and a "precision medicine" approach will define the future.*
- *Understanding SS requires a better understanding of the interactions between the immune system and neuroendocrine pathways.*

Conclusions

The origins of SS in Western medicine date back to the late 19th century, and concepts regarding the etiology and pathogenesis of SS continue to evolve. Despite the discovery of marker autoantibodies for SS in the 1980s, and more recent improvements in the classification criteria, the identification of SS in the early stages of the disease remains quite challenging. Progress in therapeutics has lagged even further behind, and there are currently many unmet clinical needs. A greater emphasis on a multidisciplinary approach toward diagnosis and management and the advent of personalized medicine will significantly impact patient care. Ultimately, better stratification of patient subsets by biomarkers and a greater understanding of the interplay between the immune and neuroendocrine systems, as well as other disease mechanisms, will facilitate the future development of more targeted therapies and, perhaps, one day, even a cure.

Acknowledgement

We are truly grateful to have Dr. Robert Fox share his almost 40 years of experience in the field of Sjögren's syndrome to provide perspective in this opening chapter on where we have been, the problems that we struggle with today, and where we are headed in the future. Dr. Fox graciously omitted any mention of his own accomplishments in the discussion but is indeed considered one of the greatest American pioneers in the field. His work in the laboratory and expertise as a clinician and educator has taught countless others, myself included, a lot about Sjögren's syndrome.

References

1. Fox R. Extraglandular manifestations of Sjogren's syndrome (SS): dermatologic, arthritis, endocrine, pulmonary, cardiovascular, gastroenterology, renal, urology, and gynecologic manifestations. In: Fox R, Fox C, eds. *Sjogren's Syndrome: Practical Guidelines to Diagnoses and Therapy.* New York City, NY: Springer; 2011.
2. Rasmussen A, Radfar L, Lewis D, Grundahl K, Stone DU, Kaufman CE, Rhodus NL, Segal B, Wallace DJ, Weisman MH, Venuturupalli S, Kurien BT, Lessard CJ, Sivils KL, Scofield RH. Previous diagnosis of Sjögren's Syndrome as rheumatoid arthritis or systemic lupus erythematosus. *Rheumatol.* 2016;55(7):1195−1201.
3. Wong Q, Levine DM, McHugh C, Laurie C, Doheny K, Lam MY, Baer AN, Challacombe S, Lanfranchi H, Schiødt M, Srinivasan M, Umehara H, Vivino FB, Zhao Y1, Shiboski SC, Daniels TE, Greenspan JS, Shiboski CH, Criswell LA. Genome-Wide association analysis reveals genetic heterogeneity of Sjögren's syndrome according to ancestry. *Arthritis Rheumatol.* 2017;69(6):1294−1305.
4. Fei H, Jiang W, Chen R, Fan L, Xu K. The genotyping of the HLA-D region and specific RFLP patterns for Chinese Han population. *Chin J Med Genet.* 1994;20:75−85.
5. Kang H-I, Fei HM, Saito I, Sawada S, Chen SL, Yi D, Chan E, Peebles C, Bugawan TL, Erlich HA. Comparison of HLA class II genes in Caucasoid, Chinese, and Japanese patients with primary Sjögren's syndrome. *J Immunol.* 1993;150:3615−3623.
6. Fox R. The incidence of pulmonary hypertension is higher in systemic lupus and Sjögren's patients than in scleroderma patients in China. *Lupus.* June 2018;27(7):1051−1052.
7. Mikulicz JH. Uber eineeigenartige symmetrische Erkrankung der Tranen- und Mundspeicheldrusen. In: Billroth GT, ed. *Beitr. Chir. Fortschr..* 1892:610−630. Stuttgart.

8. Morgan WS. The probable systemic nature of Mikulicz's disease and its relation to Sjögren's syndrome. *N Eng J Med.* 1954;251:5–9.
9. [9a] Stone JH, Zen Y, Deshpande V. IgG4-related disease. *N Engl J Med.* 2012;366(6): 539–551.[9b] Bombardieri M, De Vita S, Dörner T, Ramos-Casals M, Tzioufas A. Meeting report highlights of the 14th International symposium on Sjögren's syndrome. *Clin Exp Rheumatol.* 2018;36(112):S3–S13.
10. Hadden WB. *On "dry mouth," or Suppression of the Salivary and Buccal Secretions.* In: *Transactions of the Clinical Society of London.* Volume the 21st. Longmans: Green and Co. London; 1888:176–179.
11. Sjögren HS. Zur kenntnis der keratoconjunctvitis sicca (Keratitis folliformis be i hypofunktion der tranendrusen). *Acta Opthalmol (Copenh).* 1933;2:1–151.
12. MANTHORPE R, et al. *Proceedings of 1st International Seminar on Sjögren's -Syndrome 1986.* Copenhagen, May, 1986-Foreword. N-0608 Oslo, Norway: Scandinavian University Press Po Box 2959 Toyen, Journal Division Customer Service; 1986.
13. Morgan WS. The probable systemic nature of Mikulicz's disease and its relation to Sjögren's syndrome. *N Engl J Med.* 1954;251(1):5–10.
14. Bloch K, Buchanan W, Wohl M, Bunim J. Sjögren's syndrome: a clinical, pathological and serological study of 62 cases. *Medicine (Baltim).* 1956;44:187–231.
15. Talal N. Sjogren syndrome and pseudolymphoma. *Hosp Pract.* 1988;23(9A), 71-75, 78-80.
16. Talal N, Asofsky R, Lightbody P. Immunoglobulin synthesis by salivary gland lymphoid cells in Sjögren's syndrome. *J Clin Invest.* 1979;19:19.
17. Daniels T, Silverman S, Michalski J, Greenspan J, Sylvester R, Talal N. The oral component of Sjögren's syndrome. *Oral Surg.* 1975;39:875–885.
18. Anderson LG, Talal N. The spectrum of benign to malignant lymphoproliferation in Sjogren's syndrome. *Clin Exp Immunol.* 1972;10(2):199–221.
19. Kaltreider H, Talal N. The neuropathy of Sjögren's syndrome. Trigeminalnerve involvement. *Ann Int Med.* 1969;70(4):751–762.
20. Talal N, Zisman E, Schur P. Renal tubular acidosis, glomerulonephritis and immunologic factors in Sjögren's syndrome. *Arthritis Rheum.* 1968;11:774–780.
21. Talal N, Sokoloff L, Barth W. Extrasalivary lymphoid abnormalities in Sjögren's syndrome. *Am J Med.* 1967;43:50–55.
22. Talal N, Bunim J. The development of malignant lymphoma in Sjogren's syndrome. *Am J Med.* 1964;36:529.
23. Daniels TE, Powell M, Sylvester R, Talal N. An evaluation of salivary scintigraphy in Sjögren's syndrome. *Arthritis Rheum.* 1979;22:809–814.
24. Greenspan J, Daniels T, Talal N, Sylvester R. The histopathology of Sjögren's syndrome in labial salivary gland biopsies. *Oral Surg Oral Med Oral Pathol.* February 1974;37(2): 217–229.
25. Cremer N, Daniels T, Oshiro L, Marcus F, Claypool R, Sylvester R, Talal N. Immunological and virological studies of cultured labial biopsy cells from patients with Sjögren's syndrome. *Clin Exp Immunol.* 1974;18:213–224.
26. Ogawa N, Ogawa N, Ping L, Zhenjun L, Takada Y, Sugai S. Involvement of the interferon-γ–induced T cell–attracting chemokines, interferon-γ–inducible 10-kd protein (CXCL10) and monokine induced by interferon-γ (CXCL9), in the salivary gland lesions of patients with Sjögren's syndrome. *Arthritis Rheum.* 2002;46(10): 2730–2741.

27. Tsubota K, Xu KP, Fujihara T, Katagiri S, Takeuchi T. Decreased reflex tearing is associated with lymphocytic infiltration in lacrimal glands. *J Rheumatol*. 1996;23(2):313−320.

28. Alexander GE, Provost TT, Stevens MB, Alexander EL. Sjögren syndrome Central nervous system manifestations. *Neurology*. 1981;31(11):1391−1396.

29. Jonsson R, Kroneld U, Tarkowski A. Histological and functional features of salivary glands in rheumatic patients with oral sicca symptoms. *Scand J Rheumatol*. 1988;17(5):387−391.

30. Oxholm P, Asmussen K, Axéll T, van Bijsterveld OP, Jacobsson L, Konttinen Y, Manthorpe R, Nederfors T, JU P, Schiødt M. Sjogren's syndrome: terminology. *Clin Exp Rheumatol*. 1995;13(6):693−696.

31. Frost-Larsen K, Isager H, Manthorpe R. Sjogren syndrome treated with bromhexine: a randomized clinical study. *Br Med J*. 1978;(1):1579−1584.

32. Konttinen Y, Törnwall J, Kemppinen P, Uusitalo H, Sorsa T, Hukkanen M, Polak J. Neutral endopeptidase (EC 3.4.24.11) in labial salivary glands in healthy controls and in patients with Sjogren's syndrome. *Ann Rheum Dis*. 1996;55(8):513−519.

33. Vitali C, Bombardieri S, Moutsopoulos HM, Balestrieri G, Bencivelli W, Bernstein RM, Bjerrum KB, Braga S, Coll J, de Vita S, Drosos A, Ehrenfeld M, Hatron P, Hay E, Isenberg D, Janin A, Kalden J, Kater L, Yrjö T, Konttinen Y, Maddison P, Maini R, Manthorpe R, Meyer O, Ostuni P, Pennec Y, Prause J, Richards A, Sauvezie B, Schiødt M, Sciuto M, Scully C, Shoenfeld Y, Skopouli F, Smolen J, Snaith M, Tishler M, Todesco S, Valesini G, Venables P, Wattiaux M, Youinou P. Preliminary criteria for the classification of Sjögren's syndrome. *Arthritis Rheum*. 1993;36:340−347.

34. Pavlidis N, Karsh J, Moutsopoulos H. The clinical picture of primary Sjögren's syndrome: a retrospective study. *J Rheumatol*. 1982 Sep-Oct;9(5):685−690.

35. Ramos-Casals M1, Brito-Zerón P, Solans R, Camps MT, Casanovas A, Sopeña B, Díaz-López B, Rascón FJ, Qanneta R, Fraile G, Pérez-Alvarez R, Callejas JL, Ripoll M, Pinilla B, Akasbi M, Fonseca E, Canora J, Nadal ME, de la Red G, Fernández-Regal I, Jiménez-Heredia I, Bosch JA, Ayala MD, Morera-Morales L, Maure B, Mera A, Ramentol M, Retamozo S, Kostov B, SS Study Group, Autoimmune Diseases Study Group (GEAS) of the Spanish Society of Internal Medicine (SEMI). Systemic involvement in primary Sjogren's syndrome evaluated by the EULAR-SS disease activity index: analysis of 921 Spanish patients (GEAS-SS Registry). *Rheumatology*. February 2014;53(2):321−331.

36. Seror R, Theander E, Brun JG, Ramos-Casals M, Valim V, Dörner T, Bootsma H, Tzioufas A, Solans-Laqué R, Mandl T, Gottenberg JE, Hachulla E, Sivils KL, Ng WF, Fauchais AL, Bombardieri S, Valesini G, Bartoloni E, Saraux A, Tomsic M, Sumida T, Nishiyama S, Caporali R, Kruize AA, Vollenweider C, Ravaud P, Vitali C Mariette X, Bowman SJ, EULAR Sjögren's Task Force. Validation of EULAR primary Sjögren's syndrome disease activity (ESSDAI) and patient indexes (ESSPRI). *Ann Rheum Dis*. May 2015;74(5):859−866.

37. Sandhya P, Sharma D, Vellarikkal SK, Surin K, Jayarajan R, Verma A, Dixit V, Sivasubbu S, Danda D, Scaria V. AB0188 systematic analysis of the oral microbiome in primary SjÖgren's syndrome suggest enrichment of distinct microbes. *Ann Rheum Dis*. 2015;74:953−954.

38. Agrawal S, Srivastava R, Sharma B, Pandya S, Misra R, Aggarwal A. IL1RN* 2 allele of IL-1receptor antagonist VNTR polymorphism is associated with susceptibility to ankylosing spondylitis in Indian patients. *Clinical Rheumatol*. 2008;27(5):573−576.

39. Fox RI, Chen P, Carson DA, Fong S. Expression of a cross reactive idiotype on rheumatoid factor in patients with Sjögren's syndrome. *J Immunol*. 1986;136:477–483.
40. Zhang N, Dong Y. Primary Sjögren's syndrome in the people's Republic of China. In: *Sjögren's Syndrome*. Springer; 1987:55–60.
41. Griffith K, Chan EK, Lung CC, Hamel JC, Guo X, Miyachi K, Fritzler MJ. Molecular cloning of a novel 97 kd golgi complex autoantigen associated with Sjogren's syndrome. *Arth Rheum*. September 1997;40(9):1693–1700.
42. Chan EK, Sullivan KF, Fox RI, Tan EM. Sjögren's syndrome nuclear antigen B (La): cDNA cloning, structural domains, and autoepitopes. *J Autoimmunity*. August 1989; 2(4):321–327.
43. Martinez-Lavin M, Vaughan J, Tan E. Autoantibodies and the spectrum of Sjögren's syndrome. *Ann Intern Med*. 1979;91:185–190.
44. Wasicek C, Reichlin M. Clinical and serological differences between systemic lupus erythematosus patients with antibodies to Ro versus patients with antibodies to Ro and La. *J Clin Invest*. 1982;69(4):835–843.
45. Provost TT, Talal N, Bias W, Harley JB, Reichlin M, Alexander EL, et al. Ro (SS-A) positive Sjogren's/lupus erythematosus (SC/LE) overlap patients are associated with the HLA-DR3 and/or DRw6 phenotypes. *J Invest Dermatol*. October 1988;91(4):369–371.
46. Rosa M, Gottlieb E, Lerner MR, Steitz JA. Striking similarities are exhibited by two small Epstein-Barr virus-encoded ribonucleic acids and the adenovirus-associated ribonucleic acids VAI and VAII. *Mol Cell Biol*. September 1981;1(9):785–796.
47. Moss W, Steitz J. Genome-wide analyses of Epstein-Barr virus reveal conserved RNA structures and a novel stable intronic sequence RNA. *BMC Genomics*. 2013;14(1):543.
48. Jonsson R, Theander E, Sjöström B, Brokstad K, Henriksson G. Autoantibodies present before symptom onset in primary Sjögren syndrome. *J Am Med Assoc*. November 2013; 310(17):1854–1855.
49. Reichlin M, Harley J, Lockshin M. Serologic studies of monozygotic twins with systemic lupus erythematosus. *Arthritis Rheum*. 1992;35(4):457–464.
50. Waltuck J, Buyon J. Autoantibody-associated congenital heart block: outcome in mothers and children. *Ann Intern Med*. 1994;120(7):544–551.
51. Shiboski CH, Seror R, Criswell LA, Labetoulle M, Lietman TM, Rasmussen A, Scofield H, Vitali C, Bowman SJ, Mariette X, International Sjögren's Syndrome Criteria Working Group. 2016 American College of rheumatology/European League against rheumatism classification criteria for primary Sjögren's syndrome: aconsensus and data-driven methodology involving three international patient cohorts. *Arthritis Rheumatol*. 2017;69(1):35–45.
52. Vivino FB, Gala I, Hermann GA. Change in final diagnosis on second evaluation of labial minor salary gland biopsies. *J Rheumatol*. May 2002;29(5):938–944.
53. Gelber AC, et al. Distinct recognition of antibodies to centromere proteins in primary Sjögren's syndrome compared with limited scleroderma. *Ann Rheum Dis*. 2006;65(8): 1028–1032.
54. Tornwall J, Uusitalo H, Hukkanen M, Sorsa T, Konttinen YT. Distribution of vasoactive intestinal peptide (VIP) and its binding sites in labial salivary glands in Sjogren's syndrome and in normal controls. *Clin Exp Rheumatol*. 1994;12(3):287–292.
55. Konttinen Y, Sorsa T, Hukkanen M, Segerberg M, Kuhlefelt-Sundström M, Malmström M, Polak JM. Topology of innervation of labial salivary glands by protein gene product 9.5 and synaptophysin immunoreactive nerves in patients with Sjogren's syndrome. *J Rheumatol*. 1992;19(1):30–37.

56. Konttinen Y, Hukkanen M, Pertti Kemppinen P, Segerberg M, Sorsa T, MalmstrÖM M, Rose S, Itescu S, Polak J. Peptide-containing nerves in labial salivary glands in Sjögren's syndrome. *Arthritis Rheum.* 1992;35:815−820.
57. Zoukhri D, Hodges R, Dartt D. Lacrimal gland innervation is not altered with the onset and progression of disease in a murine model of Sjögren's syndrome. *Clin Immunol Immunopathol.* 1998;89(2):126−133.
58. Konttinen Y, Tensing EK, Laine M, Porola P, Törnwall J, Hukkanen M. Abnormal distribution of aquaporin-5 in salivary glands in the NOD mouse model for Sjogren's syndrome. *J Rheumatol.* 2005;32(6):1071−1075.
59. Stern ME, Gao J, Schwalb TA, Ngo M, Tieu DD, Chan CC, Reis BL, Whitcup SM, Thompson D, Smith JA. Conjunctival T-cell subpopulations in Sjogren's and non-Sjogren's patients with dry eye. *Invest Ophthalmol Vis Sci.* 2002;43(8):2609−2614.
60. Fox R, Stern M. Sjogren's syndrome: mechanisms of pathogenesis involve interaction of immune and neurosecretory systems. *Scand J Rheumatol Suppl.* 2002;(116):3−13.
61. Pflugfelder SC, Huang AJ, Feuer W, Chuchovski PT, Pereira IC, Tseng SC. Conjunctival cytologic features of primary Sjogren's syndrome. *Ophthalmology.* August 1990;97(8):985−991.
62. Contreras-Ruiz L, Ghosh-Mitra A, Shatos MA, Dartt DA, Masli S. Modulation of conjunctival goblet cell function by inflammatory cytokines. *Mediators Inflam.* 2013;2013:636812.
63. Pflugfelder SC. Prevalence, burden, and pharmacoeconomics of dry eye disease. *Am J Manag Care.* 2008;14(3 Suppl. l):S102−S106.
64. Reddy P, Grad O, Rajagopalan K. The economic burden of dry eye: a conceptual framework and preliminary assessment. *Cornea.* 2004;23(8):751−761.
65. Yao W, Le Q. Social-economic analysis of patients with Sjögren's syndrome dry eye in East China: a cross-sectional study. *BMC Ophthalmology.* December 2018;18(1):23.
66. Patel S, Henderson R, Bradley L, Galloway B, Hunter L. Effect of visual display unit use on blink rate and tear stability. *Optom Vis Sci.* November 1991;68:888−892.
67. Christensen L, Petersen PE, Thorn JJ, Schiødt M. Dental caries and dental health behavior of patients with primary Sjögren syndrome. *Acta Odontol Scand.* June 2001;59(3):116−120.
68. Fox P, Bowman S, Segal B, Vivino F, Murukutla N, Choueiri K, Ogale S, McLean L. Oral involvement in primary Sjögren's syndrome. *J Am Dent Assoc.* 2008;139(12):1592−1601.
69. Zero T, Brennan M, Daniels T, Papas A, Stewart C, Pinto A, Al-Hashimi I, Navazesh M, Rhodus N, Sciubba J, Singh M, Wu A, Frantsve-Hawley J, Tracy S, Fox P, Lawrence Ford T, Cohen S, Vivino F, Hammitt K for the Sjogren's Syndrome Foundation Clinical Practice Guidelines Committee. Clinical practice guidelines for oral management of Sjogren disease: dental caries prevention. *JADA.* April 2016;147(4):295−305.
70. Sullivan B, Crews L, Messmer E, Foulks G, Nichols K, Baenninger P, Geerling G, Figueiredo F, Lemp M. Correlations between commonly used objective signs and symptoms for the diagnosis of dry eye disease: clinical implications. *Acta Ophthalmol.* 2014;92:161−166.

71. Shiboski S, Shiboski C, Criswell L, Baer A, Challacombe S, Lanfranchi H, Schiodt M, Umehara H, Vivino F, Zhao Y, Dong Y, Greenspan D, Heidenreich A, Helin P, Kirkham B, Kitagawa K, Larkin G, Li M, Lietman T, Lindegaard J, McNamara N, Sack K, Shirlaw P, Sugai S, Vollenweider C, Whitcher J, Wu A, Zhang S, Zhang W, Geenspan J, Daniels T. American College of Rheumatology Classification Criteria for Sjogren's syndrome, a data driven, expert consensus approach in the Sjogren's international collaborative clinical alliance cohort. *Arthritis Care Res.* 2012;64(4): 475–487.

72. Carsons S, Vivino F, Parke A, Carteron N, Sankar V, Brasington R, Brennan M, Ehlers W, Fox R, Scofield H, Hammitt K, Birnbaum J, Kassan S, Mandel S. Treatment guidelines for rheumatologic manifestations of Sjogren's: use of biologics, management of fatigue, and inflammatory musculoskeletal pain. *Arthritis Care Res.* 2017;89(4):517–527.

73. Nocturne G, Boudaoud S, Miceli-Richard C, Viengchareun S, Lazure T, Nititham J, Taylor KE, Ma A, Busato F, Melki J, Lessard CJ, Sivils KL, Dubost JJ, Hachulla E, Gottenberg JE, Lombès M, Tost J, Criswell LA, Mariette X. Germline and somatic genetic variations of TNFAIP3 in lymphoma complicating primary Sjogren's syndrome. *Blood.* December 12, 2013;122(25):4068–4076.

74. Altorok N, et al. Genome-Wide DNA Methylation patterns in naive CD4+ T cells from patients with primary Sjögren's syndrome. *Arthritis Rheumatol.* 2014;66(3):731–739.

Diagnosis and evaluation of Sjögren's syndrome

Frederick B. Vivino, MD, MS, FACR

Chief, Division of Rheumatology, Penn Presbyterian Medical Center, Director, Penn Sjögren's Syndrome Center, Professor of Clinical Medicine, University of Pennsylvania Perelman School of Medicine, Philadelphia, PA, United States

Challenge of diagnosis

Among the various connective tissue disorders, Sjögren's syndrome (SS) has proven to be one of the most difficult to diagnose. There is typically a 3- to 4-year lag between the onset of symptoms and the time of diagnosis.[1] This phenomenon is related to multiple factors including the insidious onset of symptoms, the heterogeneity of clinical presentations, the lack of universally accepted diagnostic criteria, and a generally decreased awareness of SS when compared with other autoimmune disorders, among both the public and healthcare communities.

Nevertheless, making a correct diagnosis is crucial for several reasons. It is now generally accepted that dry eyes and dry mouth in this particular population are not trivial symptoms and, when unrecognized or untreated, can lead to some devastating and costly medical and dental complications (Table 2.1). SS is a systemic disease that involves the internal organs in roughly 25% of cases (Chapter 6) and can predispose to the development of lymphoproliferative disorders, particularly, non-Hodgkin B-cell lymphomas (Chapter 8).[2−5] SS can also be associated with a variety of other autoimmune disorders (e.g., celiac) that add to its overall morbidity. Consequently, the evaluation and management of any new health

Table 2.1 Complications of untreated dry mouth and dry eyes.

ORAL	OCULAR
Multiple cavities	Corneal melting
Loss of dentition	Corneal ulcers
Weight loss	Corneal perforation
Chronic erythematous candidiasis	Bacterial conjunctivitis
Sialolithiasis	Bacterial interstitial keratitis
Sialostenosis	Vision loss
Sleep deprivation	Photophobia
Fibromyalgia	Corneal neuropathy

Sjögren's Syndrome. https://doi.org/10.1016/B978-0-323-67534-5.00002-8

problem in a patient with suspected SS is frequently delayed or hindered among individuals without an established diagnosis. Finally, SS can significantly decrease patient quality of life and is associated with high costs and a high burden of illness (Chapter 15).[6]

Clinical presentations

In about 80% of SS patients the disease begins with some form of the sicca syndrome (from the Latin *siccus* meaning dry or thirsty) characterized by the gradual onset of dryness of the eyes, mouth, and other body parts that develops over months to years. Among the various scenarios, *keratoconjunctivitis sicca* (dry eyes) followed by other sicca symptoms is the most common clinical presentation.[7] Less frequently, xerostomia can be the presenting feature or sicca symptoms occur simultaneously. In the remaining 20% of cases, an internal organ or extraglandular manifestation will predominate and sicca symptoms may be minimal or nil at the time of initial evaluation. This atypical presentation is particularly common among SS patients who present with a neurologic manifestation (Chapters 9, 10) of the disease.[8] In pediatric patients (Chapter 5), parotitis is the most common presenting manifestation of SS.[9] Thus the spectrum of clinical presentations in SS is quite broad (Table 2.2).

As discussed later the diagnosis of SS is possible even in the absence of characteristic dryness symptoms. As the correlation between the severity of dry eyes and dry mouth and the results of objective tests is generally poor,[10,11] the physician should never be dissuaded from pursuing this diagnosis with further testing in the appropriate clinical situation even when characteristic sicca symptoms are not prominent.

Table 2.2 Spectrum of clinical presentations of Sjögren's syndrome.

Sicca syndrome	Parotitis
Rheumatoid-like arthritis	Multiple cavities
Polymyalgia rheumatica	Interstitial lung disease
Fibromyalgia	Fever of unknown origin
Demyelinating disease	Chronic fatigue syndrome
Peripheral neuropathy	Renal tubular acidosis
Autonomic neuropathy	Elevated ESR or positive ANA or RF in an asymptomatic patient
Inflammatory myositis	
Leukocytoclastic vasculitis	Corneal melt or perforation

ANA, Antinuclear antibody; ESR, Erythrocyte sedimentation rate; RF, Rheumatoid factor.

Approach to diagnosis in the clinical setting

Since the 1960s, at least 13 different sets of diagnostic and/or classification criteria have been proposed to define SS; this process reflects the challenge encountered in identifying SS patients and differentiating them from other groups with similar symptoms.

At present, no universally accepted diagnostic criteria for SS exist. Not surprisingly, physicians and other specialists sometimes use classification criteria (see later discussion) for patient diagnosis by default. This practice, however, can lead to missed diagnoses in early cases unless the provider recognizes that the classification criteria are intended for research purposes and sometimes sacrifice diagnostic sensitivity in favor of increased specificity in order to ensure uniformity of the patient group being studied. Thus a patient could still have early SS but fail to meet the classification criteria. The classification criteria also require that patients be taken off their anticholinergic drugs before measurements for dry eyes and dry mouth are performed. However, in the clinical setting, this practice is not always practical or medically advisable, and seldom done. Therefore the results of these measurements when performed in the office setting should always be interpreted in this context.

All prior attempts at diagnostic and/or classification criteria have always tried to satisfy three basic objectives: (1) documentation of objective evidence of dry eyes, (2) objective evidence of salivary gland involvement, and (3) proof of autoimmunity. Differences in criteria reflect different views of the importance of symptoms for diagnosis, the recommendations for the diagnostic studies needed to satisfy these objectives, and the definitions of abnormal test results. Ultimately, the physician's clinical judgment still remains the gold standard for diagnosis of SS in the practice setting.

Objective assessment of dry eyes

Ocular evaluation (Chapter 4) involves the Schirmer test performed without anesthesia to measure tear production (normal >10 mm/5 min minutes) as well as ocular surface staining with vital dyes (e.g., rose bengal, fluorescein, lissamine green) to look for damage to the corneal and/or conjunctival epithelium caused by dryness. These tests are best performed by a cornea specialist or other eye care provider experienced in the diagnosis and management of dry eyes. Results of staining with a single vital dye can be scored on a 0-9 scale according to the method by Van Bijsterveld.[12] At present, however, combination staining with fluorescein to detect corneal abnormalities and with lissamine green to detect conjunctival defects is considered the most sensitive way to screen for dry eyes. Findings are scored on a 0-12 scale, as described by Whitcher et al.,[13] in order to determine the "ocular surface staining score" (OSS). An OSS of 5 is equivalent to a Van Bijsterveld score of 4. Routine slit lamp examination also includes inspection of the eyelids for blepharitis (a.k.a. *meibomian gland dysfunction*), which may further contribute to ocular discomfort and cause evaporative dry eye in the SS patient.

Objective assessment of salivary gland involvement

Documentation of salivary gland involvement is most easily accomplished by office measurement of a whole mouth unstimulated salivary flow rate. The patient is asked to swallow once and then expectorate into a preweighed container (preferably after a 1-hour fast) for 5 or 15 minutes. The longer collection time can be used to maximize the chances that a specimen will be collected in patients with little or no salivary flow. The volume or weight of saliva produced (1 g saliva = 1 mL) is measured and then divided by the time of collection. A normal result would be $\geq$0.3–0.4 mL/min.[14] However, when SS is defined using classification criteria, a more stringent definition for abnormal result ($\leq$0.1 mL/min) is always used (vide infra).

Alternatively, salivary scintigraphy can easily be performed at any imaging center with nuclear medicine capabilities to screen for salivary hypofunction.[15] The patient is scanned for 60 minutes in the anterior Waters view following an intravenous injection of technetium 99m Tc sodium pertechnetate. Regions of interest are drawn around the parotid glands and submandibular/sublingual complexes in order to generate time-activity curves for each region. Isotope uptake (saliva formation) and spontaneous secretion into the oral cavity (resting function) are measured for each gland. At the 45-minute mark the patient is given a secretagogue (e.g., sugar-free lemon drop) in order to measure the stimulated function. In SS, defects in all three phases of salivary function have been observed.[16,17] Therefore scintigraphy provides not only documentation of salivary gland involvement but also a functional assessment of the salivary glands. Currently, as protocols for salivary scintigraphy are not standardized, the information provided by each study varies according to the expertise of the imaging center that performs it.

B-mode ultrasonography of the major salivary glands with various probes (5-15 MHz) has been utilized to screen for structural changes from chronic inflammation in order to provide objective evidence of salivary gland involvement.[18,19] The findings include inhomogeneity (especially the presence of hypoechoic foci), changes in glandular size, and loss of the posterior borders; various scoring systems have been developed to quantitate the changes.[20] Additionally, an ultrasound-guided core needle biopsy with a high-resolution linear array transducer may now be preferred in place of fine-needle aspiration or an open excisional biopsy as the initial procedure to determine the cause of persistent or localized salivary gland swelling.[21]

Proof of autoimmunity

Further testing to document autoimmunity is mandatory for the diagnosis of SS and helps differentiate this disorder from the other causes of dry eyes and dry mouth. This can be accomplished by serologic testing especially when one of the following three autoantibody patterns is observed: (1) anti-SSA (a.k.a. anti-Ro) positivity, (2) anti-SSA/SSB (a.k.a. anti-La) positivity, or (3) positive rheumatoid factor plus positive antinuclear antibodies $\geq$1:320 (any pattern). Isolated anti-SSB may occur in SS albeit rarely. However, it has been suggested that the majority of these patients do not exhibit the typical SS phenotype and that a positive isolated test result for anti-SSB sometimes occurs as an artifact of the assay process.[22] More recently, three tissue-specific murine autoantibodies (anti-salivary protein I, anti—parotid secretory protein, anti—carbonic anhydrase VI) were described as early disease markers in the interleukin—14α transgenic mouse model for SS.[23] Although these antibodies have been found in humans as well, their value as a diagnostic marker for SS in people has not been proven.

Patients who are seronegative or exhibit isolated anti-SSB positivity should always undergo a labial minor salivary gland biopsy to confirm the diagnosis of SS. This outpatient procedure can be utilized to document either salivary gland involvement or proof of autoimmunity; it is performed by making a small incision under local anesthesia in the lower lip through normal-appearing mucosa. At least four to five minor salivary glands or about 8 mm^2 total glandular area should be removed by blunt dissection to ensure adequate tissue sampling.[24] Hematoxylin and eosin staining characteristically reveals the focal accumulation of mononuclear cells (mostly lymphocytes) around normal-appearing glandular acini or ducts, a.k.a. *focal lymphocytic sialadenitis*. The number of *foci*, i.e., aggregates containing $\geq$50 mononuclear cells (predominantly lymphocytes), is recorded and the tissue surface area is measured using a calibrated eyepiece grid (see Ref. 25 for a detailed method description). Calculation of a *focus score* ([# foci/mm^2 tissue surface area] x 4) is essential for accurate interpretation of the biopsy, as diagnostic mistakes are frequently made.[25] A focus score of $\geq$1/4 mm^2 is the accepted histopathologic definition for salivary gland involvement in SS and is widely utilized in all the recent classification criteria (from 2002 to present) and in the clinical practice setting to facilitate SS classification or diagnosis.[26] In pediatric patients the histologic finding of any focal lymphocytic sialadenitis may be a more appropriate marker for autoimmunity or salivary gland involvement in childhood SS than the adult threshold score of $\geq$1/4 mm^2.[27]

Evolution of the classification criteria

In the research setting classification criteria should always be utilized to define SS. The goal of classification criteria is to define homogeneous populations of patients for clinical trials and other research studies. Currently, different classification criteria are used in different parts of the world to define SS.

In the modern era the first breakthrough occurred in 2002 following the publication of the American—European Consensus Group (AECG) classification criteria by Vitali and coworkers (Table 2.3).[28] These criteria were originally developed in Europe and were widely embraced because they enabled the classification of SS using a combination of symptoms and a wide variety of diagnostic tests. These criteria offered several advantages. They not only permitted a patient to be classified as having SS without a lip biopsy but also provided a pathway for the identification of SS even in patients who lacked sicca symptoms. The AECG criteria also offered case

Table 2.3 The 2002 American–European Consensus Group criteria for the classification of SS.

1. Ocular symptoms (any 1 of 3)

Dry eyes for more than 3 months
Tear use more than tid
Foreign body sensation in eyes

2. Oral symptoms (1 of 3)

Dry mouth for more than 3 months
Swollen salivary glands
Need liquids to swallow

3. Ocular signs (1 of 2)

Unanesthetized Schirmer test $\leq$ 5 mm/5 min O.U.
Positive vital dye staining $\geq$ 4 (rose bengal, fluorescein, or lissamine green)[a]

4. Oral signs (1 of 3)

Abnormal salivary scintigraphy
Abnormal parotid sialography
Abnormal sialometry (unstimulated salivary flow $\leq$ 0.1 mL/min)

5. Positive lip biopsy

Focal lymphocytic sialadenitis (focus score $\geq$ 1/4 mm^2)

6. Positive anti-SSA and/or anti-SSB antibodies

Exclusions: Prior head and neck irradiation, hepatitis C infection, graft-versus-host disease, acquired immune deficiency syndrome, preexisting lymphoma, sarcoidosis, or use of anticholinergic medications within a period of <4 half-lives of the drug.

Classification as **primary SS** requires **4 of 6 criteria including #5 or 6.**

Classification as **secondary SS** requires **established connective tissue disease** plus **one sicca symptom (#1 or 2)** plus **2 of 3 the objective tests for dry eyes and mouth (#3-5).**

Classification as SS can also be made in patients with **no sicca symptoms** if **3 of 4 objective criteria** are fulfilled (#3-6).

SS, *Sjögren's syndrome.*
[a] *Scale 0–9* [12].
Adapted from Ref. 28.

definitions for both primary SS (i.e., SS that occurs without another connective tissue disorder) and secondary SS (SS that develops later in the course of an established connective disease such as rheumatoid arthritis or lupus).

In 2012, an alternative set of classification criteria derived from data gathered through the international SS tissue registry (Sjögren's International Collaborative Clinical Alliance [SICCA]) were developed in the United States by Shiboski and colleagues,[11] and later came to be known as the ACR (American College of Rheumatology)-SICCA

Table 2.4 The 2012 ACR-SICCA criteria for the classification of SS.

1. **Serologic**: +SSA **or** SSB **or** +RF/ANA $\geq$ 1:320 (any pattern)
2. **Histologic**: +Biopsy with focal lymphocytic sialadenitis (focus score$\geq$1/4 mm^2)
3. **Ocular signs**: Ocular surface staining score[a]$\geq$3 in one eye (fluorescein and lissamine green)

Classification as **primary SS** requires fulfilling two of the three criteria.

Exclusions: Prior head and neck irradiation, hepatitis C infection, graft-versus-host disease, acquired immune deficiency syndrome, sarcoidosis, amyloidosis, IgG4-related disease.

ACR, *American College of Rheumatology;* ANA, *Antinuclear antibody;* RF, *Rheumatoid factor;* SICCA, *Sjögren's International Collaborative Clinical Alliance;* SS, *Sjögren's syndrome.*
[a] *Scale 0–12* [13].
Adapted from Ref. 11.

criteria.[11] The new criteria facilitated the classification of primary SS based entirely on results from objective tests and were simpler to follow (Table 2.4). These criteria did not offer a case definition for secondary SS as the authors suggested that this distinction may now be obsolete. Both criteria perform well in studies and demonstrate approximately $\geq$90% sensitivity and specificity for the classification of SS.[29]

Subsequently, under the auspices of the two major rheumatology professional organizations, the ACR and the European League Against Rheumatism (EULAR), a concerted effort was made to promote the uniformity of the classification criteria used around the world. In 2016 an international group of SS experts developed a hybrid model derived from the best parts of the 2002 and 2012 criteria. The new 2016 ACR-EULAR classification criteria for primary SS have been endorsed by both professional societies and proposed as the new gold standard to be used in research studies to define SS.[30] (Table 2.5).

The 2016 criteria can be applied to any individual with suspected SS who has dry eye or dry mouth symptoms as defined in 2002 [28] or an extraglandular manifestation of the disease as detailed by the EULAR Sjögren's Syndrome Disease Activity Index (ESSDAI).[31] The 2016 criteria assign different weights to 5 different tests according to the perceived level of importance. Among the various autoantibodies produced in SS, only the anti-SSA (a.k.a. anti-Ro) antibody is included because this blood test is considered the most specific for the disease. A positive lip biopsy, as defined earlier, is also weighted with equal importance. The two tests for dry eyes include the unanesthetized Schirmer test (screens for lacrimal insufficiency) and vital dye staining (e.g., fluorescein, rose bengal, lissamine green, or some combination thereof) of the ocular surface to look for dry spots. The recommended test to screen for dry mouth is simply measurement of a whole mouth unstimulated salivary flow rate. However, similar to the 2002 criteria, in order to increase the specificity of this test a more stringent cutoff of $\leq$0.1 mL/min (i.e., well below the lower limits of normal) has been utilized to define low salivary flow. If all these test results were positive then a maximum total score of 9 is obtained. However, only a score of $\geq$4 is required to classify a patient as having SS.

Table 2.5 The 2016 ACR-EULAR classification criteria for SS.

Inclusions

- anyone with dry eyes or dry mouth as defined by the 2002 criteria
- anyone with at least one extraglandular manifestation as defined by the ESSDAI clinical index

Test Item	Weight
+Lip biopsy (FS $\geq$ 1/4 mm^2)[a]	3
Anti-SSA (Ro)+	3
OSS[b] $\geq$ 5 (Van Bijsterfeld[c] $\geq$ 4) in one eye	1
Schirmer test (without topical anesthesia) $\leq$ 5 mm/5 min in one eye	1
Unstimulated whole mouth salivary flow $\leq$ 0.1 mL/min	1

Positive score for classification as SS $\geq$ 4

Exclusions: Prior head and neck irradiation, active hepatitis C infection (confirmation by PCR), graft-versus-host disease, acquired immune deficiency syndrome, sarcoidosis, amyloidosis, IgG4-related disease.

ACR, *American College of Rheumatology;* ESSDAI, *EULAR Sjögren's Syndrome Disease Activity Index;* EULAR, *European League Against Rheumatism;* FS, *focus, score;* OSS, *ocular surface staining score;* SS, *Sjögren's syndrome.*
[a] *A positive biopsy is defined as focal lymphocytic sialadenitis with a focus score $\geq$1/4 mm^2 tissue surface area.*
[b] *Scale 0–12[13] for dry eyes scoring using fluorescein/ lissamine green.*
[c] *Scale 0–9[12] for dry eyes scoring using rose bengal or other vital dye.*
Adapted from Ref. 30.

Practical diagnosis

In practical terms, given the high reported sensitivity and specificity of all the recent criteria for the classification of SS, any individual who meets the 2002, 2012, or 2016 criteria can reliably be given this diagnosis in the clinical setting. Similarly, any patient who fails to meet the classification criteria but demonstrates three out of 4 essential disease features, namely, (1) positive biopsy result, (2) anti-SSA positivity, (3) objective evidence of dry eyes, and/or (4) objective evidence of salivary gland involvement, should also be diagnosed with SS when other possibilities have been excluded. It is therefore important to complete a comprehensive diagnostic evaluation in order to distinguish between SS and its long list of mimics (Table 2.6). In equivocal cases a labial minor salivary gland biopsy is almost always helpful. See Table 2.7 for a summary of the suggested diagnostic criteria used by the author in the clinical practice setting.

Differential diagnosis

SS was once described as a benign form of lupus because of the overlapping clinical and serologic manifestations, including anti-SSA positivity.[32] Consequently, additional testing and further evaluation for lupus is sometimes required before a firm

Table 2.6 Differential diagnosis of Sjögren's syndrome.

Amyloidosis	LADD syndrome
Anxiety/depression	Medication-related dryness
Chronic sialadenitis	Mouth breathing
Diabetes mellitus	Multiple sclerosis
Dysautonomia	Radiation injury
Eosinophilia-myalgia syndrome	Sarcoidosis
Fibromyalgia	Sialadenosis
Graft-versus-host disease	Silicone breast implant disease
Hepatitis C	Systemic lupus
HIV-related diffuse infiltrative lymphocytosis syndrome	Rheumatoid arthritis
	Type V hyperlipidemia
IgG4 syndrome	Vitamin A deficiency

LADD, *Lacrimo-auriculo-dento-digital.*

Table 2.7 Suggested diagnostic criteria for Sjögren's syndrome.

1. Anti-SSA positivity *or* RF[1] + ANA ($\geq$1:320)[2] positivity **(choose 1)**
2. Positive lip biopsy (focal lymphocytic sialadenitis with FS $\geq$1/4 mm^2)
3. Objective evidence of dry eyes **(any 1)**
   a) Abnormal Schirmer test (<10 mm/5 min)
   b) Any abnormal ocular surface staining using vital dyes (i.e., rose bengal, fluorescein, lissamine green)
4. Objective evidence of salivary gland involvement **(any 1)**
   a) Abnormal whole mouth salivary flow rate (<0.3 mL/min)
   b) Abnormal scintigraphy (defect in $\geq$1 of 3 phases of salivary gland function, i.e., uptake, resting, and stimulated functions)
   c) Abnormal appearance on salivary gland ultrasonography
   d) Abnormal appearance on CT/MRI of the major salivary glands

[1] Any titer
[2] Any pattern

Clinical diagnosis requires fulfillment of ≥3 of 4, *and exclusion of prior head and neck irradiation, HIV, active hepatitis C infection (confirmation by PCR), graft-versus-host disease, acquired immune deficiency syndrome, sarcoidosis, amyloidosis, IgG4-related disease, or medications that cause dryness.*

ANA, *Antinuclear antibody;* FS, *Focus score;* RF, *Rheumatoid factor.*
Adapted from Ref. 49.

diagnosis of SS can be established. Sicca symptoms have been reported in patients with multiple sclerosis (MS) and SS patients can present with demyelinating disease of the central nervous system that mimics MS (Chapter 10).[8,33] Subtle differences in magnetic resonance images of the brain and spinal cord or documentation of other SS-related features (positive lip biopsy, cutaneous vasculitis, peripheral neuropathy, arthritis, etc.) may allow for differentiating between these two disorders.[34,35]

At present, the most common cause of dry eyes and dry mouth worldwide is medications, as over 500 prescription and/or over-the-counter drugs are known to cause these symptoms through anticholinergic or other adverse effects.[36] This list includes diuretics, opioids, tricyclic antidepressants, benzodiazepines, antipsychotics, muscle relaxants, hypnotics, antihistamines, and oral decongestants. Sicca symptoms can be significantly increased when more than one medication with the same side effects is taken concurrently.[37] Patients with unexplained severe dry eyes and risk factors for nutritional deficiencies (e.g., after certain types of bariatric surgery, celiac) should always be screened for vitamin A deficiency.

All "baby boomers" with sicca symptoms or parotidomegaly should be screened for active hepatitis C infection, which can be clinically and histologically indistinguishable from SS.[38] These patients typically exhibit one or more of the following features: abnormal liver function test results, a liver biopsy consistent with chronic active hepatitis or cirrhosis, and serum cryoglobulins. Definitive diagnosis is made by demonstration of hepatitis C viral RNA in the blood or saliva by polymerase chain reaction.[39] The HIV-induced diffuse infiltrative lymphocytosis syndrome may present in a similar fashion as hepatitis C and trigger lymphocytic infiltration of the salivary glands. However, the CD4/CD8 ratio is typically <1 compared with the ratio of >2 that would be expected in SS.[40] Individuals with persistent, symmetric, painless swelling of the lacrimal and salivary glands (previously called Mikulicz disease) should always undergo biopsy at an involved site to look for IgG4-related disease. The histopathologic examination will typically show a lymphoplasmacytic infiltrate with storiform fibrosis, obliterative phlebitis, and an abundance of IgG4 staining plasma cells.[41,42]

Patients with severe dryness and arthritis who are seronegative and whose biopsies demonstrate "chronic nonspecific sialadenitis" (i.e., acinar destruction, diffuse fibrosis, and a scattered infiltrate of lymphocytes and plasma cells; focus score <1/4 mm^2) should be evaluated for osteoarthritis and the so-called SOX (sialadenitis, osteoarthritis, xerostomia) syndrome.[43] Occasionally, sarcoidosis can cause sicca symptoms with or without parotid swelling, and a major or minor salivary gland biopsy will demonstrate noncaseating granulomas.[44] Sialadenosis or sialosis should be suspected when a patient with painless swelling of the parotid glands (usually bilateral) undergoes a CT scan of the neck, which suggests fatty infiltration of the glands. It is most frequently associated with diabetes mellitus, hyperlipidemia, alcoholism, obesity, or other eating disorders and the diagnosis can be confirmed by fine-needle aspiration or biopsy.[45–47]

Children with sicca symptoms and accelerated caries are frequently evaluated for possible SS. However, similar symptoms may also result from congenital hypoplasia of the salivary glands caused by the lacrimo-auriculo-dento-digital (LADD) syndrome, a.k.a. the Levy-Hollister syndrome.[48] This is an autosomal dominant condition with intra- and interfamilial variability that is associated with auricular abnormalities, hearing loss, abnormal tooth morphology, and anomalies of the fingers and toes. It is most reliably confirmed by genetic testing for mutations of the fibroblast growth factor and/or fibroblast growth factor receptor 2 genes. Occasionally, mild cases may go unrecognized until adulthood.

Table 2.8 Laboratory evaluation of Sjögren's syndrome.

Test	Clinical correlate
Complete blood count/differential	Leukopenia, lymphopenia, autoimmune neutropenia, thrombocytopenia
Complete metabolic panel, urinalysis	Interstitial nephritis, renal tubular acidosis, autoimmune liver disease
Erythrocyte sedimentation rate	Disease activity
Serum protein electrophoresis	Hypergammaglobulinemia, hypogammaglobulinemia, monoclonal gammopathy of unknown significance
Serum IgG, IgM, IgA	Disease activity, hypergammaglobulinemic purpura
Cryoglobulins	Disease activity, lymphoma marker
Complement C3, C4	Disease activity, lymphoma markers
Serum β2-microglobulin	Disease activity
Rheumatoid factor	Inflammatory arthritis, lymphoma marker
Anti-citrullinated cyclic peptide	Inflammatory arthritis
Anti-centromere antibody	Subset with features of limited scleroderma

Further evaluation

In addition to a comprehensive physical examination, laboratory studies are routinely performed to screen for internal organ involvement or to obtain additional information about disease activity or long-term prognosis (Table 2.8). In certain clinical situations, further testing for an associated autoimmune disease (e.g., Hashimoto thyroiditis, celiac) may also be indicated. Additional evaluation with imaging studies and/or other diagnostic tests or procedures will depend upon the results of the initial evaluation.

Conclusions

In summary, the most reliable markers for the classification and/or diagnosis of SS are anti-SSA positivity and/or a positive lip biopsy. Documentation of oral and/or ocular involvement is equally important and can be accomplished by a variety of methods. The development of new classification criteria in recent years has facilitated more clinical trials and other research in the field and also provided a framework upon which diagnostic testing can be based. Ultimately, however, in the clinical setting, the judgment of an experienced physician with knowledge of SS, its classification, and its evaluation is most often relied on to provide an SS diagnosis.

References

1. Trocchio E. The time is now for Sjögren's. *Moisture Seekers*. January 2016;34(1):12.
2. Fox R. Extraglandular manifestations of Sjögren's syndrome (SS): dermatologic, arthritis, endocrine, pulmonary, cardiovascular, gastroenterology, renal, urology, and gynecologic manifestations. In: Fox R, Fox C, eds. *Sjögren's Syndrome: Practical Guidelines to Diagnoses and Therapy*. New York City, NY: Springer; 2011.
3. Ioannidis J, Vassilios V, Moutsopoulos H. Long-term risk of mortality and lymphoproliferative disease and predictive classification of primary Sjögren's syndrome. *Arthritis Rheum*. 2002;46(3):741−747.
4. Smedby K, Vajdic C, Falster M, Engels E, Martínez-Maza O, Turner J, Hjalgrim H, Vineis P, Costantini A, Bracci P, Holly E, Willett E, Spinelli J, La Vecchia C, Zheng T, Becker N, De Sanjosé S, Chiu B, Dal Maso L, Cocco P, Maynadié M, Foretova L, Staines A, Brennan P, Davis S, Severson R, Cerhan J, Breen E, Birmann B, Grulich A, Cozen W. Autoimmune disorders and risk of non-Hodgkin lymphoma subtypes: a pooled analysis within the Interlymph Consortium. *Blood*. 2008; 111(8):4029−4038.
5. Baimpa E, Dahabreh I, Voulgarelis M, Moutsopoulos H. Hematologic manifestations and predictors of lymphoma development in primary Sjögren syndrome: clinical and pathophysiologic aspects. *Medicine (Baltim)*. 2009;88(5):284−293.
6. Vivino F. Sjögren's syndrome: clinical aspects,. *Clin Immunol*. 2017;182:48−54.
7. Akpek E, Klimava A, Thorne J, Martin D, Lekhanont K, Ostrovsky A. Evaluation of patients with dry eye for presence of underlying Sjögren's syndrome. *Cornea*. June 2009; 28(5):493−497.
8. Delalande S, de Seze J, Fauchais A, Hachulla E, Stojkovic T, Ferriby D, Dubucquoi S, Pruvo J, Vermersch P, Hatron P. Neurologic manifestations in primary Sjögren syndrome: a study of 82 patients. *Medicine (Baltimore)*. 2004;83(5):280−291.
9. Yokogawa N, Lieberman SM, Alawi F, Bout-Tabaku S, Guttenberg M, Sherry DD, Vivino FB. Comparison of labial minor salivary gland biopsies from childhood Sjögren syndrome and age-matched Controls. *J Rheumatol*. June 2014;41(6): 1178−1182.
10. Bartlett J, Keith M, Sudharshan L, Snedecor S. Associations between signs and symptoms of dry eye disease: a systematic review. *Clin Ophthalmol*. 2015;9:1719−1730.
11. Shiboski S, Shiboski C, Criswell L, Baer A, Challacombe S, Lanfranchi h, Schiodt M, Umehara H, Vivino F, Zhao Y, Dong Y, Greenspan D, Heidenreich A, Helin P, Kirkham B, Kitagawa K, Larkin G, Li M, Lietman T, Lindegaard J, McNamara N, Sack K, Shirlaw P, Sugai S, Vollenweider C, Whitch WA, Zhang S, Zhang W, Greenspan J, Daniels T. American College of rheumatology classification criteria for Sjögren's syndrome, a data driven, expert consensus approach in the Sjögren's international collaborative clinical alliance cohort. *Arthritis Care Res*. 2012;64(4): 475−487.
12. Van Bijsterveld OP. Diagnostic tests in the Sicca syndrome. *Arch Ophthalmol*. 1969;82: 10−14.
13. Whitcher JP, Shiboski CH, Shiboski SC, Heidenreich AM, Kitagawa K, Zhang S, Hamann S, Larkin G, McNamara NA, Greenspan JS, Daniels TE. Simplified quantitative method for assessing keratoconjunctivitis sicca from the Sjögren's Syndrome International Registry. *Am J Ophthalmol*. 2010;149:405−415.

14. Coulthard P, Horner K, Sloan P, Theaker E. *Oral and Maxillofacial Surgery, Radiology, Pathology and Oral Medicine (Master dentistry)*. 2nd ed. Edinburgh: Churchill Livingstone/Elsevier; 2008:212−213. p.210.

15. Vivino FB, Hermann GA. Role of nuclear scintigraphy in the characterization and management of the salivary component of Sjögren's syndrome. *Rheum Dis Clin N Am*. November 2008;34(4):973−986. ix.

16. Hermann G, Vivino F, Goin J. Scintigraphic features of chronic sialadenitis and Sjögren's syndrome: a comparison. *Nucl Med Commun*. December 1999;20(12):1123−1132.

17. Hermann G, Vivino F, Shnier D, Krumm R, Mayrin V. Diagnostic accuracy of salivary scintigraphic indices in xerostomic populations. *Clin Nucl Med*. March 1999;24(3):167−172.

18. Baldini C, Luciano N, Tarantini G, Pascale R, Sernissi J, Mosca M, Caramella D, Bombardieri S. Salivary gland ultrasonography: a highly specific tool for the early diagnosis of primary Sjögren's syndrome. *Arthritis Res Ther*. 2015;17(146).

19. Cornec D, Jousse-Joulin S, Pers J, Marhadour T, Cochener B, Boisrame-Gostrim S, Nowak E, Youinou P, Saraux A, Devauchelle-Pensec V. Contribution of salivary gland ultrasonography to the diagnosis of Sjögren's syndrome: toward new diagnostic criteria. *Arthritis Rheum*. 2013;65:216−225.

20. Jousse-Joulin S, Milic V, Jonsson M, Plagou A, Theander E, Luciano N, Rachele P, Baldini C, Bootsma H, Vissink A, Hocevar A, De Vita S, Tzioufas A, Alavi Z, Bowman S, Devauchelle-Pensec V. Is salivary gland ultrasonography a useful tool in Sjögren's syndrome? A systematic review. *Rheumatology*. 2016;55:789−800.

21. Howlett D, Menezes L, Lewis K, Moody A, Violaris N, Williams M. Sonographically guided core biopsy of a parotid mass. *Am J Roentgenol*. 2007;188:223−227.

22. Baer A, DeMarco M, Shiboski S, Lam M, Challacombe S, Daniels T, Dong Y, Greenspan J, Kirkham B, Lanfranchi H, Schiodt M, Srinivasan M, Umehara H, Vivino F, Vollenweider C, Zhao Y, Criswell L, Shiboski C, for the Sjögren's International Collaborative Clinical Alliance (SICCA) Research Groups. The SSB positive/SSA negative antibody profile is not associated with key phenotypic features of Sjögren's syndrome. *Ann Rheum Dis*. 2015;74:1557−1561.

23. Shen L, Suresh L, Lindemann M, Xuan J, Kowal P, Malyavantham K, Ambrus J. Novel autoantibodies in Sjögren's syndrome. *Clin Immunol*. 2012;145(3):251−255.

24. Fisher B, Jonsson R, Daniels T, Bombardieri M, Brown R, Morgan P, Bombardieri S, Ng W, Tzioufas A, Vitali C, Shirlaw P, Haacke E, Costa S, Bootsma H, Devauchelle-Pensec V, Radstake T, Mariette X, Richards A, Stack R, Bowman S, Barone F. Standardization of labial salivary gland histopathology in clinical trials in primary Sjögren's syndrome. *Ann Rheum Dis*. 2017;76:1161−1168.

25. Vivino FB, Gala I, Hermann GA. Change in final diagnosis on second evaluation of labial minor salary gland biopsies. *J Rheumatol*. May 2002;29(5):938−944.

26. Daniels TE, Cox D, Shiboski CH, Schiodt M, Wu A, Lanfranchi H, Umehara H, Zhao Y, Challacombe S, Lam MY, De Souza Y, Schiodt J, Holm H, Bisio PA, Gandolfo MS, Sawaki T, Li M, Zhang W, Varghese-Jacob B, Ibsen P, Keszler A, Kurose N, Nojima T, Odell E, Criswell LA, Jordan R, Greenspan JS, Sjögren's International Collaborative Clinical Alliance Research Groups. Associations between salivary gland histopathologic diagnoses and phenotypic features of Sjögren's syndrome among 1,726 registry participants. *Arthritis Rheum*. 2011;63:2021−2030.

27. Yokogawa N, Lieberman S, Sherry D, Vivino F. Features of childhood Sjögren's syndrome in comparison to adult Sjögren's syndrome: considerations in establishing child-specific diagnostic criteria. *Clin Exp Rheumatol*. 2016;34(2):343−351.

28. Vitali C, Bombardieri S, Jonsson R, Moutsopoulos HM, Alexander EL, Carsons SE, Daniels TE, Fox PC, Fox RI, Kassan SS, Pillemer SR, Talal N, Weisman MH, European Study Group on Classification Criteria for Sjögren's Syndrome. Classification criteria for Sjögren's syndrome: a revised version of the European criteria proposed by the American-European consensus group. *Ann Rheum Dis*. 2002;61:554–558.

29. Rasmussen A, Ice J, Li H, Grundahl K, Kelly J, Radfar L, Stone D, Hefner K, Anaya J, Rohrer M, Gopalakrishnan R, Houston G, Lewis D, Chodosh J, Harley J, Hughes P, Maier-Moore J, Montgomery C, Rhodus N, Farris A, Segal B, Jonsson R, Lessard C, Scofield R, Sivils K. Comparison of the American-European Consensus Group Sjögren's syndrome classification criteria to newly proposed American College of Rheumatology criteria in a large, carefully characterized sicca cohort. *Ann Rheum Dis*. January 2014; 73(1):31–38.

30. Shiboski C, Shiboski S, Seror R, Criswell L, Labetoulle M, Lietman T, Rasmussen A, Scofield H, Vitali C, Bowman S, Mariette X, The International Sjögren's Syndrome Criteria Working Group. 2016 American College of rheumatology/European League against rheumatism classification criteria for primary Sjögren's syndrome, a consensus and data-driven methodology involving three international patient cohorts. *Arthritis Rheum*. 2017;69(1):35–45.

31. Seror R, Ravaud P, Bowman SJ, Baron G, Tzioufas A, Theander E, Gottenberg JE, Bootsma H, Mariette X, Vitali C, EULAR Sjögren's Task Force. EULAR Sjögren's Syndrome Disease Activity Index: development of a consensus systemic disease activity index for primary Sjögren's syndrome. *Ann Rheum Dis*. 2010;69:1103–1109.

32. Heaton JM. Sjögren's syndrome and systemic lupus erythematosus. *Br Med J*. 1959;1: 466–469.

33. Annunziata P, De Santi L, Di Rezze S, Millefiorini E. Clinical features of Sjögren's syndrome in patients with multiple sclerosis. *Acta Neurol Scand*. 2011;124(2):109–114.

34. Kim S, Richman D, Johnson W, Hald J, Agius M. Limited utility of current MRI criteria for distinguishing multiple sclerosis from common mimickers: primary and secondary CNS vasculitis, lupus and Sjögren's syndrome. *Mult Scler*. January 2014;20(1):57–63.

35. Eckstein C, Saidha S, Levy M. A differential diagnosis of central nervous system demyelination: beyond multiple sclerosis. *J Neurol*. 2012;259(5):801–816.

36. Sreebny L, Schwartz S. A reference guide to drugs and dry mouth – 2nd edition. *Gerodontology*. 1997;14(1):33–47.

37. Nederfors T. Xerostomia: prevalence and pharmacotherapy with special reference to beta-adrenoreceptor antagonists. *Swed Dent J*. 1996;116(Suppl. l):1–70.

38. Ramos-Casals M, Muñoz S, Zerón PB. Hepatitis C virus and Sjögren's syndrome: trigger or mimic? *Rheum Dis Clin N Am*. November 2008;34(4):869–884.

39. Jorgensen C, Legouffe M, Pascal P, Cozte J, Tiszsot B, Segarra C, Bologna C, Bourrrat L, Combe B, Blanc F, Sany J. Sicca syndrome associated with hepatitis C virus infection. *Arthritis Rheum*. 1996;39(7):1166–1171.

40. Ghrenassia E, Martis N, Boyer J, Burel-Vandenbos F, Mekinian A, Coppo P. The diffuse infiltrative lymphocytosis syndrome (DILS). A comprehensive review. *J Autoimmun*. May 2015;59:19–25.

41. Yamamoto M, Harada S, Ohara M, Suzuki C, Naishiro Y, Yamamoto H, Takahashi H, Imai K. Clinical and pathological differences between Mikulicz's disease and Sjögren's syndrome. *Rheumatology*. 2005;44:227–234.

42. Stone J, Zen Y, Despande V. IgG4-related disease. *N Engl J Med*. 2012;366:539–551.

43. Kassimos D, Shirlaw P, Choy E, Hockey K, Morgan P, Challacombe S, Panayi G. Chronic sialoadenitis in patients with nodal osteoarthritis. *Br J Rheumatol.* 1997;36: 1312−1317.
44. Sack K, Carteron N, Whitcher J, Greenspan J, Daniels T. Sarcoidosis mimicking Sjögren's syndrome: histopathologic observations. *J Clin Rheumatol.* 1998;4(1):13−16.
45. Gupta S, Sodhani P. Sialadenosis of parotid gland: a cytomorphologic and morphometric study of four cases. *Anal Quant Cytol Histol.* June 1998;20(3):225−228.
46. Scully C, Bagán J, Eveson J, Barnard N, Turner F. Sialosis: 35 cases of persistent parotid swelling from two countries. *Br J Oral Maxillofac Surg.* September 2008;46(6): 468−472.
47. Jagtap S, Aramani S, Mane A, Bonde V. Sialosis: cytomorphological significance in the diagnosis of an uncommon entity. *J Cytol.* 2017;34(1):51−52.
48. Hajianpour M, Bombei H, Lieberman S, Revell R, Krishna R, Gregorsok R, Kao S, Milunsky J. Dental issues in lacrimo-auriculo-dento-digital syndrome: an autosomal dominant condition with clinical and genetic variability. *J Am Dent Assoc.* March 2017;148(3):157−163.
49. Vivino F, Bunya V, Massaro-Giordano G, Johr C, Giattino S, Schorpion A, Shafer B, Peck A, Sivils K, Rasmussen A, Chiorini J, He J, Ambrus J. Sjögren's syndrome: an update on disease pathogenesis, clinical manifestations and treatment. *Clin Immunol.* 2019; 203:81−121.

Oral manifestations and management in Sjögren's syndrome

3

Mabi L. Singh, DMD, MS[1], Adriane Kilar, DMD[2], Athena Papas, DMD, PhD[3]

[1]*Associate Professor, Div. of Oral Medicine, Department of Diagnostic Sciences, Tufts University School of Dental Medicine, Boston, MA, United States;* [2]*Massachusetts Institute of Technology, Cambridge, MA, United States;* [3]*Distinguished Professor, Johansen Professor of Dental Research, Head of the Division Oral Medicine Department of Diagnostic Sciences, Tufts University School of Dental Medicine, Boston, MA, United States*

Importance of saliva

The loss of saliva is not just a comfort issue. Qualitatively and quantitatively, saliva plays an essential role in protecting both soft and hard tissues in the oral cavity. Saliva contains 99% water and 1% proteins, minerals, and enzymes. Saliva has many effects on the teeth, oral mucosa, food, and microorganisms of the oral cavity. Saliva keeps the soft tissues moist, maintains oral homeostasis, prevents bacterial and fungal infections, and maintains caries balance.[1,2] A compromise in salivary function can lead to a subjective sensation of dryness in the mouth (xerostomia); difficulty in speech and swallowing; oral burning sensation; taste disturbances; cheilosis; recurrent oral bacterial, viral, and fungal infections; mouth sores; higher rates of dental decay; and failure of dental treatments (Fig. 3.1).[3,4] In addition to problems in the oral cavity, it has also been hypothesized that changes in oral microflora related to salivary dysfunction and other factors create a dysbiosis that may play a role in the pathogenesis of autoimmune diseases.[5]

Saliva is to the teeth what blood is to other organs. With bicarbonates, phosphates, mucins, and calcium, saliva buffers low pH in the oral cavity and protects the teeth from demineralization. Statherin, proline-rich proteins, calcium, and phosphate also promote remineralization of the dentition.

Causes of salivary hypofunction

Xerostomia due to salivary hypofunction is a common and often ignored medical complaint that can significantly affect quality of life.[6] Causative factors of salivary hypofunction include malnutrition, dehydration, use of anticholinergic medications (prescription and over the counter [OTC]), chemotherapy, and head and neck irradiation.[7] Other comorbidities that may exacerbate or cause this problem include anxiety/depression, diabetes mellitus, sarcoidosis, alcoholism, smoking, HIV, hepatitis

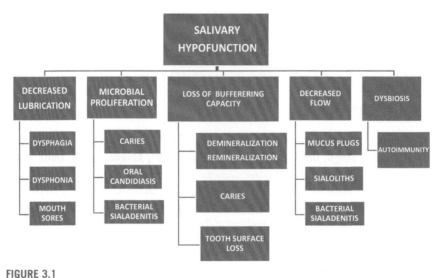

FIGURE 3.1

Consequences of salivary hypofunction in the oral cavity.

C infection, and IgG4-related disease.[8] One of the most important causes of salivary gland hypofunction is Sjögren's syndrome (SS), a chronic autoimmune, rheumatic disease characterized by lymphocytic infiltration of the salivary glands that triggers the release of cytokines and chemokines that block saliva production. SS can also cause life-threatening internal organ manifestations (Chapter 6) and lymphomas (Chapter 8).[9] Therefore proper diagnosis of SS (Chapter 2) and differentiation from other causes of xerostomia is crucial and profoundly influences the evaluation and management of other patient health problems.

Major complications and management
Treatment of xerostomia

Management strategies for dry mouth and the available products have been reviewed.[10] The treatment approach is designed according to personal need, tolerance, insurance coverage, and lifestyle. The patient's medications should be reviewed and, whenever medically feasible, intake of drugs that can cause xerostomia should be discontinued or substituted. Patients should be encouraged to eat more frequent smaller meals to stimulate saliva flow and to take small sips of water just to wet the mucosa in the mouth between drinking regular glasses of water or noncarbonated, sugar-free, nonacidic beverages during the day to maintain oral comfort. Low humidity conditions (e.g., air-conditioning, forced air heat) should be avoided, and the use of an ultrasonic cool mist humidifier in the bedroom can help alleviate nocturnal dryness. Individuals with xerostomia should also avoid the use of mouthwashes or rinses containing astringents (e.g., alcohol, witch hazel) that can aggravate dryness and oral burning.

For patients with mild symptoms, any gustatory or masticatory stimulus will improve salivary flow. A variety of OTC sugar-free gums, candies, and lozenges are available to serve this purpose. The use of xylitol-containing products is encouraged, as this artificial sweetener is superior to others for caries prevention (vide infra).

Patients with moderate to severe symptoms or who have developed complications of dry mouth should be encouraged to start systemic therapy with sialogogues. Therapeutic success depends on residual function of the salivary glands. To minimize cholinergic side effects, patients should be instructed to start this treatment at the lowest possible dose after meals (e.g., pilocarpine, 5 mg, or cevimeline, 30 mg by mouth after dinner) and advance the dosing regimen slowly as tolerated up to the daily maximal recommended divided dose (i.e., pilocarpine up to 30 mg/day and cevimeline up to 90 mg/day). This treatment may also alleviate other oral symptoms or nonoral sicca symptoms in SS. For patients with intolerable side effects from sialogogues, there are also two FDA-approved devices (Salitron®, Saliwell®) that use local electrical stimulation of the salivary glands to increase saliva production.

For patients with no salivary flow, in addition to water, a variety of OTC artificial saliva sprays and other products[10] can provide short-term relief but must be used regularly (e.g., one to two sprays every 1−2 hours while awake) for best results. Additionally, moisturizing gels and oils (coconut oil, sesame oil, olive oil) can be applied to the tongue and buccal mucosa twice a day after meals and every night at bedtime to alleviate oral symptoms. Two prescription saliva substitute powders (NeutraSal® and SalivaMAX®) are also available to be mixed with water and used as a gargle and swish for dry mouth several times per day as needed; these products may have other benefits as well (vide infra).

Caries and the loss of noncarious tooth surfaces

Even though the diagnosis of SS may positively affect patients' personal oral hygiene behavior by increasing motivation for better compliance and access to dental care, salivary hypofunction still leads to the development of dental caries and tooth surface loss. As has been reported by the Tufts Oral Medicine clinic[11] (Fig. 3.2) and the Sjögren's Syndrome Foundation, Inc. (SSF),[12] the expenditures of SS patients on dental procedures is thrice of that spent by their peers because of a higher rate of caries development.

Proliferation of cariogenic microorganisms in SS is well established. Depending on the stage of the disease, SS patients will have varying degrees of salivary hypofunction. There is clear evidence of an increase in prevalence and incidence of carious lesions both in the coronal and root surfaces of the teeth. Many studies

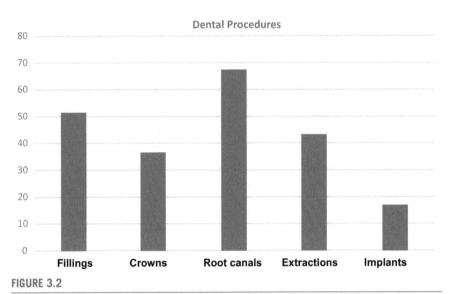

FIGURE 3.2

Percentages of Sjögren's syndrome patients who had different dental procedures performed within the past year of when the survey was conducted.

and clinical observations have shown increased clinical attachment loss of the gingival tissue and exposure of the less mineralized and easily demineralized portion of the tooth, the cervical root, resulting in a greater risk of developing carious lesions in this area. With the loss of saliva, all the tooth surfaces become vulnerable to carious lesions, including the plaque-retentive areas or non–plaque-retentive areas such as cuspal tips, incisal edges, and even the areas of the mouth that are least prone to develop carious lesions, such as the lower anterior dentition. The oral homeostasis is disturbed by qualitative and quantitative alterations of saliva, which gives rise to an increased cariogenic microbial population of 10^6 colony-forming units (CFUs) or more (normal being around 10^3 CFU). Also, the presence of various other comorbidities such as diabetes and gastroesophageal reflux disease (GERD) further increases the risk of tooth decay.

Clinical experience and studies have shown that root decay is very common among SS patients (Fig. 3.3). If the decay proceeds very deep to encircle the tooth, the tooth may have to be removed. Prosthetic crowns do not help protect the teeth from decay because the caries (decay) can occur around the margins of the crown and cause failure. When salivary flow is extremely low, even endodontically treated teeth can fail (34.5%).[13] Use of dentures among SS patients is often unsatisfactory (vide infra), and preventative measures are therefore critical.

Lack of saliva's protective functions due to hyposalivation not only increases the risk of dental caries but also plays a critical role in noncarious tooth surface loss such as erosion, abrasion, and attrition (vide infra). In addition to water, saliva contains other key components such as bicarbonates, calcium, and phosphates. These

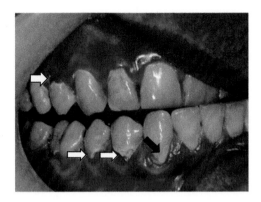

FIGURE 3.3

The arrows indicate the various stages of tooth decay in the mouth of a patient with Sjögren's syndrome. The incipient decay (*black arrow*) can be remineralized, whereas areas of established decay (*white arrows*) must be surgically restored (filled).

components protect the teeth from acid (intrinsic or extrinsic) by buffering and promoting remineralization of the demineralized tooth surfaces and by elevating the oral and plaque pH. One of the other major protective salivary functions is the formation of the acquired pellicle. The pellicle makes a barrier on the teeth against acid attack and friction caused by the mechanical abrasiveness of toothpastes and toothbrushes.[14] Therefore patients with depressed saliva secretion are at a higher risk of noncarious tooth surface loss including erosion, attrition, and abrasion.[15,16]

If patients are edentulous, oral prosthesis such as maxillary dentures can lose their palatal seal and drop. Mandibular dentures tend to be very difficult to tolerate because of their constant movement and trauma to the friable dry tissue. *Candida* can populate easily on denture surfaces. Implant-supported dentures are well tolerated and have helped patients manage their dentures. Typically, fixing the prosthesis with four implants prevents the movement that leads to trauma of the oral tissues.

SS is also associated with an increased prevalence of GERD.[17] According to the response to an SSF questionnaire by its membership, close to half the participants had GERD.[12] In addition to heartburn, patients with GERD and/or laryngopharyngeal reflux may experience other symptoms including chronic cough, dysphagia, sore throat, chest pain, hoarseness, or water brash. Gastroesophageal reflux may further increase the risk of erosion of the tooth surfaces by adding to a preexisting acidic oral environment and further overwhelming the already decreased buffering capacity of saliva. This leads to demineralization of the teeth and makes them vulnerable to secondary caries and tooth surface loss.[18]

Overview of caries prevention

The general goals of caries prophylaxis are summarized in Table 3.1. Based on our findings, we recommend the regular use of a sialogogue to prevent saliva loss early

Table 3.1 Goals of caries prophylaxis and prevention of tooth surface loss.

Avoid tooth abrasives
Control extrinsic acid exposure
Decrease ingestion of fermentable carbohydrates
Increase plaque pH
Increase oral pH
Reduce cariogenic microbial population
Use fluoride regularly
Remineralize teeth
Stimulate salivary flow

in the disease and to prevent failure of dental restorations. The use of sialogogues (pilocarpine or cevimeline) over a 4-year period doubled the salivary flow rate compared with baseline.[19] When a preventive protocol of daily fluoride toothpaste (5000 ppm, prescription strength), remineralizing mouthwash, MI Paste®, sialogogues, and fluoride varnish professionally applied every 3 months was followed, there was an 82% decrease in failures of root canals. Following this preventative protocol also had an overall positive impact on the stability of the oral cavity. Furthermore, it was found that when the stimulated salivary flow rate is <0.5 mL/min then fluoride and a remineralizing solution such as Caphosol®, NeutraSal®, or SalivaMAX® should be used along with lubricating agents because the saliva can no longer supply the necessary calcium and phosphate needed for remineralization. These strategies are discussed in detail later, and compliance with the prescribed regimen is the key to prevent carious lesions.

Fluoride

The oral medicine clinical practice guidelines published by the SSF recommend the use of a high-strength topical fluoride (any form) for caries prevention.[20] Fluoride is responsible for the formation of fluoroapatite crystals within the tooth structure, which are more resistant to acid attack and dissolve at a lower pH of 4 than the hydroxyapatite crystals (pH 5.6) in tooth enamel. Fluoride also acts as a catalyst for the remineralization of the tooth surface in the presence of supersaturated calcium and phosphate usually found in unstimulated saliva. Daily usage of OTC fluoride rinses (500 ppm), regular toothpaste with fluoride (1000–1200 ppm), or prescription-strength fluoride gels (5000 ppm) helps prevent the formation of new decay and promotes remineralization in the early stages of decay. Alternatively, fluoride varnish (22,500 ppm) applied on the teeth every 3 months by a dental professional also provides an effective means of caries prophylaxis. The frequency and type of fluoride application is dependent on the patient's risk, severity, and experience with other treatments.

Remineralizing strategies

If carious lesions are detected in the early stages of demineralization, before the formation of a cavity, remineralization is possible in the subsurface lesions. The lower the plaque pH the more pathogenic the oral microflora become so it is important to decrease the pathologic factors, increase plaque pH, and encourage diets that are low in fermentable carbohydrates (sugars and starches). Similarly, patients should be counseled to always use products for dry mouth that are sugar-free. When the stimulated saliva flow is <0.5 mL/min, it is also beneficial to introduce supersaturated calcium and phosphate via artificial saliva through products such as Caphosol®, NeutraSal®, and SalivaMAX® for mineral reuptake in the presence of trace amounts of fluoride. Other remineralizing agents such as casein phosphatase, amorphous calcium phosphate, nano-sized bioactive glass particles, and calcium sodium phosphosilicate can also help prevent caries and rebuild the tooth surfaces. Rinsing with baking soda (1 teaspoon in 8 oz of water) can create a pH of 8–8.5, which elevates the oral pH and increases plaque pH. This is even more important when GERD is present. Arginine bicarbonate and calcium carbonate (BasicBites®) have the potential to be converted into alkali or base that helps keep teeth in a healthy pH balance.[21]

Antimicrobial agents

As dental caries is a chronic disease caused by a dysbiotic biofilm, antimicrobial agents that are effective against the cariogenic microbiome may help reduce the occurrence of this complication. Fluoride at the level of 0.1 mM has an antimicrobial effect by virtue of its ability to arrest glycolysis in pathogenic *Streptococcus mutans*. Chlorhexidine rinses and fluoride varnishes likewise help reduce the cariogenic microbial population. If candidiasis is suspected, anticandidal medications should be administered for the infection because *Candida* can also create an acidic environment that is detrimental to the integrity of the tooth structure. Triclosan-containing toothpastes may also reduce caries.

Salivary stimulation

When saliva production is severely reduced in an SS patient, various forms of fluoride alone are insufficient to overcome the challenges of initiation and progression of carious lesions. Unstimulated saliva is naturally supersaturated with calcium and phosphate ions creating a concentration gradient that facilitates the reuptake of ions into the teeth, in the presence of trace amounts of fluoride, to maintain homeostasis. Usage of sialogogues, such as cevimeline HCl, 30 mg, or pilocarpine HCl, 5–7.5 mg, titrated to the maximum dose, increases the whole mouth unstimulated and stimulated salivary flow, depending on the remaining functional minor and major salivary glands. We have observed maintenance of salivary gland function over time among those who are on a stable dosage of sialogogues. The increased salivary flow washes away food debris and dead tissue, reduces microbial concentration, neutralizes plaque pH, and helps in pellicle formation, which acts as a barrier against direct acid attack on the tooth surfaces.[14]

Saliva can also be mechanically stimulated by mimicking the chewing process with wax or gum and lozenges preferably containing xylitol. Xylitol has been approved by the US FDA and the American Academy of Pediatric Dentistry as a sugar substitute. It is a naturally occurring five-carbon sugar polyol that when consumed (5–6 g) more than three times a day[22] disrupts the energy production of bacteria and causes growth inhibition,[23] as it cannot be metabolized. Also, xylitol can neutralize plaque by its ability to increase ammonia and amino acid concentrations.[24] When a stable plaque pH is maintained, a decrease in the *S. mutans* population occurs as a result of starvation, growth inhibition, development of intracellular vacuoles, and cell membrane degradation.[25] This reduces the risk and initiation of new carious lesions.

In cases of temporomandibular joint dysfunction or fatigue in the masticatory muscles, movement of gum within the oral cavity without chewing or sucking on sugar-free lozenges will also stimulate saliva flow.

Tooth surface loss

Dental caries due to low salivary flow has been widely studied and confirmed. However, the increased susceptibility of patients with xerostomia and salivary hypofunction to noncarious dental surface loss must also be addressed.

Attrition or tooth surface loss caused by antagonistic tooth-to-tooth physical contact can be a problem in SS. Additionally, the abrasive substances in oral hygiene products and the force used during mechanical oral hygiene procedures with toothbrushes may induce further physical wear, typically V-shaped defects near the gumline. Gentle brushing, the use of toothbrushes with round bristles, the application of remineralizing agents to a night/bite guard, the use of moisturizers to increase lubrication and less consumption of acidic foods will all help maintain the integrity of calcified structures. The routine use of oral hygiene products should be regularly reviewed and those that may contain abrasives or reduce oral pH should be avoided.

Erosion is the mineral dissolution of the tooth structure from intrinsic and extrinsic acid introduced to the oral cavity. In xerostomic patients, the acid buffering capacity of saliva is diminished and this results in dissolution of the tooth surface and the development of saucer-like cavitations (Fig. 3.4). Patients should be

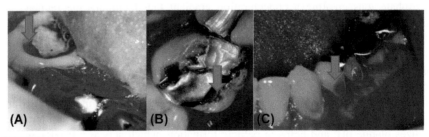

(A)   (B)   (C)

FIGURE 3.4

Loss of tooth surface (A) from the cusp, (B) around the amalgam, and (C) from the sides of the teeth due to intrinsic and extrinsic acid exposure.

Table 3.2 Acidic food and drinks that decrease oral pH.

Beverages
Coffee
Energy drinks
Fruit drinks/juices (cranberry, apple, orange, lemon)
Iced tea
Soda (including diet soda) and other carbonated beverages
Wine
Condiments
Vinegar
Salad dressing
Fruits
Apples
Berries
Citrus fruits
Cherries
Grapes
Pineapple
Plums
Other foods
American cheese
Pickled products
Sauer gummies and candies
Tomatoes

counseled to avoid acidic foods and beverages that aggravate this problem (Table 3.2). Ideally, to prevent the destructive removal of a layer of enamel or dentin, brushing should be postponed for half an hour after acid exposure. GERD should be treated in the usual manner with dietary and lifestyle modifications, histamine receptor 2 blockers, and proton pump inhibitors. Oral acid can be neutralized by rinsing with baking soda (1 teaspoon in 8 oz warm water), especially after consumption of acidic food, in the morning and before brushing. During the day, CTx2® spray or BasicBites® soft chews can also be utilized to neutralize oral acid.

Salivary gland swelling

The homeostasis of the oral cavity is maintained through the secretions from three pairs of major salivary glands and 700–1000 minor salivary glands. The major salivary glands consist of the parotid, submandibular, and sublingual glands and account for roughly 90% of saliva production. The parotid glands are situated bilaterally, inferior to the zygomatic arch, superior to the inferior border of the mandible, posterior to the masseter muscle, and anterior to the sternocleidomastoid muscle and external ear. The parotid glands are encapsulated and produce serous saliva, which drains into the oral cavity via the (parotid) Stensen ducts located opposite the second upper molars. The submandibular glands are loosely encapsulated and produce both mucous and serous saliva. They measure around 3—4 cm, are located at the posterior part of the submandibular triangle, and drain into the floor of the mouth through the Wharton duct behind the lower incisors. The sublingual glands produce mucous saliva and drain via many ducts into the floor of the mouth. Over 700 minor salivary glands are located in the submucosa in the buccal, palatal, lingual, and labial regions near the opening of the mouth and produce the remaining 10% of salivary secretions (mainly mucous).

Unilateral or bilateral swelling of the major salivary glands (especially the parotids) may be the presenting manifestation of SS and/or may occur in up to 50% of SS patients at any point during the course. Swelling can be acute and intermittent, chronic and persistent, and painful or painless depending on the acuity and cause. The presence of persistent, painless, or mild bilateral enlargement of the salivary glands, especially when cryoglobulinemia is present, should always prompt concern for non-Hodgkin B-cell lymphoma[26] (Chapter 8) and the consideration of further imaging and/or major salivary gland biopsy. In SS, however, painless bilateral swelling may also result from chronic inflammation and/or fatty infiltration (e.g., sialadenosis from chronic steroid use). SS may mimic sarcoidosis, IgG4-related diseases including Mikulicz disease, and sialadenosis related to other systemic conditions, e.g., diabetes, hyperlipidemia, or metabolic diseases.

Salivary gland obstruction
Mucus plugs

The decrease in the functionality of the serous portions of the salivary gland cells results in increased viscosity of the saliva because of an increase in mucus and decrease in water content. This resultant thick, viscous, cloudy, and gelatinous saliva in the Stensen duct or the interlobular ducts may act as a seal to occlude the draining duct. Thus the formation of mucus plugs may impede the flow of the saliva from the parotid glands into the oral cavity. The accumulation of the subsequently produced saliva in the functional part of the glands results in their acute, intermittent, painful swelling. This problem is further exacerbated by occlusion due to changes in the ductal architecture (e.g., sialostenosis) that occur as a result of chronic inflammation as well as protein leakage from blood and the presence of small sialoliths.

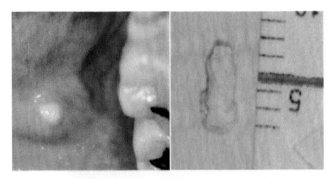

FIGURE 3.5

Salivary gland stone occluding the opening of the Stenson duct of the parotid gland.

Sialolithiasis

Another common cause of parotid gland swelling is the formation of salivary gland stones (sialoliths). Sialoliths (calculi) are composed of crystallized calcium and phosphate that can block the salivary flow from the major and minor salivary gland ducts (Fig. 3.5). Any occlusion in the duct causes acute or subacute swelling, as well as a sensation of pressure and pain. These symptoms are sometimes exacerbated by chewing, eating, or the use of sialagogues. As saliva contains high amounts of calcium and phosphate, the prior formation of mucus plugs can act as a nidus for the precipitation/crystallization of sialoliths. Sialoliths are easily identified by ultrasonography, panoramic radiography, computed tomography (CT) of the soft tissues of the neck, or magnetic resonance sialography. In our experience, CT is the best imaging technique for radiopaque and nonradiopaque sialoliths. When the blockage is cleared, the symptoms may disappear. If the blockage becomes chronic, pain and swelling in the area may get progressively worse and lead to damage of the salivary ducts and infection.

There are no guidelines for the treatment of recurrent salivary gland obstruction. However, when the symptoms resolve, in the authors' experience, further episodes can be prevented by the regular use of prescription sialagogues at maximal doses, by the use of sugar-free gums and lozenges, and by frequent milking and self-massaging of the salivary glands.

Infections

Bacterial sialadenitis

Qualitative and volumetric compromise of the saliva results in increased proliferation of noxious microbiota in the oral cavity. In situations when the duct into the mouth is occluded, microorganisms can bypass the obstruction and travel into the salivary

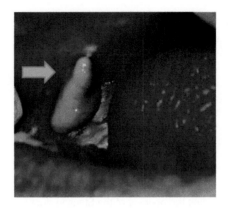

FIGURE 3.6

Purulent discharge (*arrow*) from the parotid gland of a Sjögren's syndrome patient.

glands causing infection of the glands (Fig. 3.6). If untreated, salivary gland infections can cause severe pain, swelling, difficulty opening the mouth, fevers, and erythema overlying the involved site, as well as result in abscess formation. The latter can be confirmed by salivary gland ultrasonography with color Doppler, CT, or magnetic resonance imaging. CT and magnetic resonance imaging can provide a more thorough examination of the entire salivary gland than ultrasonography where views may be limited. The glands that are well encapsulated by a fibrous tissue house the infection in a confined space, thus limiting systemic involvement. Poor oral hygiene, dehydration, malnutrition, and other chronic illnesses (e.g., diabetes) raise the risk of bacterial infections. The authors have found a wide range of microbiota in the salivary gland exudate, e.g., *Staphylococcus aureus, Klebsiella pneumoniae, Streptococcus viridans, Enterococcus, Pseudomonas, and Stenotrophomonas.* Efforts should be made to milk the involved major salivary gland in order to culture the exudate from the opening of the Stensen or Wharton duct. In cases of severe salivary gland dysfunction, it is unlikely that antibiotics will reach the infection site. In such conditions, the authors suggest the regular manual manipulation (milking) of the salivary glands when the infection is unresponsive to antibiotic therapy. The frequency of manual depletion of the abscess depends on the severity and clinical response.

Oral candidiasis

More than 20 types of *Candida* species naturally exist within the oral environment of most individuals, with *Candida albicans* being the most common. Researchers have found higher than normal total and CFU counts of *Candida*[27,28] in more than half of the patients in the SS population including both symptomatic and asymptomatic individuals.

Loss of antifungal factors in the saliva, such as histatin, chromogranin A, and immunoglobulins, promote candidal growth in susceptible patients. Lower pH and a lower rate of unstimulated and stimulated whole salivary flow also favor the proliferation of *Candida* in the oral cavity.[29] Denture wearers and people taking medications especially steroids, antibiotics, and immunosuppressants are especially vulnerable to this problem. Medical conditions that alter the immune system and the oral microenvironment (e.g., GERD, HIV, diabetes) can also predispose to oral candidiasis.

In a SS patient with severe xerostomia and mouth soreness, the classic appearance of a dry, fissured, and erythematous tongue should suggest *erythematous candidiasis* until proven otherwise. The typical signs and symptoms can include stomatopyrosis (burning sensation of the oral cavity), glossodynia (tongue soreness), an unpleasant metallic taste, erythema of the oral mucosa, and angular cheilitis (redness and cracking at the corners of the mouth) (Fig. 3.7).[29] Oral candidiasis may also present in other forms: subclinical, clinical, pseudomembranous, and chronic atrophic candidiasis.

Salivary hypofunction may result in a fissured and depapillated tongue. The penetration of *Candida* into the fissures of the tongue or other oral tissues causes irritation of the nerve endings that results in soreness and burning sensation. The white coating on the tongue can result in an unpleasant metallic taste, loss of taste, and halitosis (bad breath). In denture wearers, redness, irritation, and pain under the prosthesis can be additional clues that a candida infection is present.

Candidiasis occurs mostly on the tongue and buccal mucosa but it can also involve the roof of the mouth and the gingival tissue. In severe conditions the tonsils and esophagus may also be affected. Clinically, pseudomembranous candidiasis (thrush) may appear as a white raised lesion on the oral tissue, which can be rubbed or scraped off, with possible erythema and bleeding underneath.

Candida can ferment the available carbohydrates in the mouth and create an acidic oral environment favorable for acidogenic and aciduric bacteria. This in turn increases the virulence of *S. mutans*, resulting in an increase in dental caries. This hypothesis is supported by clinical studies that found higher candida counts and an association of *C. albicans* with the alterations of the oral bacterial composition and the virulence potential of *S. mutans* in children with early caries when compared with other groups.[30]

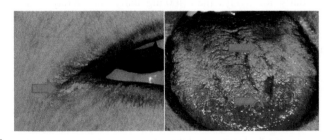

FIGURE 3.7

(A) Angular cheilitis at the corners of mouth and (B) erythematous candidiasis on the tongue of a Sjögren's syndrome patient.

Prevention and treatment of oral candidiasis

In SS patients with oral candidiasis related to salivary hypofunction, increasing the salivary flow with sialogogues and/or chewing gum or lozenges may help reduce the recurrence and severity of this problem, as the whole saliva is a better predictor of higher candidal count.[31] Physical or manual removal with a tongue brush, scraper, or powered toothbrush will help reduce the population and regrowth of *Candida* and allow for any antifungal medication to be more effective. The usage of oral products with a high pH neutralizes the acidity of the oral cavity and disrupts the conducive environment for the growth of *Candida*. Anatomic changes or the formation of deep grooves (fissuring) on the tongue hinders the ability to physically remove *Candida*, resulting in faster repopulation. Using an ultrasonic oral device to dislodge the biofilm is an effective method for clearing these areas.

Removable prosthesis should be taken out at night and soaked in a nystatin solution without sugar for disinfection. The presence of sugar in saliva provides nutrition to the microbiota, so the control of sugar intake, diet modification, and the control of medical conditions help discourage the growth of *Candida*.

Treatment of oral candidiasis in SS patients can be especially challenging and requires prolonged therapy to eradicate the infection completely. In recurrent cases, suppressive therapy is required.

Mild to moderate cases of candidiasis can be treated by clotrimazole (10 mg) troches dissolved in the mouth with small sips of water five times per day or by using miconazole, 50 mg mucoadhesive buccal tabs. The duration of treatment may vary individually and should be continued even after the symptoms of candidiasis subside. These treatments are especially useful in SS patients with little or no saliva production. Nystatin suspension, 100,000 units/mL, 5 mL four times a day, to swish and spit is also sometimes used in mild cases. However, the high concentration of fermentable sugar used to mask the flavor of nystatin may induce caries in high-risk patients with salivary hypofunction.

Moderate to severe candidiasis can be treated with oral fluconazole, 100−200 mg daily, for 14−21 days but it only works in patients who can produce saliva. Fluconazole, 100 mg three times a week, is used as a suppressive agent in recurrent cases. Itraconazole solution, 200 mg daily, or posaconazole suspension, 400 mg twice daily for 3 days then 400 mg daily for 28 days, can be used for fluconazole-refractory cases. Alternatively, voriconazole, 200 mg twice daily, or amphotericin B deoxycholate oral suspension, 100 mg/mL 4 times daily, can be used[19] depending on the individual's response.

Mucosal lesions

A variety of mucosal lesions may occur in SS patients and adversely affect oral health and patient quality of life. Decreased lubrication in the mouth due to the loss of salivary mucins can lead to increased friction of the oral tissues against each other and result in mouth sores. For example, sticking of the tongue to the palatal rugae or the teeth to the buccal mucosa causes injury to the mucosal tissue. For SS patients, even eating can lead to trauma because of the friable nature of the tissue. Depapillation (atrophic glossitis) or loss of lingual papillae and formation of deep grooves (fissuring) are common in SS patients. Cracked dry lips (cheilosis) is another frequent complaint.

Associated autoimmune oral lesions

A retrospective, multicenter cohort study reported finding other oral lesions of auto-immune nature in 12% of SS subjects. Lichen planus was most frequently observed, followed by aphthous stomatitis and chronic ulcerative stomatitis.[32]

Aphthous stomatitis (canker sores) is a common occurrence in the general population but occurs in SS patients as well (Fig. 3.8).[33] Typically, it presents as an ulceration with a central fibrinous area surrounded by a red halo. Although the primary cause is unknown, aphthous stomatitis is thought to be T-cell mediated. The three types of aphthous ulcers (minor, major, herpetiform) can be triggered by ingestion of spicy or acidic food, stress or trauma to the oral tissues, hormonal cycles, allergies, or even genetic predisposition. Infrequently, Crohn's disease can coexist with SS and not only affect the intestinal mucosa but also cause recurrent aphthous ulcerations. Normally, the ulcerations heal in 7–10 days. They are usually seen on the buccal and labial mucosa, lateral borders/ventrum of the tongue, and floor of the mouth. Symptoms range from mild discomfort to severe pain that interferes with eating and drinking. There is no cure; however, taking steroids or amlexanox may speed the healing process.

Lichen planus is a chronic inflammatory condition that affects the mucous membranes inside the mouth. It usually presents bilaterally on the buccal mucosa, the gingiva, or the tongue. It can appear lacy with erosions or ulcers that can be painful when brushing or eating; it may cause a burning sensation in the affected areas (Fig. 3.9). Lichen planus has the potential to become cancerous and must be closely monitored. In the example shown, a small lesion turned into a severe cancer in only 3 months.

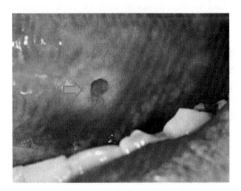

FIGURE 3.8

Aphthous ulcer (*arrow*) on the cheek.

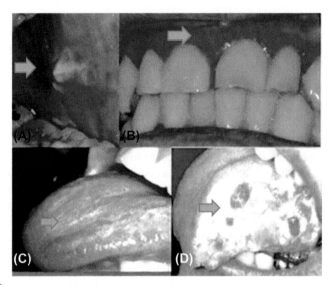

FIGURE 3.9

The arrows indicate various forms of lichen planus in a Sjögren's syndrome patient on the (A) cheek, (B) gum, (C) tongue, and (D) palate.

The association between SS and oral lichen planus is likely immune mediated, as studies have found no relationship between unstimulated or stimulated salivary flow rates and oral lichen planus.[34,35] Kenalog in Orabase is the only FDA-approved drug for this problem. However, other useful treatments include other topical steroids (e.g., clobetasol, fluocinonide) or topical calcineurin inhibitors (e.g., tacrolimus, pimecrolimus).

Glossodynia

The discomfort and even minor changes detected by the highly innervated tongue in the oral cavity can lead to the development of new parafunctional habits (e.g., frequently sticking out the tongue, constantly wetting the lips), which may worsen other oral signs and symptoms. In addition to oral candidiasis, stomatopyrosis and glossodynia in SS may be caused by or associated with dryness, inflammation of the oral mucosa, SS-associated neuropathies or vitamin B_{12} deficiency, anemia, and allergies. In "supertasters" who naturally have more taste buds and nerve endings than other individuals, the burning experience is worse. Sodium lauryl sulfate and anionic detergents found in certain toothpastes can further aggravate this problem and their use should be avoided. Restoration of salivary flow, identification and mitigation of other causative factors (e.g., faulty dentistry, allergies, dental conditions, diet), and change in oral habits and products will provide relief. When glossodynia occurs as a consequence of a neurologic problem, medications for neuropathic pain (e.g., gabapentin) are indicated.

Conclusions

Complications of untreated xerostomia in SS may include infections of the oral mucosa and salivary glands, accelerated caries, loss of dentition, salivary gland obstruction, and other problems. It is therefore critical that every SS patient with dry mouth undergoes a comprehensive oral care preventive program in the early stages of the disease before problems occur. Frequent cleanings, application of fluoride varnish every 3 months, use of sialogogues, and prescription-strength fluoride toothpaste when used daily can help preserve the teeth and oral tissues. Regular care by an oral medicine specialist can significantly improve patient quality of life and impact overall outcomes.

References

1. Lamanda A, Cheaib Z, Turgut MD, Lussi A. Protein buffering in model systems and in whole human saliva. *PLoS One*. 2007;2(2):e263.
2. van der Reijden WA, Vissink A, Veerman E, Amerongen A. Treatment of oral dryness related complaints (xerostomia) in Sjögren's syndrome. *Ann Rheum Dis*. 1999;58(8): 465—474.
3. Fenoll-Palomares C, Muñoz-Montagud JV, Sanchiz V, Herreros B, Hernández V, Mínguez M, Benages A. Unstimulated salivary flow rate, pH, and buffer capacity of saliva in healthy volunteers. *Rev Esp Enferm Dig*. 2004;96:773—783.
4. Atkinson JC, Grisius M, Massey W. Salivary hypofunction and xerostomia: diagnosis and treatment. *Dent Clin N Am*. 2005;49(2):309—326.
5. Sandhya P, Sharma D, Vellarikkal S, Surin AK, Jayarajan R, Verma A, Dixit V, Sivasubbu S, Danda D, Scaria V. AB0188 systematic analysis of the oral microbiome in primary SjÖgren's syndrome suggest enrichment of distinct microbes. *Ann Rheum Dis*. 2015;74:953—954.
6. Sreebny LM, Valdini A. Xerostomia: a neglected symptom. *Arch Intern Med*. 1987; 147(7):1333—1337.
7. Plemons JM, Al-Hashimi I, Marek CL. Managing xerostomia and salivary gland hypofunction: executive summary of a report from the American dental association council on scientific affairs. *J Am Dent Assoc*. 2014;145(8):867—873.
8. Nieuw Amerongen AV, Veerman EC. Current therapies for xerostomia and salivary gland hypofunction associated with cancer therapies. *Support Care Cancer*. 2003;11(4): 226—231.
9. Vivino F. Sjögren's syndrome: clinical aspects. *Clin Immunol*. 2017;182:48—54.
10. Vivino FB, Bunya VY, Massaro-Giordano G, Johr CR, Giattino SL, Schorpion A, Shafer B, Peck A, Sivils K, Rasmussen A0, Chiorini JA, He J, Ambrus Jr JL. Sjogren's syndrome: an update on disease pathogenesis, clinical manifestations and treatment. *Clin Immunol*. June 2019;203:81—121.
11. Keck S, Papas A, Finkelman M, Magnuson B, Singh M. *Oral health related quality of life in primary Sjögren's syndrome*. March 22, 2014. Charlotte (NC); abstract nr 1599.
12. https://www.sjogrens.org/files/articles/LivingwithSjogrens.pdf (accessed May 27, 2019).

13. Barbera K, Roomian T, Papas A. *Endodontic vs. Implant treatment outcomes in Sjögren's syndrome patients.* San Francisco (CA): IADR 2017; March 25, 2017. Abstract nr 3318.

14. Singh ML, Kugel G, Magnuson B, Papas A. Non-carious lesions due to tooth surface loss: to restore or not to restore? *Inside Dent.* 2011;7(3).

15. Buzalaf MA, Hannas AR, Kato MT. Saliva and dental erosion. *J Appl Oral Sci.* 2012; 20(5):493–502.

16. Young WG. The oral medicine of tooth wear. *Aust Dent J.* 2001;46(4):236–250. quiz 306.

17. Chang CS, Liao CH, Muo CH, Kao CH. Increased risk of concurrent gastroesophageal reflux disease among patients with Sjögren's syndrome: a nationwide population-based study. *Eur J Intern Med.* 2016;31:73–78.

18. Singh M, Magnuson B, Papas A. GERD and oral manifestations. In: DiMarino Jr AJ, Cohen S, eds. *Chapter 6: Extraesophageal manifestations of GERD.* New Jersey: Slack Incorporated; 2013.

19. Pappas PG, Kauffman CA, Andes DR, Clancy CJ, Marr KA, Ostrosky-Zeichner L, Reboli AC, Schuster MG, Vazquez JA, Walsh TJ, Zaoutis TE, Sobel JD. Clinical practice guideline for the management of candidiasis: 2016 update by the infectious diseases society of America. *Clin Infect Dis.* 2016;62(4):409–417.

20. Zero DT, Brennan MT, Daniels TE, Papas A, Stewart C, Pinto A, Al-Hashimi I, Navazesh M, Rhodus N, Sciubba J, Singh M, Wu AJ, Frantsve-Hawley J, Tracy S, Fox PC, Ford TL, Cohen S, Vivino FB, Hammitt KM. Clinical practice guidelines for oral management of Sjögren disease: dental caries prevention. *J Am Dent Assoc.* 2016; 147(4):295–305.

21. Agnello M, Cen L, Tran NC, Shi W, McLean JS, He X. Arginine improves pH homeostasis via metabolism and microbiome modulation. *J Dent Res.* 2017;96(8):924–930.

22. Milgrom P, Ly KA, Rothen M. Xylitol and its vehicles for public health needs. *Adv Dent Res.* 2009;21(1):44–47.

23. Söderling EM, Ekman TC, Taipale TJ. Growth inhibition of Streptococcus mutans with low xylitol concentrations. *Curr Microbiol.* 2008;56:382–385.

24. Soderling E, Talonpoika J, Makinen KK. Effect of xylitol-containing carbohydrate mixtures on acid and ammonia production in suspensions of salivary sediment. *Scand J Dent Res.* 1987;95:405–410.

25. Marttinen AM, Ruas-Madiedo P, Hidalgo-Cantabrana C, Saari MA, Ihalin RA, Söderling EM. Effects of xylitol on xylitol-sensitive versus xylitol-resistant Streptococcus mutans strains in a three-species in vitro biofilm. *Curr Microbiol.* 2012;65: 237–243.

26. De Vita S, Gandolfo S, Zandonella Callegher S, Zabotti A, Quartuccio L. The evaluation of disease activity in Sjögren's syndrome based on the degree of MALT involvement: glandular swelling and cryoglobulinaemia compared to ESSDAI in a cohort study. *Clin Exp Rheumatol.* 2018;112(3):150–156.

27. Medeiros CCG, Borges LGDA, Cherubini K, Salum FG, Silva RMD, de Figueiredo MAZ. Oral yeast colonization in patients with primary and secondary Sjögren's syndrome. *Oral Dis.* 2018;24:1367–1378.

28. Tzavaras E, Papas A, Singh M, Cmmino J, Corrado P, Finkelman M. *Colony forming units of Candida in Sjögren's and non-Sjögren's xerostomic population.* AADR/CADR Annual Meeting Los Angeles, (CA); 2016. Abstract nr 0792.

29. Soto-Rojas AE, Villa AR, Sifuentes-Osornio J, Alarcón-Segovia D, Kraus A. Oral manifestations in patients with Sjögren's syndrome. *J Rheumatol*. 1998;25(5):906–910.
30. Xiao J, Huang X, Alkhers N, Alzamil H, Alzoubi S, Wu T, Castillo DA, Campbell F, Davis J, Herzog K, Billings R, Kopycka-Kedzierawski D,T, Hajishengallis E, Koo H. Candida albicans and early childhood caries: a systematic review and meta-analysis. *Caries Res*. 2018;52:102–112.
31. Torres SR, Peixoto CB, Caldas DM, Silva EB, Akiti T, Nucci M, de Uzeda M. Relationship between salivary flow rates and Candida counts in subjects with xerostomia. *Oral Surg Oral Med Oral Pathol Oral Radiol Endod*. 2002;93(2):149–154.
32. Likar-Manookin K, Stewart C, Al-Hashimi I, Curtis W, Berg K, Cherian K, Lockhart PB, Brennan MT. Prevalence of oral lesions of autoimmune etiology in patients with primary Sjögren's syndrome. *Oral Dis*. 2013;19(6):598–603.
33. Błochowiak K, Olewicz-Gawlik A, Polańska A, Nowak-Gabryel M, Kociecki J, Witmanowski H, Sokalski J. Mucosal manifestations in primary and secondary Sjögren syndrome and dry mouth syndrome. *Postepy Dermatol Alergol*. 2016;33(1):23–27.
34. Larsen KR, Johansen JD, Reibel J, Zachariae C, Rosing K, Pedersen AML. Oral symptoms and salivary findings in oral lichen planus, oral lichenoid lesions and stomatitis. *BMC Oral Health*. 2017;17(1):103. https://doi.org/10.1186/s12903-017-0393-2.
35. Ramon C, Bagan JV, Milian MA, Jimenez Y, Lloria E. Quantitative analysis of saliva in patients with oral lichen planus: a study of 100 cases. *Med Oral*. 2000;5(3):187–192.

Diagnosis and management of Sjögren's syndrome related dry eye

4

Vatinee Y. Bunya, MD, MSCE[1], John A. Gonzales, MD[2], Michael E. Sulewski, MD[1], Mina Massaro-Giordano, MD[1], Stephen E. Orlin, MD[1]

[1]*Assistant Professor, Cornea & External Disease, Ophthalmology, Scheie Eye Institute, Perelman School of Medicine at the University of Pennsylvania, Philadelphia, PA, United States;* [2]*Francis I. Proctor Foundation and Department of Ophthalmology, University of California, San Francisco, CA, United States*

Introduction

Sjögren's syndrome (SS) can cause a variety of ocular manifestations, with the most common being a specific dry eye phenotype known as keratoconjunctivitis sicca (KCS), a term originally coined by Henrik Sjögren.[1] As a result, SS patients often first present to an eye care provider for dry eye symptoms and therefore it is important to consider SS as a possible underlying diagnosis in any patient with dry eyes. Ophthalmologists have a unique opportunity to screen patients with dry eyes and refer them in a timely manner for systemic SS evaluations, thereby decreasing the time to diagnosis. Dry eye can cause significant discomfort and decreased quality of life.[2] In addition, dry eye also affects visual function and can cause fluctuations in vision and blurred vision, which in turn lead to difficulties with activities of daily living such as reading and driving.[3,4]

The diagnosis and management of SS-related dry eye can pose special challenges to clinicians. Although SS patients are classically thought of as having aqueous tear-deficient dry eye, studies have shown that SS patients have both aqueous deficient and evaporative dry eye.[5] Therefore it is important to evaluate and treat these patients for both of these underlying types of dry eyes. In addition, SS patients can have dry eye that is refractory to standard therapies and may require systemic immunosuppression to control their disease. There are also special considerations regarding corneal neuropathy, contact lens wear, as well as refractive procedures and cataract surgery.

Diagnosis

Symptoms

It is important to first assess the nature of a patient's dry eye symptoms. Patients will often report foreign body sensation, burning, photosensitivity, glare, or transient blurred vision. Although there are many dry eye questionnaires available,[6] there is no single, validated survey that is universally used. However, using a short questionnaire can be helpful to evaluate a patient for dry eye symptoms. For example, a short series of questions was first proposed by Schaumberg and colleagues[7,8] for use with patients with dry eye and was later refined by Foulks et al.[9] They proposed using the following three questions: (1) How often do your eyes feel dryness, discomfort, or irritation? Would you say it is often or constantly? (Y/N), (2) When you have dryness, discomfort, or irritation, does this impact your activities (e.g., do you stop or reduce your time doing them)? (Y/N), and (3) Do you think you have dry eye? (Y/N).[9] The answer "yes" to any of these questions warrants a full ocular surface examination. Using these questions allows clinicians to quickly assess the nature of a patient's dry eye symptoms.

Ocular examination

There is a poor correlation between the severity of ocular symptoms and objective tests for dry eye.[10] Therefore regardless of the symptom severity, every SS patient should see a cornea or dry eye specialist for a comprehensive evaluation. This should include (1) measurement of tear production, (2) inspection of the eyelids for abnormalities including signs of meibomian gland dysfunction (MGD), and (3) staining of the cornea with fluorescein and the conjunctiva with lissamine green to assess the degree of ocular surface damage. It is important to determine whether the dry eye is due to aqueous tear deficiency (inadequate production of tears) or evaporative dry eye (often caused by MGD), or a combination of both. In evaporative dry eye, altered or diminished meibum secretion causes dysfunction of the outer oily layer of the tear film, which leads to increased tear evaporation from the ocular surface. Proper assessment is critical to determine the best treatment options for a given patient.

Aqueous tear deficiency can be assessed using a variety of tests, with one of the simplest and most helpful being the Schirmer test.[6] The Schirmer test measures tear production and can be performed with or without anesthesia. However, when evaluating a patient with dry eye for possible SS, it is important to perform this test without anesthesia, as this is one of the ocular criteria included in the SS classification criteria.[11] To perform the Schirmer test, the examiner carefully dries inside each lower eyelid and then the Schirmer strips are placed in the corner of the lower eyelids as far laterally as possible. The patient is then asked to close his/her eyes gently for 5 min. After the test is completed, the strips are removed and the length of the watermark line is measured in millimeters and recorded for each eye. A result of <10 mm/5 min is considered abnormal.

The presence of evaporative dry eye can be assessed through the careful evaluation of the lid blink function and lid margins, including assessment of the meibomian glands of the eyelid, which produce the lipid layer of the tear film.[6] Using the slit lamp biomicroscope, it is important to observe for the presence of incomplete blinks, as well as for evidence of blepharitis or inflammation of the eyelids. In addition, gentle pressure can be applied to the meibomian glands of each eyelid to assess the quality of the meibum that is expressed. In the normal eyelid the meibum is clear and can easily be expressed with gentle pressure. With more severe MGD the meibum thickens and is harder to express manually.

Another useful test when evaluating a patient for evaporative dry eye is the tear breakup time (TBUT) test, which examines the stability of the tear film.[6] TBUT is typically measured 30–60 seconds after administration of fluorescein dye to the eye and use of the blue cobalt filter on the slit lamp biomicroscope. The patient is instructed to blink a few times to try to evenly distribute the tear film over the surface of the eye. Next the examiner asks the patient to blink once and counts the number of seconds it takes until a dark area (signaling evaporation of tears) appears in the tear film and records this. A normal value is 10 seconds or more, with a lower value indicating increasing severity of evaporative dry eye. It is important to note that certain conditions of the cornea, such as anterior basement membrane dystrophy or Salzmann nodules can also lower TBUT and should be taken into consideration when interpreting the result.

Ocular surface staining is useful for quantifying the severity of dry eye disease, including damage to the ocular surface.[6] Two common vital dyes used for ocular surface staining include fluorescein and lissamine green. Fluorescein is typically used to evaluate the cornea, whereas lissamine green is useful for evaluating the conjunctiva. The timing of examination after dye administration is also important, as the pattern and visibility of ocular surface staining change over time. Together, these staining patterns are used to assess the ocular surface staining score (OSS) that was first described by Whitcher and colleagues.[12] It is important to note that OSS is one of the ocular criteria included in the American College of Rheumatology-European League Against Rheumatism (ACR-EULAR) SS classification criteria. By these criteria, an OSS ≥ 5 in one eye is considered clinically meaningful. Alternatively, a van Bijsterveld scale score of ≥ 4 with rose bengal staining on a 0–9 scale would also satisfy one of the ocular criteria, but is less commonly used due to the ocular stinging and burning associated with rose bengal administration.[13]

Finally, the order of tests used to examine the ocular surface is important, as certain tests can affect the results of subsequent tests. It is also important to avoid the administration of any drops before the examination of the ocular surface, as certain drops (i.e., topical anesthetics) can affect dry eye test results. For example, topical anesthetics can increase the OSS by causing a decreased blink rate, or by the ocular surface staining caused by the topical anesthetic itself. In addition, topical anesthetics may decrease the Schirmer test score, as they eliminate reflex tearing. Of note, performing the Schirmer test without anesthesia is one of the ocular criteria included in the ACR/EULAR criteria. A typical order for performing dry eye tests includes the following: (1) TBUT, (2) fluorescein staining of the cornea, (3) lissamine green staining of the conjunctiva, and (4) Schirmer test without anesthesia.

Treatment of dry eye and meibomian gland dysfunction
Overview

Once the nature of dry eye symptoms has been assessed and a complete evaluation of the ocular surface has been performed, treatment should be approached in a stepwise fashion. Although dry eye cannot be cured, effective therapies are currently available to manage symptoms and prevent complications. Management of dry eye depends on the nature and severity of the disease. Therapies should be selected depending on the degree of aqueous tear deficiency and evaporative dry eye and tailored to each patient.

Foulks et al.[9], under the auspices of the Sjögren's Syndrome Foundation, Inc., published detailed clinical practice guidelines for the management of dry eye associated with SS.[9] In that algorithm, treatment is individualized and chosen based on the presence or absence of concomitant MGD and the severity (graded levels 1—4) of the disease (Table 4.1).

For patients with mild dry eye (level 1), modifications of their environment and activities of daily living can be helpful. However, if these measures are inadequate then additional treatments can be considered. The first line of therapy for dry eye should be lubrication with artificial tears. However, as dry eye worsens to a moderate severity level (levels 2—3), patients often require additional therapies, which may include

Table 4.1 Management algorithm for Sjögren's syndrome dry eye.

Diagnosis:	Aqueous deficiency without meibomian gland disease	Dry Eye Disease	Aqueous deficiency with meibomian gland disease	GRADE	
				evidence	recommendation
				good	strong
				moderate	discretionary
				insufficient	
Treatment					
Severity Level 1	Education and environment/diet modification		Education and environment/diet modification	good	strong
	Elimination of offending systemic medication		Elimination of offending systemic medication	good	strong
	Artificial tears, gels, ointments		Artificial tears with lipid component	good	strong
			Eyelid therapy: warm compress, massage	good	strong
Severity Level 2 level 1 therapy inadequate	Omega-3 essential fatty acid supplement		Omega-3 essential fatty acid supplement	moderate	moderate strong
	Antiinflammatory therapy: cyclosporine		Antiinflammatory therapy: cyclosporine	good	moderate strong
	Antiinflammatory therapy: pulse steroids		Antiinflammatory therapy: pulse steroids	good	moderate strong
			Topical azithromycin	good	moderate strong
			Liposomal spray	good	moderate strong
			Possible oral doxycycline	good	moderate strong
			Expression of meibomian glands	good	moderate strong
	Punctal plugs		Punctal plugs	good	moderate strong
	Secretagogues		Secretagogues	good	moderate strong
	Moisture chamber spectacles		Moisture chamber spectacles	good	moderate strong
Severity Level 3 level 2 therapy inadequate	Topical autologous serum		Topical autologous serum	good	moderate strong
	Contact lenses		Contact lenses	good	moderate strong
	Permanent punctal occlusion		Permanent punctal occlusion	good	moderate strong
			(LipiFlow pulsed thermal compression)	insufficient	discretionary
			(Probing of meibomian gland)	insufficient	discretionary
Severity Level 4 level 3 therapy inadequate	Systemic antiinflammatory medication		Systemic antiinflammatory medication	moderate	discretionary
	Eyelid surgery		Eyelid surgery	good	moderate strong

[Assumes use of the International Dry Eye Workshop severity scale]

Adapted from Ref. 9.

topical anti-inflammatory drops or oral secretagogues. Once inflammation of the ocular surface is controlled, plugging of the openings (puncta) of the tear ducts using plugs or cautery can be helpful in conserving tears. Concomitant MGD can be treated with warm compresses, lid hygiene, and topical or systemic antibiotics. Patients with severe dry eye (level 4) may require topical autologous serum drops, partial closure of the interpalpebral fissure of the eyelids to reduce evaporation from the ocular surface, or scleral contact lenses. In very severe cases, systemic anti-inflammatory or immunosuppressive medications may be required to control the ocular disease.

Environmental/lifestyle modifications

For patients with mild dry eye, modifications of their activities of daily living and environment can be helpful.[14] For example, avoiding oral or topical medications that can worsen dryness is important. In addition, patients should be advised to limit certain tasks such as reading or viewing computer screens for prolonged periods, as these activities are associated with a decreased blink rate and can exacerbate symptoms.[15] It can be helpful to take frequent breaks every 20 minutes and position screens so that they are below the level of the eyes to limit evaporation from the ocular surface. Other measures that may be useful include directing heating and cooling vents away from the eyes, using eye protection such as wraparound sunglasses or moisture chamber goggles, and using a humidifier at home and at work.[14] Oral omega-3 essential fatty acid supplements may be considered; however, a large, double-blind, multicenter, randomized clinical trial did not demonstrate any benefit of the supplements over placebo for the treatment of dry eye.[16]

Lubrication

There are a large number of commercially available artificial tear options. There are important differences between artificial tears with or without preservatives. Preservatives in certain artificial tear preparations destabilize the tear film and can be toxic to the ocular surface,[17] especially if used frequently throughout the day. A general rule of thumb is that patients with mild dry eye should not use any supplemental tears with preservatives more than four times a day. SS patients with moderate-to-severe dry eye should be instructed to only use preservative-free artificial tears (Table 4.2), which typically come in single-use individual vials.

Another important consideration is the viscosity of the preparation. There are a variety of artificial tears available with different viscosities. In general, if a lubricant is more viscous, it tends to last longer but it also causes blurred vision (Table 4.3). Gels are more viscous than artificial tear solutions, and artificial tear ointments are the thickest lubricants that can be used. Therefore artificial tear ointments are typically used at bedtime to provide relief overnight because they can significantly blur vision, thereby limiting their use during the day.

There are a variety of artificial tear formulations.[9,17,18] Some preparations contain components that try to prevent ocular surface damage through the use of

Table 4.2 Preservative-free artificial tears[a].

Product	Active ingredients	Notes
Bion® Tears (Alcon/Novartis)	0.1% Dextran 70, 0.3% hypromellose 2910	
Blink® PF (Johnson & Johnson)	0.25% PEG 400	
Clear Eyes® Pure Relief™ (Prestige)	0.25% Glycerin	Preservative-free multidose bottle
FreshKote® preservative free (Focus Laboratories)	2.7% Polyvinyl alcohol, 2.0% povidone	Preservative-free multidose bottle; stored behind pharmacy counter; also contains glycerin
GenTeal® Tears (Alcon/Novartis)	0.1% Dextran 70, 0.3% hypromellose 2910	
Hylo-Forte® (AFT Pharmaceuticals)	Sodium hyaluronate 2 mg/mL	Preservative-free multidose bottle
NanoTears® TF PF (Altaire)	0.4% PEG, 0.3% PEG	
Oasis® Tears (Oasis Medical)	0.2% Glycerin	
Refresh Classic® (Allergan)	1.4% Polyvinyl alcohol, 0.6% povidone	
Refresh Optive® (Allergan)	0.5% CMC; 0.9% glycerin	
Refresh Optive Advanced® (Allergan)	0.5% CMC, 1% glycerin, 0.5% polysorbate 80	
Refresh Optive Mega-3® (Allergan)	0.5% CMC, 1% glycerin, 0.5% polysorbate 80	Also contains castor oil and flaxseed
Refresh Optive Sensitive® (Allergan)	0.5% CMC, 0.9% glycerin	
Refresh Plus® (Allergan)	0.5% CMC	
Soothe® PF (Bausch & Lomb)	0.6% PPG, 0.6% glycerin	
Systane® (Alcon/Novartis)	0.4% PEG 400, 0.3% PEG	
Systane Ultra® PF (Alcon/Novartis)	0.4% PEG 400, 0.3% PPG	
TheraTears® PF (Akorn)	0.25% CMC	

CMC, *carboxymethylcellulose*; PEG, *polyethylene glycol*; PPG, *polypropylene glycol*.
[a] *Not an exhaustive list.*

electrolytes or formulations to counteract the effects of hyperosmolarity of the tear film.[14] Other preparations try to mimic the lipid component of tears, which is thought to reduce evaporation from the ocular surface (Table 4.4). The majority of artificial tears are available over the counter, but certain preparations, such as Lacrisert® (Bausch & Lomb, Bridgewater, NJ), require a prescription. Lacrisert is a preservative-free small lubricant pellet that is placed inside the lower eyelids and it dissolves slowly to release moisture onto the ocular surface.[19]

Table 4.3 Higher viscosity artificial tears, gels, and ointments. [a]

Formulation	Product	Preservatives? Yes/No	Active ingredients
Higher viscosity artificial tears			
	Blink Gel Tears® (AMO)	Yes	0.25% PEG 400
	GenTeal® Moderate Liquid Drops (Alcon/Novartis)	Yes	0.1% Dextran 70, 0.2% glycerin, 0.3% hypromellose
	Lacrisert® (Bausch & Lomb)[b]	No	
	Oasis Tears Plus® (Oasis Medical)	No	0.2% Glycerin
	Refresh Celluvisc® (Allergan)	No	1% CMC
	Refresh Liquigel® (Allergan)	Yes	1% CMC
	Refresh Optive® Gel Drops (Allergan)	Yes	1% CMC, 0.9% glycerin
	Systane® Gel Drops (Alcon/Novartis)	Yes	0.4% PEG 400, 0.3% PPG
	TheraTears® nighttime dry eye therapy (Akorn)	No	1% CMC
Gels			
	GenTeal® Gel (Novartis)		0.3% Hypromellose
	Liposic® (Bausch & Lomb)		Carbomer
	Systane® Lubricant Eye Gel (Alcon/Novartis)		0.3% Hypromellose
Ointments			
	GenTeal® Nighttime Ointment (Alcon/Novartis)		3% Mineral oil, 94% white petrolatum
	Refresh Lacri-Lube® (Allergan)		42.5% Mineral oil, 56.8% white petrolatum
	Refresh PM® (Allergan)		42.5% Mineral oil, 57.3% white petrolatum
	Retaine PM® (Ocusoft)		20% Mineral oil, 80% white petrolatum
	Soothe® NightTime Ointment (Bausch & Lomb)		20% Mineral oil, 80% white petrolatum
	Systane® Nighttime Ointment (Alcon/Novartis)		3% Mineral oil, 94% white petrolatum

CMC, carboxymethylcellulose; PEG, polyethylene glycol; PPG, polypropylene glycol.
[a] Not an exhaustive list.
[b] Prescription-only; a dissolvable pellet is inserted inside the lower eyelid.

Table 4.4 Lipid-based artificial tears.[a]

Product	Preservatives?	Active ingredients
Refresh Optive Advanced® (Allergan)	No	1% Glycerin, 0.5% CMC, 0.5% polysorbate 80
Retaine MGD® (Ocusoft)	No	0.5% Light mineral oil, 0.5% mineral oil
Soothe XP® (Bausch & Lomb)	Yes	1% Light mineral oil, 4.5% mineral oil
Systane Balance® (Alcon/Novartis)	Yes	0.6% PPG, mineral oil
Systane Complete® (Alcon/Novartis)	Yes	0.6% PPG, mineral oil
Tears Again® (Ocusoft)	Yes	Liposomal soy lecithin, vitamin A palmitate, vitamin E

CMC, *carboxymethylcellulose*; PPG, *polypropylene glycol*.
[a] *Not an exhaustive list.*

It is important to note that none of the various artificial tear preparations is superior to others. Patients often need to try several different preparations to find one that is most soothing. Tear selection should be individualized to the patient's specific needs.

Oral secretagogues

Oral secretagogues, such as pilocarpine and cevimeline, stimulate the secretion of saliva from the salivary glands. Although not FDA approved for the treatment of dry eye, there is some evidence that oral secretagogues may be effective in reducing dry eye symptoms and/or ocular surface staining.[20–22] However, they seem to have a greater benefit for the relief of dry mouth symptoms, with sweating being the predominant side effect.[9]

Topical anti-inflammatory medications

There is increasing evidence that inflammation of the ocular surface plays an important role in dry eye disease.[23] Therefore controlling inflammation is thought to play an important role in the treatment of dry eye. Topical steroids can be useful for short periods in alleviating dry eye symptoms, although possible complications such as cataract formation, infection, and secondary glaucoma limit their long-term use[24,25] A short 2-3-week course of topical steroids can be considered in select patients during severe flare-ups.

Topical cyclosporine is thought to decrease inflammation by several mechanisms including through the inhibition of T-lymphocyte activation.[26,27] The recommended treatment dose is one drop to each eye twice daily. The most common side effect is stinging upon instillation, which can be alleviated by instilling a drop of artificial tears 5 minutes before each dose, refrigeration of the drug, or the concurrent use of a topical steroid for the first 2 weeks.[28]

Topical lifitegrast was approved by the FDA for the treatment of dry eye. Lifitegrast decreases inflammation by blocking the interaction between intercellular adhesion molecule 1 and lymphocyte function—associated antigen 1.[29] In four, large, multicellular, randomized clinical trials, lifitegrast was shown to be effective in improving the signs and symptoms of dry eye.[29] The side effects of lifitegrast include transient ocular irritation and dysgeusia. Further studies are needed to explore the effectiveness of combination therapy such as the concomitant use of topical cyclosporine and topical lifitegrast.

Conservation of tears

Once inflammation of the ocular surface is controlled, blocking the drainage of tears through the openings of the tear ducts (puncta) of each eyelid can be useful. Punctal occlusion using plugs or cautery can be helpful in conserving tears and retaining moisture on the ocular surface.[30] This procedure is typically performed in a stepwise fashion beginning with the inferior lacrimal canaliculi.

Management of severe dry eye

Patients with severe ocular surface disease (level 4) may require additional measures. Topical autologous serum drops contain a variety of substances that are beneficial to the ocular surface, including vitamin A and growth factors, and are a useful treatment option in patients with severe dry eye.[31,32] Partial closure of the interpalpebral fissure using surgical methods or botulinum toxin can help reduce evaporation from the ocular surface. Large-diameter scleral contact lenses can be helpful in patients with severe ocular surface disease by providing a fluid reservoir over the cornea.[33] Patients with filaments or mucus strands on the surface of the cornea (i.e. filamentary keratitis) may benefit from topical *N*-acetylcysteine drops, which can be obtained from a compounding pharmacy. Finally, patients with severe dry eye may require systemic anti-inflammatory medications or immunosuppressants to control their ocular disease.

Treatment of eyelid disease

It is important to treat concomitant MGD or blepharitis in SS patients. First-line treatment for MGD should include the use of warm compresses, eyelid massage, and eyelid scrubs.[34] Patients should apply warm compresses that utilize moist heat, such as using a washcloth with warm tap water. A typical recommendation is to apply warm compresses twice a day for 5 minutes with gentle lid massage to encourage flow from the meibomian glands. Additional measures that are helpful in controlling MGD include eyelid hygiene; the use of topical antibiotics, such as erythromycin ointment or azithromycin drops; and the use of oral antibiotics, such as doxycycline or azithromycin.[34,35] Patients with refractory MGD may be candidates for new treatments such as meibomian gland probing, intense pulsed light treatment, or continuous controlled thermal compression (LipiFlow® System, TearScience, Morrisville, NC). However, these treatments are often not covered by insurance and must be paid for out of pocket.

Special considerations
Contact lenses

SS patients with mild dry eye can typically wear soft or rigid contact lenses safely. It is important that the contact lens has a proper fit and moves freely on the ocular surface with each blink to avoid hypoxia and subsequent corneal neovascularization. There is some evidence that certain materials have a higher oxygen transmission rate and may therefore be preferred over other contact lens materials,[36,37] although further studies are needed.[38] Patients with dry eye often do better with a more frequent replacement schedule, such as using daily disposable soft contact lenses instead of daily-wear contacts that are changed every 2–4 weeks. Patients with moderate-to-severe dry eye with significant corneal staining should be advised not to wear standard contact lenses because they will likely exacerbate their symptoms. Instead, these patients may benefit from wearing a therapeutic contact lens such as a large-diameter rigid scleral lens, as described in the Treatment section.

Corneal neuropathy, neuropathic pain, and dry eye

While dry eye is often considered the hallmark ocular feature of SS, significant changes in the cornea lie below the clinically observable ocular surface. Studies indicate that some features of ocular discomfort may be mediated by pathologic changes in the subbasal nerve plexus of the cornea.[39]

Prior studies investigating small fiber peripheral sensory neuropathies in SS patients have provided clues on the possible pathophysiologic mechanisms that mediate and modulate ocular surface discomfort in this population. The hallmark feature that characterizes small fiber neuropathies is the sensation of burning. This may occur in a length-dependent fashion and affect the distal extremities such as the feet or in a non–length-dependent fashion and cause burning of the face or trunk.[40] The pain elicited may arise from non-painful stimuli (allodynia) or an especially exuberant response to painful stimuli (hyperalgesia). Small fiber neuropathies are common in SS but are challenging to diagnose. On examination, there is sometimes a loss of pinprick and temperature sensation but no deficit in strength, light touch sensation, proprioception, or deep tendon reflexes. Nerve conduction studies in such patients are typically unremarkable.[41] Skin biopsy, although invasive, may show reduced intraepidermal nerve fiber density and pathologic changes including axonal swelling.[42] This diagnosis should be considered whenever patients complain of symptoms consistent with neuropathic pain.

The assessment of neuropathic pain typically involves inquiring about symptoms such as burning or electric shocks. Questionnaires have been developed that are useful in identifying patients with neuropathic body pain and include tools such as the Neuropathic Pain Symptom Inventory and the Leeds Assessment of Neuropathic Symptoms and Signs.[43,44] Identification of small fiber neuropathic pain is important, as effective non-opioid treatments exist.[45,46]

Interestingly, non-ocular small fiber neuropathic symptoms may sometimes precede the development of ocular or oral sicca symptoms in SS patients.[45] In ophthalmology the use of corneal *in vivo* confocal microscopy has also provided a non-invasive means to identify this phenomenon in the eye. Various studies have demonstrated pathologic structural changes in the subbasal nerve plexus of patients with dry eye that are consistent with a diagnosis of corneal neuropathy. These abnormalities include a reduction in the number and density of the subbasal nerves, reduced caliber of individual nerves, increased tortuosity, increased nerve beading, and a decrease in corneal mechanical sensation as measured by esthesiometry.[47,48] In addition, perineural dendritic cells are also found in the corneal neuropathy of dry eye[49,50] and diabetes.[51] Other corneal features seen in SS patients include keratocyte activation, thinner epithelium, and a reduction in epithelial cell density compared to non-SS dry eye patients, suggesting that corneal neuropathy is associated with concomitant epitheliopathy.[52] Currently, it is unknown whether the corneal neuropathy in SS is a primary process in itself, secondary to a reduction in tear production and an increase in inflammatory mediators on the ocular surface, or a combination of both. While a decreased density of nerve fibers may be associated with a reduction in neurotrophic factors that maintain corneal nerve health, decreased tear lacritin (a glycoprotein produced by the lacrimal gland) has been correlated with a reduced density and length of corneal nerve fibers and increased dry eye symptoms in SS patients.[53]

There is evidence that modulating ocular surface inflammation may help improve corneal nerve morphology. For example, six months of topical cyclosporine A (0.05%) application has been associated with a reduction in the number of perineural dendritic cells and an increase in the density of the subbasal nerve plexus in SS patients.[54] Topical autologous platelet lysate has also been associated with a reduction in perineural dendritic cells and an improvement in the density of nerve fibers.[55] Patients with neuropathic ocular pain are becoming increasingly distinguished from other patients with dry eye and have advanced to neuropathic pain—modulating medications because lubricating the ocular surface is frequently insufficient in providing relief from the ocular discomfort mediated by neuropathic pain.[56–58]

Ocular refractive surgery

Because SS patients often have difficulty wearing contact lenses due to discomfort from dry eye, undergoing refractive surgery may be an attractive alternative. However, refractive surgery may exacerbate ocular surface disease in SS and can be contraindicated in certain patients. Studies regarding refractive surgery outcomes in SS patients are lacking,[59] and more research is needed. At the present time, however, it is recommended that special consideration be given to SS patients in this clinical situation; every effort should be made to assess and improve ocular surface disease before proceeding with any type of refractive surgery.

Refractive surgery using laser vision correction was first introduced in the 1980s and with significant technologic advances, the success and precision of the surgery have made it one of the most common operations performed in the United States today. However, even though the success of the surgery is remarkably high with reports of over 97% patient satisfaction,[60,61] the operation is still not without risk.

One of the most common refractive surgery procedures performed is *laser in situ keratomileusis* (LASIK). During LASIK surgery, a thin-hinged flap is made in the superficial cornea with either a microkeratome (oscillating blade) or a femtosecond laser. The flap is then retracted and the underlying cornea is ablated with an excimer laser to correct the appropriate refractive error. The flap is repositioned and is self-adherent without requiring sutures. However, with the creation of the flap, the corneal nerves supplying sensation to the superficial cornea are transected, thereby interrupting the critical reflex arc that is needed for the stimulation of natural tear production.[62] Because a 4-5-mm hinge is left intact, not all the corneal nerves are cut and with time they do regenerate. However, in patients with a compromised tear film to begin with, particularly in those with SS, this interruption can be critical and cause significant exacerbation of dry eye symptoms and clinical findings.

Another refractive surgery procedure is *photorefractive keratectomy* (PRK). During PRK the surface of the cornea is ablated with a laser without creating a flap, thereby avoiding severing of the corneal nerves. Therefore this may be a viable option for patients with mild-to-moderate dry eyes. However, PRK is contraindicated in patients with severe ocular surface disease. The creation of a larger central corneal abrasion during the procedure can result in delayed surface healing in patients with severe dry eye. This delayed healing can lead to significant corneal scarring and persistent haze, which can compromise the final visual acuity. In addition, there are conflicting reports as to whether PRK or LASIK induces less dry eye[63], and further studies are needed. It is possible that a newer refractive procedure, *small incision lenticule extraction* (SMILE), which has less impact on the corneal nerves, may induce less postoperative dry eye but, again, further studies are needed.[64]

There are special preoperative and postoperative considerations for SS patients undergoing refractive surgery. A careful preoperative history and clinical evaluation is critical in assessing patients with SS before considering refractive surgery.[64] Patients with mild dry eyes may only be symptomatic when wearing their contact lenses and are asymptomatic without them. If these patients have minimal or no ocular surface staining then they may be suitable candidates for surgery. However, there have been case reports of SS patients with well-controlled disease preoperatively who developed severe, refractory dry eye after LASIK.[65] Careful instruction about maximizing the ocular surface health before and immediately after surgery with treatments such as artificial tears, punctal occlusion, and low-dose topical cyclosporine or lifitegrast therapy to stimulate tear production is essential. Patients who are more symptomatic might benefit from autologous serum tear supplementation.

Postoperatively, the clinical findings of post-LASIK dry eye syndrome include decreased functional visual acuity, decreased Schirmer test values, rapid TBUT, staining of the ocular surface, and decreased corneal sensation.[64] Post-LASIK dry eye can be a major reason for dissatisfaction among patients after the procedure[66] and can often be more difficult to manage than dry eye not associated with refractive surgery.

Therefore certain SS patients may not be suitable candidates for any form of laser vision correction. Other alternatives for these patients include Intacs, or implantable contact lenses. Intacs are intrastromal spacers that alter the curvature of the cornea, thereby adjusting the refractive power.[67] Although less invasive than LASIK surgery, stromal dissection of the cornea is still necessary and some corneal sensation interruption is inevitable. In addition, Intacs have limitations in that they can only correct lower powers of myopia or nearsightedness. Implantable contact lenses (a.k.a. phakic intraocular lenses) have the capacity to correct a full range of myopia and are noncorneal procedures with very little risk to the ocular surface.[68] However, they do involve intraocular surgery with all of its inherent risks such as infection, glaucoma, and cataract formation.

Dry eye continues to be a major complication of refractive surgery, and careful preoperative evaluation and management can mitigate some of these issues. Careful patient selection is critical and the potential risks should be reviewed in detail. Studies regarding SS patients and refractive surgery are lacking, and more research is needed. It is important to note that not everybody is a suitable candidate for refractive surgery and high-risk patients such as those with SS and moderate-to-severe dry eye should be dissuaded from undergoing such operations and should seek alternatives.

Cataract surgery

Cataract surgery is the most common procedure performed in Medicareage patients in the United States and is expected to steadily increase as the population ages.[69] However, patients of any age can develop cataracts that interfere with their visual function and limit their ability to perform and fully enjoy the activities of daily living. Cataract surgery with implantation of an intraocular lens has made considerable advances in the past 25 years with a very high success rate. However, performing this usually routine procedure on patients with SS poses more of a challenge for the surgeon and the patient because there is a higher risk of complications.

All patients undergoing cataract surgery should receive a comprehensive preoperative evaluation, which includes a detailed history and a comprehensive eye examination including a detailed assessment of the ocular surface. Patients with SS-related dry eye may potentially develop numerous postoperative complications including poor healing incisions, corneal epithelial erosions, infection, stromal melting, or postoperative inflammation.[70] In addition, cataract surgery has been shown to induce or exacerbate dry eye.[71,72] Therefore SS patients should be followed more closely postoperatively to assess healing and proactively monitor for complications.

One of the most important considerations in SS patients is to identify and treat any ocular surface disease issues aggressively before and immediately after surgery.[63,70] Treatments to optimize the ocular surface may include increased lubrication, management of concomitant eyelid disease such as MGD, topical anti-inflammatory medications, and punctal occlusion/cautery. Patients are often also treated with antibiotic drops preoperatively and postoperatively to prevent infection (for at least 1 week postoperatively unless there are surface defects that might necessitate longer therapy). Topical nonsteroidal anti-inflammatory drugs should be avoided in SS patients because of the rare complication of corneal melting, which is higher in patients with severe ocular surface disease.[70,73]

In patients with more advanced dry eyes undergoing cataract surgery, there may be a need for more aggressive measures, especially if the postoperative course is complicated by delayed corneal wound healing or persistent corneal epithelial defects. In addition to the measures described above, other helpful treatment options to consider include the application of a bandage contact lens to protect the delicate surface epithelium of the cornea, amniotic membrane overlays, and temporary partial or complete tarsorrhaphies (lid closure) to reduce evaporation from the ocular surface.

In summary, cataract surgery in patients with SS can pose an increased threat to normal wound healing. A good understanding of the ocular surface risks is paramount for maximizing the outcomes in these patients. It is important to aggressively treat patients with SS-related dry eye before and immediately after surgery to avoid complications. Although SS patients with moderate-to-severe dry eyes are at a higher risk for complications, most have excellent outcomes with proper preparation and timely interventions.

Conclusions

In conclusion, it is helpful to take a stepwise approach to treatment when managing SS-related dry eye and to tailor therapy to each individual patient. Although SS poses special challenges, there are effective treatment strategies for its management. It is important to be aware that corneal neuropathy can exacerbate ocular surface disease and discomfort in SS patients. Careful consideration should be given to any SS patient considering wearing contact lenses or undergoing ocular surgery such as refractive or cataract surgery.

References

1. Sjögren H. Zur Kenntnis der Keratoconjunctivitis sicca. *Acta Ophthalmol.* 1933; 11(Suppl. 2):1−151.
2. Uchino M, Schaumberg DA. Dry eye disease: impact on quality of life and vision. *Curr Ophthalmol Rep.* 2013;1(2):51−57.
3. Ramos-Casals M, Brito-Zeron P, Siso-Almirall A, Bosch X. Primary Sjögren syndrome. *BMJ.* 2012;344:e3821.
4. Segal B, Bowman SJ, Fox PC, et al. Primary Sjögren's Syndrome: health experiences and predictors of health quality among patients in the United States. *Health Qual Life Outcomes.* 2009;7:46.

5. Shimazaki J, Goto E, Ono M, et al. Meibomian gland dysfunction in patients with Sjögren syndrome. *Ophthalmology*. 1998;105(8):1485−1488.

6. Wolffsohn JS, Arita R, Chalmers R, et al. TFOS DEWS II Diagnostic methodology report. *Ocul Surf*. 2017;15(3):539−574.

7. Schaumberg DA, Sullivan DA, Buring JE, Dana MR. Prevalence of dry eye syndrome among US women. *Am J Ophthalmol*. 2003;136(2):318−326.

8. Schaumberg DA, Dana R, Buring JE, Sullivan DA. Prevalence of dry eye disease among US men: estimates from the Physicians' Health Studies. *Arch Ophthalmol*. 2009;127(6): 763−768.

9. Foulks GN, Forstot SL, Donshik PC, et al. Clinical guidelines for management of dry eye associated with Sjögren disease. *Ocul Surf*. 2015;13(2):118−132.

10. Bartlett JD, Keith MS, Sudharshan L, Snedecor SJ. Associations between signs and symptoms of dry eye disease: a systematic review. *Clin Ophthalmol*. 2015;9: 1719−1730.

11. Shiboski CH, Shiboski SC, Seror R, et al. 2016 American College of Rheumatology/European League against Rheumatism classification criteria for primary Sjögren's syndrome: a consensus and data-driven methodology involving three international patient cohorts. *Ann Rheum Dis*. 2017;76(1):9−16.

12. Whitcher JP, Shiboski CH, Shiboski SC, et al. A simplified quantitative method for assessing keratoconjunctivitis sicca from the Sjögren's Syndrome International Registry. *Am J Ophthalmol*. 2010;149(3):405−415.

13. van Bijsterveld OP. Diagnostic tests in the Sicca syndrome. *Arch Ophthalmol*. 1969; 82(1):10−14.

14. Jones L, Downie LE, Korb D, et al. TFOS DEWS II management and therapy report. *Ocul Surf*. 2017;15(3):575−628.

15. Cardona G, Garcia C, Seres C, et al. Blink rate, blink amplitude, and tear film integrity during dynamic visual display terminal tasks. *Curr Eye Res*. 2011;36(3):190−197.

16. Dry Eye A, Management Study Research G, Asbell PA, et al. n-3 fatty acid supplementation for the treatment of dry eye disease. *N Engl J Med*. 2018;378(18):1681−1690.

17. Moshirfar M, Pierson K, Hanamaikai K, et al. Artificial tears potpourri: a literature review. *Clin Ophthalmol*. 2014;8:1419−1433.

18. Murube J, Paterson A, Murube E. Classification of artificial tears. I: composition and properties. *Adv Exp Med Biol*. 1998;438:693−704.

19. Wander AH, Koffler BH. Extending the duration of tear film protection in dry eye syndrome: review and retrospective case series study of the hydroxypropyl cellulose ophthalmic insert. *Ocul Surf*. 2009;7(3):154−162.

20. Vivino FB, Al-Hashimi I, Khan Z, et al. Pilocarpine tablets for the treatment of dry mouth and dry eye symptoms in patients with Sjögren syndrome: a randomized, placebo-controlled, fixed-dose, multicenter trial. P92-01 Study Group. *Arch Intern Med*. 1999;159(2):174−181.

21. Tsifetaki N, Kitsos G, Paschides CA, et al. Oral pilocarpine for the treatment of ocular symptoms in patients with Sjögren's syndrome: a randomised 12 week controlled study. *Ann Rheum Dis*. 2003;62(12):1204−1207.

22. Ono M, Takamura E, Shinozaki K, et al. Therapeutic effect of cevimeline on dry eye in patients with Sjögren's syndrome: a randomized, double-blind clinical study. *Am J Ophthalmol*. 2004;138(1):6−17.

23. Wei Y, Asbell PA. The core mechanism of dry eye disease is inflammation. *Eye Contact Lens*. 2014;40(4):248−256.

24. Marsh P, Pflugfelder SC. Topical nonpreserved methylprednisolone therapy for keratoconjunctivitis sicca in Sjögren syndrome. *Ophthalmology.* 1999;106(4): 811−816.

25. Hong S, Kim T, Chung SH, et al. Recurrence after topical nonpreserved methylprednisolone therapy for keratoconjunctivitis sicca in Sjögren's syndrome. *J Ocul Pharmacol Ther.* 2007;23(1):78−82.

26. Waldmeier PC, Zimmermann K, Qian T, et al. Cyclophilin D as a drug target. *Curr Med Chem.* 2003;10(16):1485−1506.

27. Matsuda S, Koyasu S. Mechanisms of action of cyclosporine. *Immunopharmacology.* 2000;47(2−3):119−125.

28. Sheppard JD, Scoper SV, Samudre S. Topical loteprednol pretreatment reduces cyclosporine stinging in chronic dry eye disease. *J Ocul Pharmacol Ther.* 2011;27(1):23−27.

29. Lollett IV, Galor A. Dry eye syndrome: developments and lifitegrast in perspective. *Clin Ophthalmol.* 2018;12:125−139.

30. Balaram M, Schaumberg DA, Dana MR. Efficacy and tolerability outcomes after punctal occlusion with silicone plugs in dry eye syndrome. *Am J Ophthalmol.* 2001;131(1): 30−36.

31. Tsubota K, Goto E, Fujita H, et al. Treatment of dry eye by autologous serum application in Sjögren's syndrome. *Br J Ophthalmol.* 1999;83(4):390−395.

32. Kojima T, Ishida R, Dogru M, et al. The effect of autologous serum eyedrops in the treatment of severe dry eye disease: a prospective randomized case-control study. *Am J Ophthalmol.* 2005;139(2):242−246.

33. Pullum K, Buckley R. Therapeutic and ocular surface indications for scleral contact lenses. *Ocul Surf.* 2007;5(1):40−48.

34. Geerling G, Tauber J, Baudouin C, et al. The international workshop on meibomian gland dysfunction: report of the subcommittee on management and treatment of meibomian gland dysfunction. *Investig Ophthalmol Vis Sci.* 2011;52(4):2050−2064.

35. Kashkouli MB, Fazel AJ, Kiavash V, et al. Oral azithromycin versus doxycycline in meibomian gland dysfunction: a randomised double-masked open-label clinical trial. *Br J Ophthalmol.* 2015;99(2):199−204.

36. Szczesna-Iskander DH. Comparison of tear film surface quality measured in vivo on water gradient silicone hydrogel and hydrogel contact lenses. *Eye Contact Lens.* 2014; 40(1):23−27.

37. Varikooty J, Keir N, Richter D, et al. Comfort response of three silicone hydrogel daily disposable contact lenses. *Optom Vis Sci.* 2013;90(9):945−953.

38. Russo PA, Bouchard CS, Galasso JM. Extended-wear silicone hydrogel soft contact lenses in the management of moderate to severe dry eye signs and symptoms secondary to graft-versus-host disease. *Eye Contact Lens.* 2007;33(3):144−147.

39. Galor A, Moein HR, Lee C, et al. Neuropathic pain and dry eye. *Ocul Surf.* 2018;16(1): 31−44.

40. Holland NR, Crawford TO, Hauer P, et al. Small-fiber sensory neuropathies: clinical course and neuropathology of idiopathic cases. *Ann Neurol.* 1998;44(1):47−59.

41. Mori K, Iijima M, Sugiura M, et al. Sjögren's syndrome associated painful sensory neuropathy without sensory ataxia. *J Neurol Neurosurg Psychiatry.* 2003;74(9):1320−1322.

42. Pencina MJ, D'Agostino RB, Vasan RS. Statistical methods for assessment of added usefulness of new biomarkers. *Clin Chem Lab Med.* 2010;48(12):1703−1711.

43. Bouhassira D, Attal N, Fermanian J, et al. Development and validation of the neuropathic pain symptom inventory. *Pain.* 2004;108(3):248−257.

44. Bennett M. The LANSS Pain Scale: the Leeds assessment of neuropathic symptoms and signs. *Pain*. 2001;92(1–2):147–157.
45. Birnbaum J, Lalji A, Saed A, Baer AN. Biopsy-proven small-fiber neuropathy in primary Sjögren's syndrome: neuropathic pain characteristics, autoantibody findings, and histopathological features. *Arthritis Care Res (Hoboken)*. 2019;71(7):936–948.
46. Fisher BA, Brown RM, Bowman SJ, Barone F. A review of salivary gland histopathology in primary Sjögren's syndrome with a focus on its potential as a clinical trials biomarker. *Ann Rheum Dis*. 2015;74(9):1645–1650.
47. Benitez-Del-Castillo JM, Acosta MC, Wassfi MA, et al. Relation between corneal innervation with confocal microscopy and corneal sensitivity with noncontact esthesiometry in patients with dry eye. *Investig Ophthalmol Vis Sci*. 2007;48(1):173–181.
48. Tuominen IS, Konttinen YT, Vesaluoma MH, et al. Corneal innervation and morphology in primary Sjögren's syndrome. *Investig Ophthalmol Vis Sci*. 2003;44(6):2545–2549.
49. Resch MD, Marsovszky L, Nemeth J, et al. Dry eye and corneal Langerhans cells in systemic lupus erythematosus. *J Ophthalmol*. 2015;2015:543835.
50. Marsovszky L, Nemeth J, Resch MD, et al. Corneal Langerhans cell and dry eye examinations in ankylosing spondylitis. *Innate Immun*. 2014;20(5):471–477.
51. Leppin K, Behrendt AK, Reichard M, et al. Diabetes mellitus leads to accumulation of dendritic cells and nerve fiber damage of the subbasal nerve plexus in the cornea. *Investig Ophthalmol Vis Sci*. 2014;55(6):3603–3615.
52. Gabbriellini G, Baldini C, Varanini V, et al. In vivo confocal scanning laser microscopy in patients with primary Sjögren's syndrome: a monocentric experience. *Mod Rheumatol*. 2015;25(4):585–589.
53. McNamara NA, Ge S, Lee SM, et al. Reduced levels of tear lacritin are associated with corneal neuropathy in patients with the ocular component of Sjögren's syndrome. *Investig Ophthalmol Vis Sci*. 2016;57(13):5237–5243.
54. Levy O, Labbe A, Borderie V, et al. Increased corneal sub-basal nerve density in patients with Sjögren syndrome treated with topical cyclosporine A. *Clin Exp Ophthalmol*. 2017; 45(5):455–463.
55. Fea AM, Aragno V, Testa V, et al. The effect of autologous platelet lysate eye drops: an in vivo confocal microscopy study. *BioMed Res Int*. 2016;2016:8406832.
56. Galor A, Batawi H, Felix ER, et al. Incomplete response to artificial tears is associated with features of neuropathic ocular pain. *Br J Ophthalmol*. 2015;100(6):745–749.
57. Galor A, Covington D, Levitt AE, et al. Neuropathic ocular pain due to dry eye is associated with multiple ccomorbid chronic pain syndromes. *J Pain*. 2016;17(3):310–318.
58. Galor A, Zlotcavitch L, Walter SD, et al. Dry eye symptom severity and persistence are associated with symptoms of neuropathic pain. *Br J Ophthalmol*. 2015;99:665–668.
59. Simpson RG, Moshirfar M, Edmonds JN, et al. Laser in situ keratomileusis in patients with collagen vascular disease: a review of the literature. *Clin Ophthalmol*. 2012;6: 1827–1837.
60. Bailey MD, Mitchell GL, Dhaliwal DK, et al. Patient satisfaction and visual symptoms after laser in situ keratomileusis. *Ophthalmology*. 2003;110(7):1371–1378.
61. McGhee CN, Craig JP, Sachdev N, et al. Functional, psychological, and satisfaction outcomes of laser in situ keratomileusis for high myopia. *J Cataract Refract Surg*. 2000; 26(4):497–509.
62. Ambrosio Jr R, Tervo T, Wilson SE. LASIK-associated dry eye and neurotrophic epitheliopathy: pathophysiology and strategies for prevention and treatment. *J Refract Surg*. 2008;24(4):396–407.

63. Gomes JAP, Azar DT, Baudouin C, et al. TFOS DEWS II iatrogenic report. *Ocul Surf.* 2017;15(3):511–538.

64. Toda I. Dry eye after LASIK. *Investig Ophthalmol Vis Sci.* 2018;59(14). DES109-D115.

65. Liang L, Zhang M, Zou W, Liu Z. Aggravated dry eye after laser in situ keratomileusis in patients with Sjögren syndrome. *Cornea.* 2008;27(1):120–123.

66. Patryn EK, Vrijman V, Nieuwendaal CP, et al. Indications for and outcomes of tertiary referrals in refractive surgery. *J Refract Surg.* 2014;30(1):54–61.

67. Park J, Gritz DC. Evolution in the use of intrastromal corneal ring segments for corneal ectasia. *Curr Opin Ophthalmol.* 2013;24(4):296–301.

68. Pineda 2nd R, Chauhan T. Phakic intraocular lenses and their special indications. *J Ophthalmic Vis Res.* 2016;11(4):422–428.

69. Schein OD, Cassard SD, Tielsch JM, Gower EW. Cataract surgery among Medicare beneficiaries. *Ophthalmic Epidemiol.* 2012;19(5):257–264.

70. Afsharkhamseh N, Movahedan A, Motahari H, Djalilian AR. Cataract surgery in patients with ocular surface disease: an update in clinical diagnosis and treatment. *Saudi J Ophthalmol.* 2014;28(3):164–167.

71. Cetinkaya S, Mestan E, Acir NO, et al. The course of dry eye after phacoemulsification surgery. *BMC Ophthalmol.* 2015;15:68.

72. Li XM, Hu L, Hu J, Wang W. Investigation of dry eye disease and analysis of the pathogenic factors in patients after cataract surgery. *Cornea.* 2007;26(9 Suppl. 1):S16–S20.

73. Wolf EJ, Kleiman LZ, Schrier A. Nepafenac-associated corneal melt. *J Cataract Refract Surg.* 2007;33(11):1974–1975.

Approach to children with Sjögren's syndrome

Scott M. Lieberman, MD, PhD[1], Sara M. Stern, MD[2], Matthew L. Basiaga, DO, MSCE[3]

[1]*Associate Professor of Pediatrics, Stead Family Children's Hospital and Carver College of Medicine, University of Iowa, Iowa City, IA, United States;* [2]*Assistant Professor of Pediatrics, University of Utah School of Medicine, Salt Lake City, UT, United States;* [3]*Senior Associate Consultant, Mayo Clinic, Rochester, MN, United States*

Introduction

Sjögren's syndrome (SS) may present at any age during childhood (range <1−18 years), with a median age at diagnosis of 12 years.[1,2] The presentation may be different than that in adults, although female predominance is present in both (male: female ratio of 1:6 for children with SS).[1−3] As is evident later, a lack of well-defined diagnostic criteria or longitudinal studies has hampered our understanding of SS in children. We presume that this is a chronic disease with similar pathophysiologic features to SS in adults and, thus, expect that over time these children will progress to more classic adult-type SS features. Therefore SS in children may be an early presentation of adult SS or, alternatively, disease in adults may actually begin earlier in life but with nonspecific features resulting in diagnostic delay. This is supported by the observation that serologic evidence of autoimmunity was found many years before diagnosis of SS in a Scandinavian population.[4,5] Another study using a questionnaire-based approach found that many adults diagnosed with SS actually recalled symptoms before the age of 20 years, with some recalling symptoms before age 10 years.[6]

Clinical manifestations

Clinical manifestations of children with SS vary widely. Many children present with parotitis or have frequent/extensive dental caries. Many have sicca symptoms; however, this may need to be elicited through careful and thorough questioning due to the lack of awareness that their symptoms represent dryness. Other children have neither parotitis nor sicca symptoms. The manifestations described in the following are based on our clinical experience as well as a review of relevant medical literature,[3] a case series not included in the review,[2] and our ongoing retrospective study of children with SS.[1]

Sjögren's Syndrome. https://doi.org/10.1016/B978-0-323-67534-5.00005-3

Glandular manifestations

Parotitis

The most common presenting symptom in childhood SS is parotid enlargement. Reported in approximately 60% of children at diagnosis, this may be the sole presenting manifestation. Parotid enlargement is often episodic and may cause parotid pain and fever. In some children, parotid swelling may be persistent and other salivary glands including submandibular and sublingual glands may be affected. Some children may present with frequent or recurrent oral lesions, such as ranulas, that suggest salivary gland disease and prompt consideration of SS as a cause.[3,7] Parotid involvement typically affects both glands but may be unilateral or bilateral during any given episode of acute parotitis. The failure to recognize parotid enlargement as a presenting symptom of childhood SS, false reassurance by lack of other systemic features, or lack of oral or ocular dryness likely leads to underdiagnosis of the disease. Any child presenting with recurrent or persistent parotitis deserves a thorough evaluation for SS and should be monitored for disease evolution.

Every child with salivary gland enlargement, particularly when unilateral or at the first episode, should be carefully evaluated to rule out other causes besides SS (Table 5.1). Highest on the differential diagnosis for recurrent parotitis in SS are idiopathic recurrent parotitis and/or infection (Table 5.1). Idiopathic recurrent parotitis, also called juvenile recurrent parotitis, is most often described in men and younger children.[8,9] The cause of recurrent parotitis in this population is not well understood, but it may be due to partial duct obstruction predisposing to duct dilation and infection.[10] The histopathologic descriptions of idiopathic recurrent parotitis includes periductal lymphocytic infiltration.[11] Children with this diagnosis lack serum autoantibodies; however, initial

Table 5.1 Causes of parotid enlargement in children[a].

Immune Mediated: Childhood Sjögren's syndrome, sarcoidosis, IgG4-related disease, immune dysregulation associated with immune deficiency (IgA deficiency, combined variable immune deficiency)
Idiopathic recurrent parotitis
Infection:
Bacterial: *Staphylococcus, Streptococcus, Haemophilus influenzae, Klebsiella, Pseudomonas, Actinomyces*
Mycobacterial: Tuberculosis, nontuberculosis
Viral: Human immunodeficiency virus, Epstein-Barr virus, cytomegalovirus, hepatitis C virus, influenza virus, parainfluenzavirus, coxsackievirus, parvovirus, mumps virus
Sialolithiasis
Anorexia Nervosa
Cystic Fibrosis
Malformation, lymphatic or vascular
Tumors, benign or malignant
Pneumoparotitis

[a] *Summarized from Refs. 49–51.*

descriptions predate the routine testing for anti-Ro/SSA or anti-La/SSB autoantibodies. Thus whether idiopathic recurrent parotitis is a distinct entity or rather seronegative SS or a *forme fruste* of SS is unclear at present. Long-term studies of children with idiopathic recurrent parotitis are warranted. Parotitis, as the presenting manifestation of childhood SS, can also occur at any age but most commonly in young children.[1,2] For example, in one study, nearly all children with SS under age 7 years presented with parotitis, whereas fewer than half of the teenagers had this manifestation.[1]

Oral/ocular sicca symptoms

Although sicca symptoms are often considered the hallmark of adult SS, these symptoms are rarely the reason children seek medical attention.[2] At diagnosis, many children have signs or symptoms suggestive of oral or ocular dryness, but they may not perceive these symptoms as dry mouth or dry eyes. Therefore children often answer "no" when asked if they have dry eyes or dry mouth. This underscores the need to ask specific questions aimed at identifying sicca symptoms in children (the need to drink liquid to aid in swallowing foods, the need for frequent drinks throughout the day or overnight, frequent or extensive dental caries despite adequate hygiene, frequent foreign body sensation or grittiness in their eyes, nonspecific ocular irritation with or without redness, the need to use eye drops for ocular irritation, or photophobia). Oral manifestations have been reported in children as early as 1−2 years of age.[1,12] Evidence that may suggest salivary gland dysfunction includes increased dental decay and tooth extraction,[13,14] halitosis, and/or difficulty swallowing food. Increased periodontitis as reported in some adults[15,16] has not been formally demonstrated in children, but its risk could potentially increase with disease duration. Thus maximizing oral health care is of utmost importance.

Clinicians may notice decreased salivary pooling on examination as a sign of salivary gland dysfunction. Ocular dryness is much less commonly reported in children with SS. However, in our experience, children can be asymptomatic but can still exhibit evidence of a decreased tear meniscus or evidence of ocular surface damage on ophthalmologic examination. Ultimately, signs of ocular or oral dryness may be present in up to two-thirds of children with SS even when the sensation of dryness is not appreciated. This means that at presentation, approximately one-third of children with SS will have no symptoms of dryness regardless of the extensive questioning, as mentioned earlier (Table 5.2). This lack of profound sicca symptoms at diagnosis is one of the key differences between childhood SS and adult SS.

Gynecologic manifestations

Vaginal irritation occurs in approximately 5% of children with SS.[1] This may include vulvovaginitis or pruritis. The incidence of dyspareunia has not been described but should be discussed in sexually active teenagers with SS. The overall prevalence of gynecologic manifestations in children with SS may be underestimated because children are less likely to voluntarily report symptoms, and specific questions regarding vaginal irritation are often not elicited during routine clinic visits. In addition, vaginal examinations are often deferred in children.

Table 5.2 Clinical characteristics of children with Sjögren's syndrome[a].

Clinical characteristics	Percentage
Glandular	
Recurrent parotitis	53–62
Dry eyes	35–62
Dry mouth	34–65
Both dry eyes and dry mouth	40–42
No sicca symptoms	27–32
Extraglandular	
Arthralgia and/or arthritis	21–55
Lymphadenopathy	8–46
Fever	9–23
Neurologic	3–23
Kidney	7–19
Hematologic	4–18
Rash	6–15
Weight loss	10
Pulmonary	8
Vaginitis	5
Myositis	2

[a] *Ranges represent reported values from Refs. 1–3 values without ranges are from Ref. 1.*

Extraglandular manifestations

Constitutional symptoms

Constitutional symptoms are common, especially during periods of active disease. Fatigue is common in adolescents with SS in our experience, although reports have not formally quantified this. One study of Japanese children with SS reported easy fatigability in 30%.[17] Lymphadenopathy is reported in up to 46%, fever in up to 23%, and weight loss in 10% (Table 5.2). These symptoms are prevalent in many diseases and by themselves are not specific for childhood SS. If they persist without a clear cause, childhood SS should be considered in the differential diagnosis, particularly, when other signs are present.

Neurologic manifestations

Neurologic manifestations occur in up to 23% of children with SS.[2] Peripheral neuropathy presents with paresthesia, painful dysesthesia, mononeuritis multiplex, cranial neuropathy, and autonomic neuropathy. Central nervous system features may include meningoencephalitis that may mimic acute disseminated encephalomyelitis or demyelinating disease that may mimic multiple sclerosis. The association of SS with neuromyelitis optica (NMO) spectrum disorders is well established in adults and has been reported in children with SS.[18,19] Although not a common feature in pediatric SS, NMO may be life threatening if not quickly managed. Headaches, cognitive dysfunction, and mood disorders including depression and anxiety may also occur in children with SS.

Renal manifestations

Renal involvement occurs in up to 19% of children with SS and can lead to significant morbidity. Onset and progression of kidney disease may be indolent, and patients may have minimal symptoms until the disease has progressed to cause significant renal dysfunction or even hypokalemic paralysis. Kidney disease in children with SS may manifest as renal tubular acidosis (more commonly distal), diabetes insipidus, nephrocalcinosis, or renal insufficiency.[20,21] Biopsies most commonly demonstrate tubulointerstitial nephritis.

Cutaneous manifestations

Skin manifestations of SS occur in up to 15% of children. Rashes may include purpura, annular erythema, cutaneous lupus, erythema nodosum, or cutaneous vasculitis.[1−3] The frequency of cryoglobulinemic vasculitis is not known, but in our experience, this is quite rare. Raynaud phenomenon may occur in the context of SS, and nonspecific xerosis with or without pruritis may also occur.

Gastrointestinal manifestations

The frequency of gastrointestinal manifestations in children with SS is not clear. The inclusion of abdominal pain in the first proposed child-specific diagnostic criteria suggests that nonspecific gastrointestinal complaints may be relatively common.[22] Cases of hepatitis and gastritis have been reported.[22−24] In these cases, hepatitis presented with persistently elevated levels of transaminases prompting liver biopsy, which demonstrated lymphocytic infiltration suggesting autoimmune hepatitis. Primary biliary cirrhosis is rare in children and has not been reported in children with SS. Despite having exocrine gland function, pancreatitis or glandular insufficiency has been rarely reported in children with SS. In two children with SS, pancreatitis developed in the context of hyperlipoproteinemia associated with autoantibodies to lipoprotein lipase.[25,26]

Musculoskeletal manifestations

Arthralgias are common in children being evaluated by pediatric rheumatologists and occur in approximately half of the children with SS.[1] Arthritis is less common but may occur in up to approximately one-third of children.[1] In our experience, some children with a diagnosis of juvenile idiopathic arthritis early in childhood may later be diagnosed with SS. Whether this represents the same pathophysiologic process or is the coincidental occurrence of two distinct disease processes with shared immune dysregulation remains unclear. Myalgias or other nonspecific musculoskeletal pain may occur, especially in the context of fatigue. Myositis is less common.

Pulmonary manifestations

Pulmonary manifestations are not commonly reported in children with SS but may occur.[1,27] Interstitial and resultant restrictive lung disease and pulmonary hypertension have been reported.[28] A persistent cough, dyspnea, or decreased endurance warrants further evaluation for chronic lung disease or unrelated infectious causes, especially if the child is on immunosuppressive therapy.

Hematologic manifestations

Autoimmune cytopenias, including autoimmune hemolytic anemia, leukopenia, lymphopenia, and thrombocytopenia, may occur in up to 18% of children with SS.[1] Polyclonal hypergammaglobulinemia is common especially in children with positive rheumatoid factor (RF), and this presumably represents B-cell hyperactivity, which is a known feature of SS. Whether these children are at greater risk for developing monoclonal B-cell populations and subsequent lymphoma is not well understood (see the Long-Term Prognosis section).

Evaluation
Challenge of diagnosis

Childhood SS is likely underdiagnosed for many reasons. As highlighted earlier, presentation of the disease in children is usually different than that in adults.[2] The lack of sicca symptoms at presentation and the general notion that SS is a disease of middle-aged women likely prevent pediatric rheumatologists and other practitioners from strongly considering this diagnosis in many clinical situations. In our experience the clinical presentation of pediatric SS can be separated into three broad categories: (1) recurrent parotitis, (2) sicca symptoms, and (3) extraglandular manifestations. Recurrent parotitis is now widely recognized as a manifestation of children with SS, although initially other causes should be considered (Table 5.1). Sicca symptoms most often prompt the consideration of testing for SS; however, this is by far the least common category in which children present. The third category, extraglandular manifestations, includes the many children (approximately half) who present without overt parotitis or sicca symptoms; symptoms may range from nonspecific musculoskeletal pain with or without fatigue to any of the other manifestations noted earlier (Table 5.2). In many of these children, consideration of systemic lupus erythematosus (SLE) leads to testing for antinuclear antibodies (ANAs) that may then reveal a positive anti-SSA/Ro antibody, thus prompting further workup for SS. Unfortunately, in the absence of formal child-specific diagnostic criteria, the algorithm for further diagnostic testing in childhood SS remains unclear. The lack of well-defined normal values for lacrimal and salivary gland functional studies, imaging, or histologic assessment renders these diagnostic studies difficult to interpret. In some children, especially younger children, cooperation with testing may be insufficient to allow accurate quantitation of tears, saliva, or ocular surface damage. Thus a combination of factors, including the infrequency with which tests for oral and ocular assessment are routinely performed in children,[1] leaves many oral or ocular healthcare providers reluctant to do further studies as part of the diagnostic process.

Adult classification criteria in pediatric Sjögren's syndrome

The iterations of the criteria for the classification of SS in adults have not been adequate for the diagnosis of SS in children,[1,2,23,29] and the lack of routine testing of lacrimal and salivary gland function and ocular surface damage in children may have contributed to the relatively low sensitivity of these adult criteria. As gland dysfunction is likely a later manifestation that occurs progressively over years (or decades) after the initiation of an autoimmune attack on lacrimal and salivary glands, children may not routinely have evidence of lacrimal and/or salivary hypo-function at diagnosis. Thus diagnostic criteria for childhood SS may require the development of a new set of tests designed specifically for children. These more spe-cific tests will hopefully increase the sensitivity and specificity in diagnosing SS at an earlier stage. Child-specific criteria or child-specific modifications to the adult criteria have been suggested, but, when retrospectively tested, none of these criteria have performed well enough thus far to be routinely used.[2,22,23,29] Development of additional criteria is underway, but currently no validated child-specific diagnostic criteria for SS exist.

Diagnostic algorithm

First and foremost, diagnosis of childhood SS requires a high index of suspicion. In our opinion, workup for SS should be considered for any child presenting with classic SS symptoms (dry eyes, dry mouth, recurrent parotitis), any child being worked up for SLE, and any child presenting with the extraglandular manifestations described earlier or those included in the European League Against Rheumatism Sjögren's Syndrome Disease Activity Index (ESSDAI).[27,30]

The optimal evaluation for childhood SS requires a multidisciplinary team. This begins with a comprehensive history and physical examination by a pediatric rheu-matologist, along with additional evaluations by ocular and oral medicine specialists with experience in diagnosing pediatric SS. In some cases the ocular or oral medi-cine specialists may be the first to encounter the child, depending on the symptoms. An overview of diagnostic testing for childhood SS is presented in Table 5.3.

Ocular testing for dry eye assessment should include quantitation of tear produc-tion (Schirmer I test), ocular surface staining with lissamine green (for conjunctival damage) and fluorescein (for corneal damage), and quantitation of salivary produc-tion through measurement of an unstimulated whole mouth salivary flow rate, as routinely performed during workup in adults. Of note, the value of an assessment by an experienced clinician, particularly when dealing with younger or anxious chil-dren, cannot be overestimated.

Laboratory testing and imaging also add valuable information to the evaluation that not only provides support for the diagnosis of SS but also helps rule out diseases (see later) that can mimic SS. Relevant laboratory tests (Table 5.3) include anti-SSA/Ro (including Ro52 and Ro60) antibodies, anti-SSB/La antibodies, ANA with titer (by immunofluorescence with Hep2 cells), RF, serum IgG, complete blood count (CBC) with differential, complete metabolic panel to screen for kidney and liver ab-normalities, urinalysis with microscopic evaluation, and urine protein/creatinine quantitation if proteinuria is evident on dipstick. Use of erythrocyte sedimentation rate, C-reactive protein, complements C3 and C4, and serum amylase (if levels are elevated, then verify it is not of pancreatic origin by checking serum lipase)

Table 5.3 Relevant testing for diagnosis or characterization of Sjögren's syndrome in children.

Test	Significance/Notes
Tests for exocrine gland inflammation	
Salivary gland biopsy	Labial minor salivary gland or major salivary gland
Imaging[a]	Salivary gland US, MRI, CT
Serum amylase[a]	Elevated amylase levels with normal lipase suggests salivary origin
Tests for autoimmunity and/or B-cell hyperactivity[b]	
Anti-SSA antibodies (Ro52, Ro60)	Positive in 75%−80% of children with Sjögren's syndrome
Anti-SSB antibodies (La)	Positive in 43%−65% of children with Sjögren's syndrome
ANA	Positive in 83%−96% of children with Sjögren's syndrome
Rheumatoid factor	Positive in 67%−73% of children with Sjögren's syndrome
Serum IgG	Elevated in 60% of children with Sjögren's syndrome
Tests for gland dysfunction	
Unstimulated whole saliva	May be normal early in disease
Schirmer test	May be normal early in disease
Ocular surface staining	Fluorescein for cornea, lissamine green for conjunctiva
Tests that may provide additional supportive evidence[a]	
CBC with differential	Autoimmune cytopenias may occur
Complete metabolic panel	Kidney inflammation, RTA, hepatitis may occur
Complements (C3, C4)	Low C3 or C4 may occur
Urinalysis	Kidney inflammation, RTA may occur
ESR and CRP	May be elevated chronically or with flares of parotitis

ANA, *antinuclear antibody;* CBC, *complete blood count;* CRP, *C-reactive protein;* ESR, *erythrocyte sedimentation rate;* RTA, *renal tubular acidosis;* US, *ultrasonography.*
[a] *Abnormal test results may support diagnosis and may be followed up for response to treatment or to indicate disease flare.*
[b] *Ranges of percentages represent reported values from Refs. 1−3.*

analyses further documents the inflammatory nature of the condition and assesses disease activity. Other laboratory tests to consider will depend on additional manifestations—cryoglobulins if vasculitis or other suggestive manifestations exist and serum protein electrophoresis or immunofixation electrophoresis if hypergammaglobulinemia is present to ensure polyclonality. Additional testing for other closely related autoimmune diseases (e.g., celiac, autoimmune thyroid disease) that can coexist with SS may be warranted in certain clinical situations.

Imaging is used to verify the presence of salivary glands and characterize the degree of salivary gland changes. Ultrasonography, CT scan, and MRI have all been used to satisfy these objectives in the evaluation of childhood SS.[31,32]

Ultrasonography provides a safe and easy method to test for parotid and submandibular integrity, with no ionizing radiation or sedation needed in children; the value of this study and its interpretation depend on the experience of the ultrasonographer. CT and MRI studies may be superior for the evaluation of salivary gland masses.[31] The presence of inhomogeneity or discrete hypoechoic lesions on ultrasonography or T2 hyperintense lesions on MRI may be evident early in disease development, and the lesion sizes may increase with time following symptom onset or diagnosis. Lesions may become more discretely cystic in appearance often with increasing echogenicity in later stages, and calcifications, glandular atrophy, and adipose deposition may occur. Whether any such features are specific for childhood SS has not been formally evaluated. These findings are most likely not disease specific but, rather, reflect chronic inflammation found in SS and other conditions that affect the salivary glands. Sialoendoscopy is another diagnostic technique that is occasionally used to evaluate children with parotid swelling related to salivary duct obstruction. Its value in the diagnosis of childhood SS remains unclear.[33] Minor salivary gland biopsy is an important diagnostic study that can be used to demonstrate the characteristic salivary gland inflammation in a child with suspected SS, particularly when the child is seronegative. It should always be performed by an experienced oral medicine specialist or otorhinolaryngologist and read by an experienced oral pathologist. Histopathologic examination may reveal focal lymphocytic sialadenitis typical of SS; however, the extent of sialadenitis may be less in children than that typically seen in adults (see the Salivary gland histopathologic examination in children section).[34] Moreover, histopathologic examination may reveal an alternate diagnosis such as sarcoidosis or IgG4-related disease as the explanation for the patient's symptoms. Parotid, submandibular gland, or lacrimal gland biopsy may occasionally be warranted in select cases where there is marked persistent swelling and suspicion of malignancy or other causes.

Differential diagnosis of childhood Sjögren's syndrome

In any child with dry eyes, dry mouth, or other sicca symptoms who is being evaluated for SS, other causes of dryness should also be considered, including side effects of medications or genetic causes (e.g., lacrimo-auriculo-dento-digital syndrome) resulting in the absence of major salivary glands.[33] Ultrasonography of the salivary gland may be used to confirm the presence or absence of major salivary glands in these children (and their parents or siblings),[35] and it should be performed early in the diagnostic process to prevent additional unnecessary testing such as a minor salivary gland biopsy; the latter cannot be justified when the presence of sicca symptoms is explained by the lack of major salivary glands.

As alluded to earlier, parotid swelling is a common feature in children with SS, and other causes including various infectious agents and/or immunodeficiency syndromes need to be excluded before the diagnosis of SS is confirmed (Table 5.1). Appropriate laboratory testing and imaging should be performed based on clinical suspicion.

For children who present with extraglandular manifestations, the evaluation should include consideration and additional testing for other systemic diseases that can mimic childhood SS, including childhood lupus, juvenile idiopathic arthritis, childhood sarcoidosis, IgG4-related disease, other granulomatous diseases that may affect lacrimal and salivary glands (e.g., granulomatosis with polyangiitis), malignancy, or atypical infections that may prompt workup for immune deficiencies.

Salivary gland histopathologic examination in children

One of the earliest objective features of SS is the development of focal lymphocytic sialadenitis. As SS in children may be an early form of the adult disease, many pediatric rheumatologists consider the presence of focal lymphocytic sialadenitis on minor salivary (or major salivary) gland biopsy to be a key finding for diagnosis. However, the definition of positive result in a salivary gland biopsy has not been formally established in children. The cutoff of one or more mononuclear cell foci per 4 mm^2 of tissue that is currently used to define a positive biopsy result in adults is supported by correlation with SS-specific features.[36] However, in adults the value of biopsy as a stand-alone test in patients without any objective evidence of sicca or extraglandular manifestations to suggest SS is highly questionable, as a study of labial minor salivary gland biopsies in healthy adults without a diagnosis of SS revealed that up to 15% still met the definition of a positive biopsy result.[37] This suggests that either the development of nonspecific focal lymphocytic sialadenitis may occur in adults due to other causes not related to autoimmune disease or many cases of subclinical SS exist in the "normal" population that are undiagnosed.

The presence of focal sialadenitis may be much less likely in healthy children than that in the aforementioned report in healthy adults. In a study of labial minor salivary gland histologic findings in children, the presence of any focal sialadenitis (focus score >0 foci/4 mm^2) in non-SS control specimens was exceedingly rare—present in only 1 of 8 control specimens.[34] In the specimens from children diagnosed with SS, 8 of 12 specimens met the positive biopsy definition used in adults, but all 12 had evidence of focal lymphocytic sialadenitis (focus scores ranged from 0.4 to 2.7/4 mm^2).[34] Notably, in that study the phenotypic and serologic features of SS did not correlate with focus scores as noted previously in adults. Although no similar studies have evaluated histologic findings in non-SS controls, two other reports noted a subset of children with SS having evidence of focal lymphocytic sialadenitis not meeting the adult positive biopsy criteria. In one report of eight children with SS, five of the eight children had focus scores meeting adult definitions, but all specimens had some degree of lymphocytic infiltration.[38] In another study, 11 of 26 samples had focus scores of at least 1 focus per 4 mm^2, but all samples had features suggestive of SS.[39] Thus further study is warranted to better define positive lip biopsy scores in children or perhaps to devise a graded scoring system for diagnosis.

Making the diagnosis

As no validated criteria exist for the diagnosis of SS in children, making the diagnosis may best be accomplished by demonstrating evidence of the key features of

SS: (1) evidence of inflammation of lacrimal and/or salivary glands (imaging and/or histopathologic examination), (2) evidence of serologic autoimmunity (including anti-SSA/Ro, anti-SSB/La, ANA, RF, hypergammaglobulinemia), and (3) glandular dysfunction (decreased tears or saliva or ocular surface damage). In any case lacking clear serologic evidence of disease (ideally positive anti-SSA/Ro antibodies), a labial minor salivary gland biopsy should be strongly considered to evaluate for characteristic focal lymphocytic sialadenitis or to suggest other potential diagnoses. Fig. 5.1 depicts a preliminary algorithm that summarizes our approach toward the diagnosis of childhood SS. International efforts are currently underway to formally define diagnostic criteria for pediatric Sjögren's.

Management

Treatment of SS in children is best accomplished by a multidisciplinary team including oral and ocular healthcare providers, other specialists as needed, and the pediatric rheumatologist as coordinator. Other professionals including social workers as well as physical and occupational therapists can be important assets to the team and are often needed to help address the social, emotional, and developmental concerns for a growing child with a chronic disease. Treatment algorithms are not well established for pediatric SS. As such, our approach is generally to follow the recent adult guidelines[40] with child-relevant additions or changes as noted in the following.

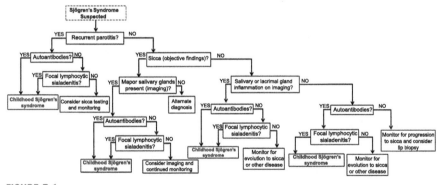

FIGURE 5.1

Proposed preliminary diagnostic algorithm for children suspected of having Sjögren's syndrome. Consider Sjögren's syndrome in any child with recurrent parotitis, sicca symptoms, or extraglandular manifestations as described in the text. For any child in whom anti-SSA/Ro antibody assay results are negative, a combination of anti-SSB/La, antinuclear antibodies, and/or rheumatoid factor may be suggestive of Sjögren's syndrome but additional testing such as labial minor salivary gland biopsy may be warranted to confirm the diagnosis. Additional details of specific tests are included in the text.

Recurrent parotitis

Children with recurrent episodes of parotitis may benefit from brief courses of corticosteroids to speed the resolution of acute parotid inflammation once it has begun. Dosing can vary from 0.5 to 2 mg/kg/dose given daily for 1–3 weeks as a constant or tapering dose depending on the duration. Alternatively, pulse-dose methylprednisolone (30 mg/kg/dose up to 1 g/dose given daily for one to three doses at the start of swelling) may be used. Therapies to prevent recurrent flares of acute parotitis may include use of immunomodulatory medications such as hydroxychloroquine (up to 5 mg/kg/dose given daily) or methotrexate (1 mg/kg/dose up to 25 mg given weekly).[41–43] Of note, none of these therapies has been studied in a formal clinical trial. The use of sialagogues at low doses, if tolerated, may help promote salivary flow and prevent transient plugging of ducts by viscous salivary secretions, which may be an additional contributor to or the cause of episodes of recurrent acute parotitis in childhood SS. Whether any of these treatments prevent accrual of glandular damage or modulate the chronic inflammation has not been formally assessed.

Dry mouth

Similar to the approach followed in adults, sicca symptoms may be managed in children with SS using a variety of gustatory or masticatory stimulants (including over-the-counter sugar-free gums, candies, and lozenges). Replacement therapy with artificial saliva (e.g., one to two sprays every 1–2 hours while awake) may also provide transient relief from symptoms. When symptoms are severe or persist, pharmacologic sialagogues may be prescribed. Pilocarpine was effective in one study of 4 children with SS in Japan.[44] When pilocarpine is not tolerated, cevimeline may provide improvement in symptoms. Of note, when sicca symptoms are limited to only one exocrine organ (e.g., dry mouth but not dry eyes), the increased fluid production promoted by sialagogue therapy may lead to intolerable side effects that outweigh the benefits of the treatment (e.g., excessive tearing in a child treated for dry mouth).

Keratoconjunctivitis sicca

Similar to adults the use of artificial tears is a mainstay of treatment for children with symptoms or features of dry eye disease. In addition to the use of artificial tears for dry eyes, children with evidence of inflammatory changes of the ocular surface may benefit from the use of topical antiinflammatory agents. Brief courses of topical corticosteroids may help, but as SS is a chronic inflammatory disease, consideration should be given for the use of other immunomodulatory agents used in adults to treat dry eye disease, including topical cyclosporine and lifitegrast. Use of these agents should not be withheld in children with the potential for ocular surface damage that may progress to threaten vision.

Other organs

Use of immunomodulatory agents besides those noted earlier may be warranted. Specifically, depending on the clinical manifestations, children with SS may benefit from the use of abatacept, rituximab, mycophenolate mofetil, azathioprine, and belimumab. Although tumor necrosis factor inhibitors are not recommended for the treatment of sicca symptoms, they may still be effective in managing severe or erosive arthritis in children with SS.[45]

Preventive therapy

As SS in children likely represents a chronic autoimmune disease that will progress over time to include features typical of adult SS, the ultimate goal in the treatment of SS is to prevent progression of disease. Unfortunately, no studies have been performed to evaluate the efficacy of medications in slowing the progression of inflammation in children with SS. Discussion regarding the likelihood of progression over time and the potential risks and benefits of chronic immunomodulatory therapy should be open and should reflect the latest data available to support the use of systemic immunomodulatory therapies for the treatment of specific manifestations. At minimum, children should be monitored regularly by both oral and ocular healthcare providers so that therapies can be instituted at the first signs of progression of disease. Dental examinations and treatments (including regular cleanings and fluoride treatments) should be performed at least every 6 months but more frequent visits (up to every 3 months) may be necessary for children with dry mouth symptoms or frequent dental caries. A major effort to preserve dentition should be instituted and the use of prescription-grade fluoride-containing toothpaste should be discussed; children may benefit from the use of such toothpaste before going to bed so that the extra fluoride may take effect overnight. Ocular examinations should be performed at least yearly but may need to be more regular for children with ocular signs or symptoms. Some pediatric rheumatologists offer chronic immunomodulatory therapy such as with hydroxychloroquine in the hope of preventing progression of inflammation-associated damage to exocrine glands over time. Although no clear data exists to support the use of these medications for such purposes, the short-term risks are minimal and retrospective studies have suggested that the use of hydroxychloroquine may be associated with fewer extraglandular manifestations.[46]

Long-term prognosis

As noted earlier, no large cohort studies have reported long-term outcomes or disease course for children diagnosed with SS. We assume that this chronic inflammatory disease will progress to cause similar outcomes as in adults with SS, including marked dryness of the eyes and/or mouth as well as other extraglandular manifestations and/or sequela including pain, fatigue, and disability. Malignancies, especially mucosa-associated lymphoid tissue lymphomas, have been reported in children with SS[47,48] however, the relative risk in this population is unknown. Notably, development of lymphoma may precede the diagnosis of SS or occur in a child with established disease. No long-term outcome studies have been reported, so whether children with SS have the same increased risk of developing lymphoma over their lifetime as observed in adults, presumably related to prolonged chronic B-cell stimulation, is not known. Whether the risk factors for lymphoma identified in adults with SS similarly represent an increased risk of lymphoma in children with SS has also not been evaluated. Until more specific data-driven guidelines are established, it is advisable to regularly monitor any child with SS and chronic hypergammaglobulinemia for transition from polyclonal to monoclonal gammopathy by repeat testing with serum protein electrophoresis or serum immunofixation, along with evaluation for hematologic abnormalities. Similarly, any persistent abnormal glandular swelling (lymph node, salivary gland, or others) in a child warrants further imaging and a biopsy in cases where malignancy is suspected.

Conclusions

SS in children most commonly presents with recurrent episodes of acute parotitis, presumably in the setting of indolent chronic parotitis. Symptoms of dryness may not be perceived by the child early on and may rarely lead the child to seek medical care. In some children, SS begins with extraglandular manifestations. Diagnosis requires a high index of suspicion and a multidisciplinary approach including laboratory tests, imaging, histopathologic examination, and functional studies. The diagnostic criteria used for adults tend not to be highly sensitive for use in diagnosing children, but no child-specific diagnostic criteria have yet been developed and validated. Additional study is required to fill the many gaps in our knowledge of disease manifestations, most appropriate diagnostic tests, effective treatments, and prognosis. Of special importance in children is the possibility of defining a treatment regimen that prevents the progression of early SS autoimmunity to SS with complete glandular dysfunction as is common in adults. International collaborative efforts are underway to better understand SS in children.

References

1. Basiaga M, Stern SM, Mehta J, Lieberman SM. A better understanding of childhood Sjögren syndrome: evaluation of the 2016 ACR/EULAR classification criteria for use in diagnosing Sjögren syndrome in children. *Arthritis & Rheumatology*. 2018;70(Suppl. 10). abstract #476.
2. Yokogawa N, Lieberman SM, Sherry DD, Vivino FB. Features of childhood Sjögren's syndrome in comparison to adult Sjögren's syndrome: considerations in establishing child-specific diagnostic criteria. *Clin Exp Rheumatol*. 2016;34(2):343–351.
3. Means C, Aldape MA, King E. Pediatric primary Sjögren syndrome presenting with bilateral ranulas: a case report and systematic review of the literature. *Int J Pediatr Otorhinolaryngol*. 2017;101:11–19.
4. Jonsson R, Theander E, Sjöstrom B, Brokstad K, Henriksson G. Autoantibodies present before symptom onset in primary Sjögren syndrome. *J Am Med Assoc*. 2013;310(17): 1854–1855.

5. Theander E, Jonsson R, Sjöstrom B, Brokstad K, Olsson P, Henriksson G. Prediction of Sjögren's syndrome years before diagnosis and identification of patients with early onset and severe disease course by autoantibody profiling. *Arthritis Rheum.* 2015;67(9): 2427–2436.

6. Bjerrum K, Prause JU. Primary Sjögren's syndrome: a subjective description of the disease. *Clin Exp Rheumatol.* 1990;8(3):283–288.

7. Lieberman SM, Lu A, McGill MM. Oral lesions as presenting feature of childhood Sjögren syndrome. *Int J Pediatr Otorhinolaryngol.* 2018;113:303–304.

8. Leerdam CM, Martin HC, Isaacs D. Recurrent parotitis of childhood. *J Paediatr Child Health.* 2005;41(12):631–634.

9. Garavello W, Redaelli M, Galluzzi F, Pignataro L. Juvenile recurrent parotitis: a systematic review of treatment studies. *Int J Pediatr Otorhinolaryngol.* 2018;112:151–157.

10. Katz P, Hartl DM, Guerre A. Treatment of juvenile recurrent parotitis. *Otolaryngol Clin N Am.* 2009;42(6):1087–1091.

11. Ericson S, Zetterlund B, Ohman J. Recurrent parotitis and sialectasis in childhood. Clinical, radiologic, immunologic, bacteriologic, and histologic study. *Ann Otol Rhinol Laryngol.* 1991;100(7):527–535.

12. De Oliveira MA, De Rezende NP, Maia CM, Gallottini M. Primary Sjögren syndrome in a 2-year-old patient: role of the dentist in diagnosis and dental management with a 6-year follow-up. *Int J Paediatr Dent.* 2011;21(6):471–475.

13. Christensen LB, Petersen PE, Thorn JJ, Schiodt M. Dental caries and dental health behavior of patients with primary Sjögren syndrome. *Acta Odontol Scand.* 2001;59(3): 116–120.

14. Maarse F, Jager DH, Forouzanfar T, Wolff J, Brand HS. Tooth loss in Sjögren's syndrome patients compared to age and gender matched controls. *Med Oral Patol Oral Cir Bucal.* 2018;23(5):e545–e551.

15. Boutsi EA, Paikos S, Dafni UG, Moutsopoulos HM, Skopouli FN. Dental and periodontal status of Sjögren's syndrome. *J Clin Periodontol.* 2000;27(4):231–235.

16. Jorkjend L, Johansson A, Johansson AK, Bergenholtz A. Periodontitis, caries and salivary factors in Sjögren's syndrome patients compared to sex- and age-matched controls. *J Oral Rehabil.* 2003;30(4):369–378.

17. Tomiita M, Saito K, Kohno Y, Shimojo N, Fujikawa S, Niimi H. The clinical features of Sjögren's syndrome in Japanese children. *Acta Paediatr Jpn.* 1997;39(2): 268–272.

18. Kornitzer JM, Kimura Y, Janow GL. Primary Sjögren syndrome in a child with a neuromyelitis optica spectrum disorder. *J Rheumatol.* 2016;43(6):1260–1261.

19. Gmuca S, Lieberman SM, Mehta J. Pediatric neuromyelitis optica spectrum disorder and Sjögren syndrome: more common than previously thought? *J Rheumatol.* 2017;44(6): 959–960.

20. Pessler F, Emery H, Dai L, Wu YM, Monash B, Cron RQ, Pradhan M. The spectrum of renal tubular acidosis in paediatric Sjögren syndrome. *Rheumatology.* 2006;45(1): 85–91.

21. Bogdanovic R, Basta-Jovanovic G, Putnik J, Stajic N, Paripovic A. Renal involvement in primary Sjögren syndrome of childhood: case report and literature review. *Mod Rheumatol.* 2013;23(1):182–189.

22. Bartunkova J, Sediva A, Vencovsky J, Tesar V. Primary Sjögren's syndrome in children and adolescents: proposal for diagnostic criteria. *Clin Exp Rheumatol.* 1999;17(3): 381–386.

23. Schuetz C, Prieur AM, Quartier P. Sicca syndrome and salivary gland infiltration in children with autoimmune disorders: when can we diagnose Sjögren syndrome? *Clin Exp Rheumatol*. 2010;28(3):434—439.

24. Kashiwagi Y, Hatsushika T, Tsutsumi N, Go S, Nishimata S, Kawashima H. Gastrointestinal and liver lesions in primary childhood Sjögren syndrome. *Clin Rheumatol*. 2017; 36(6):1433—1435.

25. Ashraf AP, Beukelman T, Pruneta-Deloche V, Kelly DR, Garg A. Type 1 hyperlipoproteinemia and recurrent acute pancreatitis due to lipoprotein lipase antibody in a young girl with Sjögren's syndrome. *J Clin Endocrinol Metab*. 2011;96(11):3302—3307.

26. Lilley JS, Linton MF, Kelley JC, Graham TB, Fazio S, Tavori H. A case of severe acquired hypertriglyceridemia in a 7-year-old girl. *J Clin Lipidol*. 2017;11(6):1480—1484.

27. Kobayashi I, Okura Y, Ueki M, Tozawa Y, Takezaki S, Yamada M, Ariga T. Evaluation of systemic activity of pediatric primary Sjögren's syndrome by EULAR Sjögren's syndrome disease activity index (ESSDAI). *Mod Rheumatol*. 2018:1—4.

28. Zhang X, Zeng X. Severe pulmonary hypertension in pediatric primary Sjögren syndrome: a case report. *J Clin Rheumatol*. 2007;13(5):276—277.

29. Houghton K, Malleson P, Cabral D, Petty R, Tucker L. Primary Sjögren's syndrome in children and adolescents: are proposed diagnostic criteria applicable? *J Rheumatol*. 2005;32(11):2225—2232.

30. Seror R, Bowman SJ, Brito-Zeron P, Theander E, Bootsma H, Tzioufas A, Gottenberg JE, Ramos-Casals M, Dorner T, Ravaud P, Vitali C, Mariette X, Asmussen K, Jacobsen S, Bartoloni E, Gerli R, Bijlsma JW, Kruize AA, Bombardieri S, Bookman A, Kallenberg C, Meiners P, Brun JG, Jonsson R, Caporali R, Carsons S, De Vita S, Del Papa N, Devauchelle V, Saraux A, Fauchais AL, Sibilia J, Hachulla E, Illei G, Isenberg D, Jones A, Manoussakis M, Mandl T, Jacobsson L, Demoulins F, Montecucco C, Ng WF, Nishiyama S, Omdal R, Parke A, Praprotnik S, Tomsic M, Price E, Scofield H, K.L.S., Smolen J, Laque RS, Steinfeld S, Sutcliffe N, Sumida T, Valesini G, Valim V, Vivino FB, Vollenweider C. EULAR Sjögren's syndrome disease activity index (ESSDAI): a user guide. *RMD Open*. 2015;1(1):e000022.

31. Friedman E, Patino MO, Udayasankar UK. Imaging of pediatric salivary glands. *Neuroimaging Clin N Am*. 2018;28(2):209—226.

32. Nieto-Gonzalez JC, Monteagudo I, Bello N, Martinez-Estupinan L, Naredo E, Carreno L. Salivary gland ultrasound in children: a useful tool in the diagnosis of juvenile Sjögren's syndrome. *Clin Exp Rheumatol*. 2014;32(4):578—580.

33. Francis CL, Larsen CG. Pediatric sialadenitis. *Otolaryngol Clin N Am*. 2014;47(5): 763—778.

34. Yokogawa N, Lieberman SM, Alawi F, Bout-Tabaku S, Guttenberg M, Sherry DD, Vivino FB. Comparison of labial minor salivary gland biopsies from childhood Sjögren syndrome and age-matched controls. *J Rheumatol*. 2014;41(6):1178—1182.

35. Hajianpour MJ, Bombei H, Lieberman SM, Revell R, Krishna R, Gregorsok R, Kao S, Milunsky JM. Dental issues in lacrimo-auriculo-dento-digital syndrome: an autosomal dominant condition with clinical and genetic variability. *J Am Dent Assoc*. 2017; 148(3):157—163.

36. Daniels TE, Cox D, Shiboski CH, Schiodt M, Wu A, Lanfranchi H, Umehara H, Zhao Y, Challacombe S, Lam MY, De Souza Y, Schiodt J, Holm H, Bisio PA, Gandolfo MS, Sawaki T, Li M, Zhang W, Varghese-Jacob B, Ibsen P, Keszler A, Kurose N, Nojima T, Odell E, Criswell LA, Jordan R, Greenspan JS. Sjögren's International

Collaborative Clinical Alliance Research G. Associations between salivary gland histopathologic diagnoses and phenotypic features of Sjögren's syndrome among 1,726 registry participants. *Arthritis Rheum.* 2011;63(7):2021−2030.

37. Radfar L, Kleiner DE, Fox PC, Pillemer SR. Prevalence and clinical significance of lymphocytic foci in minor salivary glands of healthy volunteers. *Arthritis Rheum.* 2002; 47(5):520−524.

38. Saad Magalhaes C, de Souza Medeiros PB, Oliveira-Sato J, Custodio-Domingues MA. Clinical presentation and salivary gland histopathology of paediatric primary Sjögren's syndrome. *Clin Exp Rheumatol.* 2011;29(3):589−593.

39. Stiller M, Golder W, Doring E, Biedermann T. Primary and secondary Sjögren's syndrome in children–a comparative study. *Clin Oral Investig.* 2000;4(3):176−182.

40. Vivino FB, Carsons SE, Foulks G, Daniels TE, Parke A, Brennan MT, Forstot SL, Scofield RH, Hammitt KM. New treatment guidelines for Sjögren's disease. *Rheum Dis Clin N Am.* 2016;42(3):531−551.

41. Baszis K, Toib D, Cooper M, French A, White A. Recurrent parotitis as a presentation of primary pediatric Sjögren syndrome. *Pediatrics.* 2012;129(1):e179−e182.

42. Singer NG, Tomanova-Soltys I, Lowe R. Sjögren's syndrome in childhood. *Curr Rheumatol Rep.* 2008;10(2):147−155.

43. Ostuni PA, Ianniello A, Sfriso P, Mazzola G, Andretta M, Gambari PF. Juvenile onset of primary Sjögren's syndrome: report of 10 cases. *Clin Exp Rheumatol.* 1996;14(6): 689−693.

44. Tomiita M, Takei S, Kuwada N, Nonaka Y, Saito K, Shimojo N, Kohno Y. Efficacy and safety of orally administered pilocarpine hydrochloride for patients with juvenile-onset Sjögren's syndrome. *Mod Rheumatol.* 2010;20:486−490.

45. Pessler F, Monash B, Rettig P, Forbes B, Kreiger PA, Cron RQ. Sjögren syndrome in a child: favorable response of the arthritis to TNFalpha blockade. *Clin Rheumatol.* 2006; 25(5):746−748.

46. Demarchi J, Papasidero S, Medina MA, Klajn D, Chaparro Del Moral R, Rillo O, Martire V, Crespo G, Secco A, Catalan Pellet A, Amitrano C, Crow C, Asnal C, Pucci P, Caeiro F, Benzanquen N, Pirola JP, Mayer M, Zazzetti F, Velez S, Barreira J, Tamborenea N, Santiago L, Raiti L. Primary Sjögren's syndrome: extraglandular manifestations and hydroxychloroquine therapy. *Clin Rheumatol.* 2017;36(11):2455−2460.

47. Collado P, Kelada A, Camara M, Zeft A, Flagg A. Extranodal marginal zone B cell lymphoma: an unexpected complication in children with Sjögren's syndrome. *Reumatol Clin.* 2018;14(4):227−229.

48. Tesher MS, Esteban Y, Henderson TO, Villanueva G, Onel KB. Mucosal-associated lymphoid tissue (MALT) lymphoma in association with pediatric primary Sjögren syndrome: 2 cases and review. *J Pediatr Hematol Oncol.* 2018;Oct 26. https://doi.org/10.1097/MPH.0000000000001321 [Epub ahead of print].

49. Iro H, Zenk J. Salivary gland diseases in children. *GMS Curr Top Otorhinolaryngol, Head Neck Surg.* 2014;13:Doc06.

50. Lennon P, Silvera VM, Perez-Atayde A, Cunningham MJ, Rahbar R. Disorders and tumors of the salivary glands in children. *Otolaryngol Clin N Am.* 2015;48(1):153−173.

51. Wilson KF, Meier JD, Ward PD. Salivary gland disorders. *Am Fam Physician.* 2014; 89(11):882−888.

Extraglandular abnormalities in Sjögren's syndrome

Chadwick R. Johr, MD

Co-Director, Penn Sjögren's Center, Assistant Professor of Clinical Medicine, Rheumatology, Penn Presbyterian Medical Center, University of Pennsylvania Perelman School of Medicine, Philadelphia, PA, United States

Fatigue and fever

After dry eyes and dry mouth, fatigue is the next most common symptom of Sjögren's syndrome (SS), occurring in ~75% of patients.[1–4] For many, it is disabling and adversely affects work, relationships, and overall quality of life. It can also be a source of frustration, as friends and family repeatedly note that the fatigued patient, who feels terrible, appears just fine. It is often the most troublesome symptom. The cause of fatigue in SS is generally unknown and is felt to be intrinsic to the disease itself.[2,3,5,6] However, for any individual SS patient, one should also consider other potential causes/contributors of fatigue (Table 6.1). Fatigue in SS is particularly challenging because, with scant evidence for useful treatments, it can be difficult to manage and tends to persist over time.[2]

Less common than fatigue, fevers have been noted in 6%–13% of SS patients in most large cohorts at the time of initial evaluation,[7–9] although they can occur at any time during the disease course. They tend to be low grade and can be associated with

Table 6.1 Causes of fatigue in Sjögren's syndrome.

- Fibromyalgia
- Depression/anxiety
- Hypothyroidism
- Sleep apnea
- Restless legs syndrome
- Musculoskeletal pain causing frequent awakening
- Nocturia causing frequent awakening
- Mouth/throat dryness causing frequent awakening
- Anemia
- Vitamin B_{12} deficiency
- Vitamin D deficiency
- Celiac disease
- Medication side effects

flulike symptoms. Fevers that are persistent and/or associated with night sweats and/or weight loss should prompt an evaluation for non-Hodgkin lymphoma (NHL) and other forms of cancer.

CLINICAL PEARLS ON FATIGUE AND FEVER IN SS

- Fatigue affects most SS patients.
- It is one of the most troublesome symptoms.
- Persistent fevers when associated with night sweats and/or weight loss should prompt evaluation for lymphoma.

Musculoskeletal manifestations

As with dryness and fatigue, musculoskeletal symptoms in SS are found in a majority of patients, can be a presenting feature, and are a significant contributor to diminished quality of life (Table 6.2). Arthralgias are the most common rheumatic symptom but arthritis has been described in up to 35% of patients in some SS populations.[10] The most common pattern of joint involvement is a symmetric polyarthralgias/polyarthritis of the metacarpophalangeal, proximal interphalangeal, wrist, and/or knee joints; however, other joints can be affected as well (Table 6.3).[10–13] This pattern is indistinguishable from that typically found in rheumatoid arthritis (RA) making it difficult to tell whether a patient with SS and inflammatory arthritis has concurrent RA or SS alone because the two disorders may coexist. Patients with SS that presents as inflammatory polyarthritis may frequently be misdiagnosed as having RA in the early stages. Less commonly, oligoarthritis or monoarthritis may occur.

The natural history of RA is to cause joint deformity and erosive bone damage on the margins of affected joints. As a general rule, this is not the case with SS. As such, finding marginal erosions on joint imaging is highly suggestive of concurrent RA and should prompt consideration for more aggressive treatment. Rheumatoid factor (RF) positivity is similarly common in both RA and SS and is not useful in distinguishing concurrent RA from SS alone. Anticyclic citrullinated protein antibody (ACPA) positivity is far more frequent in RA than SS but, like RF, its presence does not reliably distinguish between SS and SS + RA.[14] Interestingly, both RF[15] and ACPA[14,15] have been shown to be significant risk factors for the development of RA in SS.

Table 6.2 Musculoskeletal manifestations of Sjögren's syndrome.

Feature	Prevalence (%)
Arthralgias	50–75[7,10,30]
Myalgias	≤70[21]
Inflammatory arthritis	10–39[7,10,12,30,65]
Inflammatory myopathy	<2[7,19,20]

Table 6.3 Frequency of joint involvement in Sjögren's syndrome.

Location (n=152)	Patients, n (%)
Proximal IP joint	57 (35)
MCP joint	57 (35)
Wrist	49 (30)
Elbow	25 (16)
Knee	17 (10)
Ankle	16 (10)
Shoulder	9 (7)
MTP joint	8 (6)
Distal IP joint	5 (4)

Modified from a systematic literature review focused on systemic manifestations of SS.[11]
IP, interphalangeal; MCP, metacarpophalangeal; MTP, metatarsophalangeal.

Fibromyalgia is another condition known to both mimic and occur alongside SS. It is a chronic disorder characterized by widespread arthralgias, myalgias, fatigue, sleep disturbances, and alterations in mood. Although most patients have joint pain, inflammatory arthritis is not a feature of fibromyalgia. Fibromyalgia has been noted in up to 30% of SS patients yet it is described in only ~2% of the general population.[3,16−18] In SS patients who have chronic fatigue and diffuse musculoskeletal pain without evidence of synovitis on examination consider concurrent fibromyalgia.

Inflammatory myopathy is rare in SS, occurring in less than 2% of patients.[7,19,20] It is typically mild and can present with weakness, myalgias, or no symptoms at all.[21] Elevation of muscle enzyme levels in SS-associated myositis is typically lower than that observed in polymyositis and dermatomyositis.[21]

MUSCULOSKELETAL PEARLS IN SS

- Can be the presenting feature of SS
- Pattern of joint involvement same as in RA
- Marginal erosions on joint imaging strongly suggest presence of concurrent RA and warrant more aggressive treatment

---

Pulmonary manifestations

The two main pulmonary manifestations of SS, in broad strokes, are airways disease and interstitial lung disease (ILD) but a variety of other diseases have also been described (Table 6.4). Pulmonary disease in SS has been associated with decreased quality of life and increased mortality.[22−25] Because of the associated morbidity, routine screening is strongly encouraged in all patients with chronic respiratory symptoms.

Table 6.4 Pulmonary manifestations of Sjögren's syndrome.

Feature	Frequency (approximate percentage)
Symptoms (of 260 SS patients with detailed notes)	
Airway dryness (nose, mouth, throat)	
Dyspnea	60
Cough	50
Sputum	≤15
Chest pain	5
Hoarseness	
Pulmonary function test results (of 163 SS patients with pulmonary function test results reported)	
Restrictive pattern	60
Obstructive pattern	20
High-resolution CT scan findings (of 526 SS patients with CT scan results reported)	
Bronchiectasis/bronchiolectasis	50
Ground-glass opacities	50
Nodules	25
Interlobular septal thickening	25
Reticular pattern	20
Cysts/bullae	20
Airspace consolidation	15
Honeycombing	15
Nonseptal linear/platelike opacities	10
Mosaic perfusion/attenuation	5
Tree-in-bud opacities	5
Emphysema/air trapping	5
Pleural thickening/effusion	5
Histopathologic findings (of 146 SS patients with histopathologic results)	
Nonspecific interstitial pneumonia	45
Usual interstitial pneumonia	15
Lymphocytic interstitial pneumonia	15
Organizing pneumonia	10
Amyloidosis	5
Lymphoma	5
Pseudolymphoma	<5
Noncaseating granuloma	≤5
Cystic disease	1
Other manifestations	
Venous thromboembolism	<5
Pulmonary hypertension	<5

Modified from a systematic literature review focused on systemic manifestations of SS.[11]

The most common respiratory symptoms in SS are dyspnea and cough. Chronic cough has been reported in up to 60% and can be dry or productive.[26] Potential causes of chronic cough in SS may include xerotrachea, airway hyperreactivity, bronchiectasis, ILD, and gastroesophageal reflux.[27] Respiratory tract dryness along with decreased mucociliary clearance and immunosuppression may also contribute to the increased rates of sinusitis, bronchitis, and pneumonia observed in this population.[27]

Evaluation for underlying lung disease in SS may include pulmonary function testing (PFT), high-resolution computed tomographic (HRCT) scanning of the chest, and lung biopsy. The overall diagnostic yield of such testing was 16% in a systematic literature review of 4897 unselected SS patients (Table 6.4).[11] Among those with abnormal PFT results, a restrictive pattern was most common, noted in ~60%, and an obstructive pattern in ~20%. Of those with HRCT findings, the most common were bronchiectasis/bronchiolectasis and ground-glass opacities each noted in about 50%. Of those who underwent lung biopsy, the most common histopathologic finding was nonspecific interstitial pneumonia (NSIP) (Fig. 6.1).

Airways disease in SS, manifested mainly by cough and sometimes dyspnea, is due to dryness from exocrine gland dysfunction and/or lymphocytic infiltration of the trachea, bronchi, and bronchioles.[27] Related HRCT findings may include bronchiectasis/bronchiolectasis, airway wall thickening, nodules, tree-in-bud opacities, mosaic attenuation, air trapping, and subsegmental atelectasis.[26,27] Although obstruction may be noted in PFT results, the effect on respiratory function is generally inconsequential and thus airway disease in SS is not a significant contributor to mortality.[27]

ILD in SS usually presents with chronic cough and shortness of breath. Less commonly, it can mimic infectious pneumonia. In one study the clinical presentation was acute/subacute in 50%, insidious in 25%, and asymptomatic in the remaining

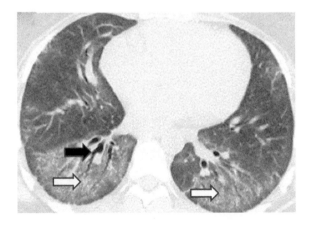

FIGURE 6.1

High-resolution chest CT of Sjögren's syndrome patient with nonspecific interstitial pneumonia. Lower lobe predominant ground-glass opacities (*white arrows*) and bronchiectasis (*black arrow*) are noted.[23]

25%.[22] The onset of ILD preceded the diagnosis of SS in about a quarter of cases.[22] Factors at SS diagnosis that predicted later development of ILD included old age, esophageal involvement, and Raynaud phenomenon (RP).[22] PFT typically reveals a restrictive pattern, along with a decreased diffusing capacity of carbon monoxide.[27] The most prevalent pattern on HRCT is that of NSIP with bibasilar symmetric reticular changes, traction bronchiectasis, and ground-glass opacities.[27] Although lymphocytic interstitial pneumonia (LIP) is not the most common pattern seen in SS-related ILD, it has a strong association with SS.[28,29] The HRCT pattern typical of LIP consists of cysts, nodules, ground-glass opacities, and thickening of the interlobular septa[27] (Fig. 6.2). Regardless of the underlying pattern, ILD is a significant cause of mortality in SS.

PULMONARY PEARLS IN SS

- Chronic cough occurs in ~50% patients and contributes to decreased quality of life.
- Airways disease is common in SS.
- ILD occurs in ~10% of patients, and the most common pattern is NSIP.
- Lung involvement is associated with increased mortality in SS.
- PFTs and HRCT are required in SS patients with chronic respiratory symptoms.

Renal manifestations

For many, the first thing that comes to mind when considering renal disease in a rheumatology patient is glomerulonephritis (GN), an often dramatic process with impressive hypertension and acute kidney injury. Although this may be

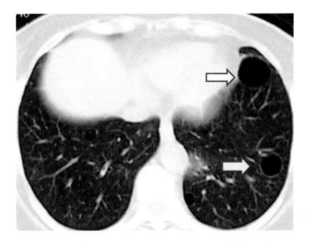

FIGURE 6.2

High-resolution chest CT of Sjögren's syndrome patient with lymphocytic interstitial pneumonia. Lower lobe predominant subpleural cysts are noted (*arrows*).[23]

Table 6.5 Clinical clues for renal disease in SS.

History
Polyuria/polydipsia
Muscle weakness
Nephrolithiasis and/or nephrocalcinosis

Laboratory abnormalities
Hypokalemia
Elevated creatinine levels (chronic kidney disease)
Non-anion gap metabolic acidosis
Elevated urine pH levels
Proteinuria

characteristic of systemic lupus erythematosus (SLE) and granulomatosis with polyangiitis, it is not the norm in SS. A medical history of nephrolithiasis, serum potassium level just below the lower limit of normal, and polyuria in a patient with dry mouth who frequently drinks water may be the evidence of renal involvement in SS that can be easily glossed over without a second thought. The most common renal manifestations in SS tend to be subtle and so they are often underappreciated (Table 6.5). This is true both clinically and in the medical literature. Retrospective studies estimate the prevalence of renal disease in SS as only 5%.[30–33] However, prospective studies specifically looking for evidence of renal disease in SS report a prevalence as high as 50%.[33] Identifying renal disease in SS requires vigilance and a high index of suspicion.

Tubulointerstitial nephritis

The most common renal pathology in SS is tubulointerstitial nephritis (TIN). TIN has been found in 50%–98% of SS kidney biopsies[32–36] and is characterized by inflammation of the interstitium. The inflammation is mostly lymphocytic and can be diffuse or patchy and variable in degree[34,37,38] (Fig. 6.3). This lymphocytic inflammation is similar to that found in other involved organs such as the salivary glands and respiratory tract.[34,38] It is important to note that the histopathology of TIN is nonspecific and can be due to causes other than SS (Table 6.6). Unlike the acute interstitial nephritis that one might observe from a drug reaction, interstitial nephritis in SS is a chronic process. The resultant tissue injury, fibrosis, and atrophy may lead to elevations in serum creatinine levels, low range proteinuria, and renal tubular acidosis (RTA).[37,38] Due to its slow progression, chronic kidney disease in SS patients may be incorrectly attributed to other coincident diagnoses such as hypertension or diabetes mellitus. The low-molecular-weight proteinuria of TIN may be easily missed, as it is not detected with routine dipstick testing.[38] Sometimes the only clue for TIN is a slight electrolyte disturbance caused by concurrent RTA.

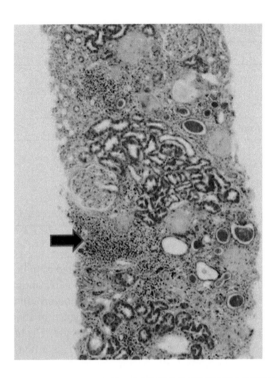

FIGURE 6.3

Hematoxylin and eosin—stained renal biopsy specimen showing lymphocytic infiltration (arrow) due to Sjögren's —related tubulointerstitial nephritis.

Modified from Ref. [42].

Renal tubular acidosis

The inflammation from TIN can lead to tubular dysfunction manifesting as RTA. The most common type is distal RTA (dRTA) or type 1 which has a prevalence of ~10—40% in SS patients according to prospective and cross-sectional studies.[29,33,39,40] The alpha-intercalated cells of the distal tubules are responsible for secreting hydrogen ions into the urine to help maintain the body's proper acid-base balance. Inflammation, typically from TIN, causes a decrease in alpha-intercalated cell function, which in turn leads to a decrease in hydrogen ion secretion into the urine and a resultant non-anion gap metabolic acidosis.[38] In order to maintain electroneutrality, other cations are secreted into the urine in place of the hydrogen ions resulting in hypokalemia, hypercalciuria, and hyperphosphaturia. The electrolyte disturbances of dRTA are typically minimal and asymptomatic, although they can occasionally lead to sequelae (Table 6.7). Sometimes dysfunction of the proximal rather than the distal tubule may be the cause of RTA (type 2) in SS. However, proximal RTA is rare, noted in only about 3%—4% of SS patients with renal involvement[36,41] (Table 6.7).

Table 6.6 Causes of tubulointerstitial nephritis.

Autoimmune diseases
Sjögren's syndrome
IgG4-related disease (increased staining for IgG4+ plasma cells and storiform fibrosis)
Sarcoidosis (noncaseating granulomas)
Tubulointerstitial nephritis and uveitis syndrome

Infections
Pyelonephritis
Tuberculosis
Leptospirosis
Hantavirus

Drugs
Nonsteroidal antiinflammatory drugs
β-Lactam antibiotics
Allopurinol
Chinese herbs containing aristolochic acid

Malignancies
Lymphoma
Leukemia

Modified from Ref. 38.

Table 6.7 Renal dysfunction and sequelae in Sjögren's syndrome.

TIN → Renal scarring/atrophy → CKD → ESRD (in ∼5%−10% of those with CKD)
TIN → Intercalated cell dysfunction → Decreased hydrogen ion secretion → non-anion gap metabolic acidosis (dRTA)
dRTA → Hypokalemia → Muscle cramps +/or periodic paralysis
dRTA → Hypercalciuria and hyperphosphaturia → Nephrolithiasis +/or nephrocalcinosis
TIN → Proximal tubule dysfunction → Decreased bicarbonate ion reabsorption → Non-anion gap metabolic acidosis (pRTA)
pRTA → Decreased bicarbonate, phosphate, small proteins, amino acids, glucose, and urate reabsorption (Fanconi syndrome)
pRTA → Decreased phosphate reabsorption → osteomalacia, nephrolithiasis +/or nephrocalcinosis
Chronic metabolic acidosis (RTA) → Bone loss +/or osteomalacia
MPGN → AKI → ESRD
TIN → Principle cell (cells of collecting duct) dysfunction → Decreased ability to concentrate urine (diabetes insipidus) → Polyuria/nocturia → polydipsia

AKI, acute kidney injury; CKD, chronic kidney disease; dRTA, distal renal tubular acidosis; ESRD, end-stage renal disease; MPGN, membranoproliferative glomerulonephritis; pRTA, proximal renal tubular acidosis; TIN, tubulointerstitial nephritis.

Other renal manifestations

In SS, clinically significant GN is far less common than TIN, with a prevalence estimated at ~2% according to two prospective cohorts.[7,39] The largest study to date of kidney biopsy samples from SS patients with renal disease found TIN in 98% and GN in only 23% (largely concurrent with TIN).[34] Membranoproliferative glomerulonephritis (MPGN) is the most common subtype noted. This is typically an immunocomplex-mediated vasculitis associated with hypocomplementemia and cryoglobulinemia.[32,34,38,42] Other forms of GN are less common. The presentation of GN in SS, as in SLE, is typically acute. When diagnosing MPGN in an SS patient, it is also important to evaluate for other causes of MPGN, such as SLE, infective endocarditis, viral infections (human immunodeficiency virus, hepatitis B and C), and monoclonal gammopathy (e.g., multiple myeloma).[38]

Another renal manifestation of note is diabetes insipidus (DI). DI has been reported in ~15–30% of SS patients and can be seen alongside other forms of renal involvement.[35,39,42] It is often not clinically apparent, as hypernatremia is avoided by drinking plenty of water, an ordinary habitual activity in most SS patients.

RENAL PEARLS IN SS

- TIN occurs most frequently.
- RTA is common in SS and can lead to bone loss, renal calculi, and periodic paralysis.
- GN is unusual in SS and, unlike TIN, tends to present acutely.
- Renal disease in SS is typically asymptomatic and insidious; regular screening with serum creatinine assay, serum electrolyte assay, and urine testing is recommended.
- A renal biopsy should be considered in all SS patients with significant evidence of renal disease.

Gastrointestinal manifestations

A variety of gastrointestinal (GI) manifestations have been reported in SS (Table 6.8). These may arise from lymphocytic infiltration of the GI mucosa or exocrine glands, autonomic neuropathy, or the development of associated autoimmune diseases that occur with increased prevalence in SS. Vasculitis of the GI tract may also occur but rarely (Chapter 7).

Esophageal/gastric

Dysphagia, the sensation of food getting "stuck" in the throat or chest, is commonly reported in SS.[43,44] Esophageal issues such as dryness, dysmotility, and reflux have all been identified as causes (Table 6.9). Persistent dysphagia that fails to respond to empirical treatment warrants evaluation with endoscopy and barium swallow plus video esophagram; infrequently, manometry may also be required.

Gastroesophageal reflux is another common manifestation, occurring in a majority of SS patients.[43] It may have multiple potential causes and, in turn, may be a

Table 6.8 Gastrointestinal manifestations reported in SS.

Manifestation	Approximate % prevalence in SS (and/or comment)
Esophageal	
Dysphagia	30–80[43,44]
Gastroesophageal reflux	60[43]
Gastric	
Gastroparesis	30–50[46,47]
Dyspepsia	20[44]
Nausea	$\leq$5[44]
Chronic atrophic gastritis	25–80 of those undergoing endoscopy[44,81]
Helicobacter pylori infection	Controversial association with SS[44,52]
Intestinal	
Abdominal pain	$\leq$40[44]
Constipation	20[82]
Chronic diarrhea	$\leq$10[44]
Celiac disease	1–14[49–51]
Vasculitis	A few case reports
Pancreatic	
Exocrine insufficiency	40–60[52,83,84]
Pancreatitis	A few case reports[85–89]
Hepatic	
Elevated liver enzyme levels	10–40[52–55]
Primary biliary cholangitis	<5
Autoimmune hepatitis	<5
Sclerosing cholangitis	A few case reports[85–89]
Hepatitis C infection	

SS, *Sjögren's syndrome.*

Table 6.9 Causes of dysphagia in Sjögren's syndrome.

- Mouth and esophageal dryness
- Esophageal dysmotility
- Esophageal reflux
- Esophageal webs
- Achalasia
- Zenker diverticulum

Table 6.10 Causes and effects of gastroesophageal reflux disease in Sjögren's syndrome.[45]

Causes
Diminished saliva
Esophageal dysmotility
Sphincter relaxation
Delayed gastric emptying time
Side effects of medications

Effects
Dysphagia
Chronic cough
Hoarseness
Heartburn
Nausea
Chest pain

contributing factor to symptoms such as dysphagia, chronic cough, and hoarseness (Table 6.10).[45]

Another upper GI problem commonly reported in SS is gastroparesis.[46,47] This and other examples of dysmotility are felt to reflect dysfunction of the underlying autonomic nervous system.[46–48] The diagnosis of gastroparesis should be considered in any SS patient with chronic nausea, vomiting, anorexia, early satiety, and/or weight loss and who has unremarkable results of upper endoscopy.

Intestinal

Chronic diarrhea occurs in up to 10% of SS patients and has an assortment of potential causes (Table 6.11).[44] One of the most important causes is celiac disease that, according to some studies, seems to be more prevalent in SS patients than in the general population.[49–51] The diagnosis of celiac should also be considered in any patient with unexplained weight loss or multiple vitamin deficiencies.

Table 6.11 Causes of chronic diarrhea in Sjögren's syndrome.

- Cholinergic side effect of pilocarpine or cevimeline
- Excessive use of dry mouth lozenges containing xylitol or sorbitol
- Food hypersensitivity
- Celiac disease
- Small intestinal bacterial overgrowth syndrome
- Inflammatory bowel disease
- Lymphocytic colitis

Hepatic

Abnormalities in liver function test results are not unusual in SS occurring in up to 40% of patients.[52–55] Drug toxicity and nonalcoholic fatty liver disease should be considered early in the evaluation.[52] Testing for chronic hepatitis C virus (HCV) infection should be carried out in any patient with persistent sicca symptoms and abnormal elevation of liver enzyme levels because HCV infection can cause a clinical syndrome mimicking SS[56] and it is also highly prevalent in the United States[57] and certain European populations.[58]

Autoimmune liver diseases may be associated with SS and include primary biliary cholangitis (PBC) and chronic active autoimmune hepatitis (AIH). In PBC, autoimmune mononuclear cell infiltration leads to destruction of small- and medium-sized bile ducts with resultant cholestasis.[59] Although patients may note fatigue and pruritus, about half are asymptomatic at diagnosis.[60] Antimitochondrial antibody testing is highly sensitive and specific for PBC[59,60] and should be considered in any SS patient with elevated levels of alkaline phosphatase, bilirubin, or γ-glutamyltransferase. PBC is not common in SS, occurring in only 2%–5%.[7,12,53,61] On the other hand, and of interest, SS has been reported in up to one-third of known PBC patients.[62,63] The prognosis of PBC is generally positive with only a minority of treated patients evolving to cirrhosis.[64]

AIH is perhaps less common than PBC, having been reported in about 1% of patients in a large SS registry[12] and up to 4% in other studies.[52] It is characterized by immune-mediated destruction of hepatocytes, increased serum aminotransferase levels, increased serum autoantibodies, and nonspecific findings on liver biopsy.[64] As with PBC, the onset is typically insidious. Symptoms and signs may include fatigue, arthralgias, rash, anorexia, jaundice, and hepatosplenomegaly.[64] SS patients with AIH frequently test positive for antinuclear antibodies and anti—smooth muscle antibodies. As with PBC, the prognosis of AIH when treated is generally good with a 10-year survival rate of greater than 90%.[64]

GI PEARLS IN SS

- GI symptoms is SS may have multiple causes and require a thorough evaluation to determine the underlying cause.
- Gastroparesis may explain chronic nausea, vomiting, anorexia, early satiety, and/or weight loss in a SS patient with normal upper endoscopy.
- Elevations in the levels of alkaline phosphatase, bilirubin, or γ-glutamyltransferase in SS should prompt an evaluation for PBC.
- Chronic abdominal pain, nausea, and/or bloating in SS should trigger a workup for celiac disease.

Hematologic abnormalities

Cytopenias

Hematologic manifestations are common in SS (Table 6.12). Cytopenias affect 30% −60%[65] and are usually mild and asymptomatic.[66] They are often due to the underlying SS itself but medication side effects and other causes should be considered. Anemia is seen in almost half of the SS patients and is typically an anemia of chronic disease[65] that is normocytic and normochromic.[66] Leukopenia is less common. Neutropenia can be associated with an increased risk of infections.[67] An increased risk of developing NHL has been associated with both neutropenia and lymphopenia.[68] Thrombocytopenia is the least frequent cytopenia and like the others is typically mild and clinically silent. Pancytopenia rarely occurs in SS.[65]

Table 6.12 Hematologic abnormalities in SS.

Manifestation	Approximate percentage of SS (%)
Cytopenias	
Any cytopenia	30−60[65]
Bicytopenia	5−10[65]
Pancytopenia	1[65]
Anemia	15−45[7,12,31,65,66]
Severe anemia (Hb <9 g/L)	4[66]
Hemolytic anemia	1[65]
Leukopenia	10−25[7,31,65,66]
Severe (<2000/mm^3)	0.2[66]
Neutropenia	5−30[31,65−67]
Severe neutropenia (<500/mm^3)	2[67]
Lymphopenia	10[31,65,66]
Eosinophilia	10[66]
Thrombocytopenia	5−15[12,31,65,66]
Moderate (<100 K/mm^3)	3[66]
Severe (<50 K/mm^3)	0.4[66]
Immunoglobulin and other abnormalities	
Elevated ESR	20[66]
Severe (>100 mm/h)	4[66]
Hypergammaglobulinemia	20−50[7,12,65,66]
Hypogammaglobulinemia	5−15[65,66]
Monoclonal immunoglobulinemia	10−20[31,66,69]
Cryoglobulinemia	10−20[7,30,31,65,66,70,71]
Low C3	10−15[12,30,31,65]
Low C4	5−20[7,12,30,31,65]

ESR, *erythrocyte sedimentation rate*; Hb, *hemoglobin*; SS, *Sjögren's syndrome*.

Immunoglobulin abnormalities

As SS is characterized by infiltration of lymphocytes into affected tissues and B-cell hyperactivity, it is not surprising to note findings related to active B cells in the blood. Hypergammaglobulinemia, as noted in serum protein electrophoresis (SPEP) or an increase in quantitative IgG levels, is present in up to half of the SS patients.[7,12,65,66] Interestingly, hypogammaglobulinemia can also be found but far less commonly, and immunodeficiencies were noted in only ~1% of SS patients, according to one series.[66] Hypergammaglobulinemia is a common contributor to an elevation in the erythrocyte sedimentation rate, which is reported in ~20% of SS patients.[66]

Other somewhat common immunoglobulin abnormalities include monoclonality and cryoglobulinemia. SPEP will show the presence of monoclonal immunoglobulins in ~10%−20% of SS patients.[31,66,69] The monoclonal component is typically IgG and less frequently IgM followed by other subtypes.[69] Cryoglobulinemia is noted in ~10−20% of SS patients as well.[7,30,31,65,66,70,71] Most frequently, this is a so-called "mixed" type made of both monoclonal IgM and polyclonal IgG.[70,71]

Immunoglobulin and complement abnormalities have noteworthy clinical significance in SS. Cryoglobulinemia and low C4 levels are each markers of poor prognosis. These, along with the presence of monoclonal immunoglobulins, are independent risk factors for the development of NHL (Chapter 8).[70,72] In patients suspected of having SS who have significant objective evidence of dryness but do not meet the SS classification criteria, the presence of hypergammaglobulinemia and low C4 levels have each been shown to help predict meeting the SS classification upon repeat evaluation 2−3 years later. Also, of note, the presence of cryoglobulinemia is associated with cutaneous vasculitis.[71]

HEMATOLOGIC/ONCOLOGIC PEARLS IN SS

- Cytopenias in SS are common and typically mild.
- Anemia occurs in up to half of the SS patients and is typically anemia of chronic disease.
- Cryoglobulinemia and low C4 levels are important markers of NHL development and poor prognosis in SS; yearly screening for these findings is recommended.
- In patients suspected of having SS who do not meet SS classification criteria, hypergammaglobulinemia and low C4 have been shown to help predict future diagnosis.

Dermatologic manifestations

About half of SS patients experience dry skin (xeroderma)[73] as well as other less common dermatologic manifestations. The xeroderma is often associated with pruritus, both of which may be adequately controlled with an effective skin care regimen. Chronic pruritus in SS may be associated with dermatographic urticaria, which is sometimes triggered by exposure to tartrazine dyes and/or salicylates.[74,75] Chronic pruritus that persists despite appropriate treatment should prompt an evaluation for primary biliary cirrhosis and/or lymphoma.

Raynaud's phenomenon (RP) typically manifests as sudden-onset well-demarcated color changes of the distal fingers and/or toes induced by cold exposure. The classically described pattern of color change is white to blue/purple then to red; however, the vast majority of patients describe only one or two such changes. RP can be painful and attacks last up to 30 minutes before resolving completely. It is known to occur in up to one-third of SS patients,[7,12,30,65] particularly in those who are anti-centromere antibody positive (Table 6.13).[76]

Annular erythema occurs in about 10% of SS patients and appears as ring-shaped erythema with wide raised borders and central pallor[77] (Fig. 6.4). It looks just like subacute cutaneous lupus erythematosus (SCLE), and as with SCLE, it is associated with SSA positivity.[77]

Purpura, both palpable and nonpalpable, is also noted in about 10% of SS patients.[7] Biopsy will typically reveal small vessel vasculitis, either leukocytoclastic or lymphocytic.[78] Nonvasculitic petechiae and purpura may also occur due to

Table 6.13 Dermatologic manifestations of SS.

Manifestation	Approximate percentage of SS (%)
Common	
Dry skin (with or without chronic pruritus)	50[73]
Raynaud phenomenon	15–30[7,12,30,65]
Annular erythema	10[77]
Purpura (vasculitis)	10[7]
Less common (with clear association to SS)	
Maculopapular rash (vasculitis)[73]	
Urticaria (vasculitis)[73]	
Cutaneous ulcers (vasculitis)[73]	
Localized cutaneous amyloidosis[73,90]	
Less common (with unclear association to SS)[73]	
Lichen planus	
Erythema nodosum–like lesions	
Vitiligo	
Alopecia	
Sweet syndrome	
Granulomatous panniculitis	
Erythema multiforme–like lesions	
Erythema elevatum diutinum	
Erythema perstans–like lesions	
Subcorneal pustular dermatosis	
Anetoderma	

SS, Sjögren's syndrome.
Modified from Ref. 73.

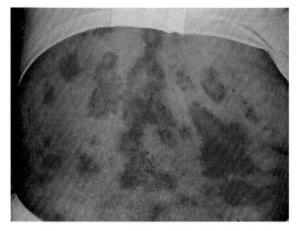

FIGURE 6.4

Erythematous polycylic rash typical of annular erythema in a patient with Sjögren's syndrome.[77]

thrombocytopenia or hypergammaglobulinemia. In addition to purpura, cutaneous vasculitis in SS may appear as urticaria, cutaneous ulcerations, and/or a maculopapular rash.[72] Cutaneous vasculitis is generally located on the lower extremities and is a marker for more severe disease and poor prognosis.[73,79]

DERMATOLOGIC PEARLS IN SS

- Common manifestations include xeroderma, purpura, and RP.
- Chronic pruritus in SS refractory to treatment should prompt further evaluation for PBC and/or lymphoma.
- Cutaneous vasculitis in SS is associated with more severe disease and poor prognosis.

Conclusions

The extraglandular manifestations of SS are myriad, affect virtually every organ system, and occur with varying frequency. Some are subtle, whereas others may be life threatening and influence long-term prognosis. When extraglandular involvement precedes the hallmark symptoms of SS, this diagnosis may go unrecognized for months to years. Every SS patient should be carefully assessed and monitored for the risk of non-Hodgkin B-cell lymphoma. Having a solid appreciation of the breadth and depth of the extraglandular manifestations of SS is essential to making a timely diagnosis and preventing serious morbidity and mortality.

References

1. Vivino FB. Sjögren's syndrome: clinical aspects. *Clin Immunol.* 2017;182:48−54.
2. Haldorsen K, Bjelland I, Bolstad AI, Jonsson R, Brun JG. A five-year prospective study of fatigue in primary Sjögren's syndrome. *Arthritis Res Ther.* 2011;13(5):R167.
3. Giles I, Isenberg D. Fatigue in primary Sjögren's syndrome: is there a link with the fibromyalgia syndrome? *Ann Rheum Dis.* 2000;59(11):875−878.
4. Sjögren's Syndrome Foundation, Inc. Living with Sjögren's: summary of major findings. Sjögren's Quarterly Spring 2017;12(2): 6-8.
5. Karageorgas T, Fragioudaki S, Nezos A, Karaiskos D, Moutsopoulos HM, Mavragani CP. Fatigue in primary Sjögren's syndrome: clinical, laboratory, psychometric, and biologic associations. *Arthritis Care Res.* 2016;68(1):123−131.
6. Theander L, Strömbeck B, Mandl T, Theander E. Sleepiness or fatigue? Can we detect treatable causes of tiredness in primary Sjögren's syndrome? *Rheumatology.* 2010; 49(6):1177−1183.
7. Skopouli F, Dafni U, Ioannidis J, Moutsopoulos H. Clinical evolution, and morbidity and mortality of primary Sjögren's syndrome. *Semin Arthritis Rheum.* 2000;129(5):296−304.
8. García-Carrasco M, Ramos-Casals M, Rosas J, Pallarés L, Calvo-Alen J, Cervera R, Font J, Ingelmo M. Primary Sjögren syndrome: clinical and immunologic disease patterns in a cohort of 400 patients. *Medicine.* 2002;81(4):270−280.
9. Zhao Y, Li Y, Wang L, Li XF, Huang CB, Wang GC, Zhang XW, Zhang ZL, Zhang X, Xiao WG, Dai L, Wang YF, Hu SX, Li HB, Gong L, Liu B, Sun LY, Zhang MJ, Zhang X, Li YZ, Du DS, Zhang SH, Sun YY, Zhang FC. Primary Sjögren syndrome in Han Chinese: clinical and immunological characteristics of 483 patients. *Medicine.* 2015;94(16): e667.
10. Fauchais AL, Ouattara B, Gondran G, Lalloué F, Petit D, Ly K, Lambert M, Launay D, Loustaud-Ratti V, Bezanahari H, Liozon E, Hachulla E, Jauberteau MO, Vidal E, Hatron PY. Articular manifestations in primary Sjögren's syndrome: clinical significance and prognosis of 188 patients. *Rheumatology.* 2010;49(6):1164−1172.
11. Ramos-Casals M, Brito-Zeron P, Seror R, Bootsma H, Bowman S, Dorner T, Gottenberg J-E, Mariette X, Theander E, Bombardieri S, De Vita S, Mandl T, Ng WF, Kruize A, Tzioufas A, Vitali C, EULAR Sjögren Syndrome Task Force. Characterization of systemic disease in primary Sjögren's syndrome: EULAR-SS Task Force recommendations for articular, cutaneous, pulmonary and renal involvements. *Rheumatology.* 2015;54(12):2230−2238.
12. Malladi AS, Sack KE, Shiboski SC, Shiboski CH, Baer AN, Banushree R, Dong Y, Helin P, Kirkham BW, Li M, Sugai S, Umehara H, Vivino FB, Vollenweider CF, Zhang W, Zhao Y, Greenspan JS, Daniels TE, Criswell LA. Primary Sjögren's syndrome as a systemic disease: a study of participants enrolled in an international Sjögren's syndrome registry. *Arthritis Care Res.* 2012;64(6):911−918.
13. Mirouse A, Seror R, Vicaut E, Mariette X, Dougados M, Fauchais AL, Deroux A, Dellal A, Costedoat-Chalumeau N, Denis G, Sellam J, Arlet JB, Lavigne C, Urbanski G, Fischer-Dumont D, Diallo A, Fain O, Mékinian A, Club Rhumatismes Inflammation and SNFMI. Arthritis in primary Sjögren's syndrome: characteristics, outcome and treatment from French multicenter retrospective study. *Autoimmun Rev.* 2019;18(1):9−14.

14. Payet J, Belkhir R, Gottenberg JE, Bergé E, Desmoulins F, Meyer O, Mariette X, Seror R. ACPA-positive primary Sjögren's syndrome: true primary or rheumatoid arthritis-associated Sjögren's syndrome? *RMD Open.* 2015;1(1):e000066.

15. Yang H, Bian S, Chen H, Wang L, Zhao L, Zhang X, Zhao Y, Zeng X, Zhang F. Clinical characteristics and risk factors for overlapping rheumatoid arthritis and Sjögren's syndrome. *Sci Rep.* 2018;8(1):6180.

16. Ostuni P, Botsios C, Sfriso P, Punzi L, Chieco-Bianchi F, Semerano L, Grava C, Todesco S. Fibromyalgia in Italian patients with primary Sjögren's syndrome. *Jt Bone Spine.* 2002;69(1):51–57.

17. Torrente-Segarra V, Corominas H, Sanchez-Piedra C, Fernandez-Castro M, Andreu JL, Martinez-Taboada V, Olive A, Rosas J, Sanchez-Alonso F, Sjögrenser Study Group of the Spanish Society of Rheumatology. Fibromyalgia prevalence and associated factors in primary Sjögren's syndrome patients in a large cohort from the Spanish Society of Rheumatology registry (Sjögrenser). *Clin Exp Rheumatol.* 2017;35(Suppl. 105(3)):28–34.

18. Choi B, Oh HJ, Lee Y, Song YW. Prevalence and clinical impact of fibromyalgia in patients with primary Sjögren's syndrome. *Clin Exp Rheumatol.* 2016;34(2 Suppl. 96): S9–S13.

19. Colafrancesco S, Priori R, Gattamelata A, Picarelli G, Minniti A, Brancatisano F, D'Amati G, Giordano C, Cerbelli B, Maset M, Quartuccio L, Bartoloni E, Carubbi F, Cipriani P, Baldini C, Luciano N, De Vita S, Gerli R, Giacomelli R, Bombardieri S, Valesini G. Myositis in primary Sjögren's syndrome: data from a multicentre cohort. *Clin Exp Rheumatol.* 2015;33(4):457–464.

20. Martinez VA, Leal CA, Moreno DC. Hematological changes as the initial manifestation of primary Sjögren's syndrome. *Rev Colomb Reumatol.* 2018;25(1):55–58.

21. Espitia-Thibault A, Masseau A, Néel A, Espitia O, Toquet C, Mussini JM, Hamidou M. Sjögren's syndrome-associated myositis with germinal centre-like structures. *Autoimmun Rev.* 2017;16(2):154–158.

22. Roca F, Dominique S, Schmidt J, Smail A, Duhaut P, Lévesque H, Marie I. Interstitial lung disease in primary Sjgoren's syndrome. *Autoimmun Rev.* 2017;16(1):48–54.

23. Lopez Velazquez M, Highland KB. Pulmonary manifestations of systemic lupus erythematosus and Sjögren's syndrome. *Curr Opin Rheumatol.* 2018;30(5):449–464.

24. Palm O, Garen T, Berge Enger T, et al. Clinical pulmonary involvement in primary Sjögren's syndrome: prevalence, quality of life and mortality–a retrospective study based on registry data. *Rheumatology.* 2013;52:173–179.

25. Belenguer R, Ramos-Casals M, Brito-Zeron P, et al. Influence of clinical and immunological parameters on the health-related quality of life of patients with primary Sjögren's syndrome. *Clin Exp Rheumatol.* 2005;23:351–356.

26. Kampolis C, Fragkioudaki S, Mavragani C, Zormpala A, Samakovli A, Moutsopoulos H. Prevalence and spectrum of symptomatic pulmonary involvement in primary Sjögren's syndrome. *Clin Exp Rheumatol.* 2018;36(3):94–101.

27. Flament T, Bigot A, Chaigne B, Henique H, Diot E, Marcharnd-Adam S. Pulmonary manifestations of Sjögren's syndrome. *Eur Respir Rev.* 2016;25:110–123.

28. Liebow AA, Carrington CB. Diffuse pulmonary lymphoreticular infiltrations associated with dysproteinemia. *Med Cclinics North Am.* 1973;57:809–843.

29. Both T, Hoorn E, Zietse R, van Laar J, Dalm V, Brkic Z, Versnel M, van Hagen P, van Daele P. Prevalence of distal renal tubular acidosis in primary Sjögren's syndrome. *Rheumatology.* 2015;54(5):933–939.

30. Ramos-Casals M, Solans R, Rosas J, Camps MT, Gil A, Del Pino-Montes J, Calvo-Alen J, Jiménez-Alonso J, Micó ML, Beltrán J, Belenguer R, Pallarés L, GEMESS Study Group. Primary Sjögren syndrome in Spain: clinical and immunologic expression in 1010 patients. *Medicine.* 2008;87(4):210−219.

31. Ramos-Casals M, Brito-Zerón P, Solans R, Camps M, Casanovas A, Sopeña B, Díaz-López B, Rascón F, Qanneta R, Fraile G, Pérez-Alvarez R, Callejas J, Ripoll M, Pinilla B, Akasbi M, Fonseca E, Canora J, Nadal M, de la Red G, Fernández-Regal I, Jiménez-Heredia I, Bosch J, Ayala M, Morera-Morales L, Maure B, Mera A, Ramentol M, Retamozo S, Kostov B, SS Study Group, Autoimmune Diseases Study Group (GEAS) of the Spanish Society of Internal Medicine (SEMI). Systemic involvement in primary Sjögren's syndrome evaluated by ESSDAI: analysis of 921 Spanish patients (GEAS-SS Registry). *Rheumatology.* 2014;53(2):321−331.

32. Goules A, Tatouli I, Moutsopoulos H, Tzioufas A. Clinically significant renal involvement in primary Sjögren's syndrome, clinical presentation and outcome. *Arthritis Rheum.* 2013;65(11):2945−2953.

33. Jain A, Srinivas B, Emmanuel D, Jain V, Parameshwaran S, Negi V. Renal involvement in primary Sjögren's syndrome: a prospective cohort study. *Rheumatology Int.* 2018; 38(12):2251−2262.

34. Jasiek M, Karras A, Le Guern V, Krastinova E, Mesbah R, Faguer S, Jourde-Chiche N, Fauchais A, Chiche L, Dernis E, Moulis G, Fraison J, Lazaro E, Jullien P, Hachulla E, Le Quellec A, Rémy P, Hummel A, Costedoat-Chalumeau N, Ronco P, Vanhille P, Meas-Yedid V, Cordonnier C, Ferlicot S, Daniel L, Seror R, Mariette X, Thervet E, François H, Terrier B. A multicenter study of 95 biopsy-proven cases of renal disease in primary Sjögren's syndrome. *Rheumatology.* 2017;56(3):362−370.

35. Bossini N, Savoldi S, Franceschini F, Mombelloni S, Baronio M, Cavazzana I, Viola B, Valzorio B, Mazzucchelli C, Cattaneo R, Scolari F, Maiorca R. Clinical and morphological features of kidney involvement in primary Sjögren's syndrome. *Nephrol Dial Transplant.* 2001;16(12):2328−2336.

36. Maripuri S, Grande J, Osborn T, Fervenza F, Matteson E, Donadio J, Hogan M. Renal involvement in primary Sjögren's syndrome in a clinicopathologic study. *Clin J Am Soc Nephrol.* 2009;4(9):1423−1431.

37. Evans R, Laing C, Ciurtin C, Walsh S. Tubulointerstitial nephritis in primary Sjögren's syndrome: clinical manifestations and response to treatment. *BMC Muscoskelet Disord.* 2016;17:2.

38. Francois H, Mariette X. Renal involvement in primary Sjögren's syndrome. *Nat Rev Nephrol.* 2016;12(2):82−93.

39. Aasarod K, Haga H, Berg KJ, Hammerstrom J, Jorstad S. Renal involvement in primary Sjögren's syndrome. *QJM.* 2000;93(5):297−304.

40. Pertovaara M, Korpela M, Kouri T, Pasternack A. The occurrence of renal involvement in primary Sjögren's syndrome: a study of 78 patients. *Rheumatology.* 1999;38(11):1113−1120.

41. Ren H, Wang W, Chen X, Zhang W, Pan X, Wang X-L, Lin Y, Zhang S, Chen N. Renal involvement and follow up of 130 patients with primary Sjögren's syndrome. *J Rheumatol.* 2008;35(2):278−284.

42. Evans R, Zdebik A, Ciurtin C, Walsh SB. Renal involvement in primary Sjögren's syndrome. *Rheumatology.* 2015;54(9):1541−1548.

43. Mandl T, Ekberg O, Wollmer P, Manthorpe R, Jacobsson LT. Dysphagia and dysmotility of the pharynx and oesophagus in patients with primary Sjögren's syndrome. *Scand J Rheumatol.* 2007 Sep-Oct;36(5):394−401.

44. Ebert EC. Gastrointestinal and hepatic manifestations of Sjögren syndrome. *J Clin Gastroenterol*. 2012;46(1):25−30.

45. Chang CS, Liao CH, Muo CH, Kao CH. Increased risk of concurrent gastroesophageal reflux disease among patients with Sjögren syndrome: a nationwide population-based study. *Eur J Med*. 2016;31:73−78.

46. Hammar O, Ohlsson B, Wollmer P, Mandl T. Impaired gastric emptying in primary Sjögren's syndrome. *J Rheumatol*. 2010;37(11):2313−2318.

47. Imrich R, Alevizos I, Bebris L, Goldstein D, Holmes C, Illei G, Nikolov N. Predominant glandular cholinergic dysautonomia in patients with primary Sjögren's syndrome. *Arthritis Rheum*. 2015;67(5):1345−1352.

48. Park K, Park S, Jackson M. The inhibitory effects of antimuscarinic autoantibodies in the sera of primary Sjögren syndrome patients on the gastrointestinal motility. *Mol Immunol*. 2013;56:583−587.

49. Szodoray P, Barta Z, Lakos G, Szakáll S, Zeher M. Coeliac disease in Sjögren's syndrome–a study of 111 Hungarian patients. *Rheumatol Int*. 2004;24(5):278−282.

50. Iltanen S, Collin P, Korpela M, Holm K, Partanen J, Polvi A, Mäki M. Celiac disease and markers of celiac disease latency in patients with primary Sjögren's syndrome. *Am J Gastroenterol*. 1999;94(4):1042−1046.

51. Lazarus M, Isenberg D. Development of additional autoimmune diseases in a population of patients with primary Sjögren's syndrome. *Ann Rheum Dis*. 2005;64(7):1062−1064.

52. Retamozo S, Brito-Zeron P, Morcillo C, Kostov B, Acar-Denizli N, Ramos-Casals M. Chapter 15: digestive involvement in primary Sjögren's syndrome. In: Manuel Ramos-Casals R, et al., eds. *The Digestive Involvement in Systemic Autoimmune Diseases*. vol. 13. 2017:271−292.

53. Montano-Loza AJ, Crispin-Acuna JC, Remes-Troche JM, Uribe M. Abnormal hepatic biochemistries and clinical liver disease in patients with primary Sjögren's syndrome. *Ann Hepatol*. 2007;6(3):150−155.

54. Csepregi A, Szodoray P, Zeher M. Do autoantibodies predict autoimmune liver disease in primary Sjögren's syndrome? Data of 180 patients upon a 5 year follow-up. *Scand J Immunol*. 2002;56(6):623−629.

55. Abraham S, Begum S, Isenberg D. Hepatic manifestations of autoimmune rheumatic diseases. *Ann Rheum Dis*. 2004;63(2):123−129.

56. Haddad J, Deny P, Munz-Gotheil C, Ambrosini J, Trinchet J, Pateron D, Mal F, Callard P, Beaugrand M. Lymphocytic sialadenitis of Sjögren's syndrome associated with chronic hepatitis C virus liver disease. *Lancet*. 1992;339(8789):321−323.

57. *U.S. Department of Health and Human Services: Centers for Disease Control and Prevention. Hepatitis C: Why people born from 1945−65 should get tested*; 2016. publication # 220401 www.cdc.gov/knowmore hepatitis.

58. Ramos-Casals M, Muñoz S, Medina F, Jara L, Rosas J, Calvo-Alen J, Brito-Zerón P, Forns X, Sánchez-Tapias J, HISPAMEC Study Group. Systemic autoimmune diseases in patients with hepatitis C virus infection: characterization of 1020 cases (The HISPAMEC Registry). *J Rheumatol*. 2009;36(7):1442−1448.

59. Gershwin ME. Pathogenesis of primary biliary cholangitis (primary biliary cirrhosis). In: Robson KM, ed. *UpToDate*. Waltham: Mass; 2017. https://www.uptodate.com/contents/pathogenesis-of-primary-biliary-cholangitis-primary-biliary-cirrhosis.

60. Poupon R. Clinical manifestations, diagnosis, and prognosis of primary biliary cholangitis (primary biliary cirrhosis). In: Robson KM, ed. *UpToDate*. Waltham:

Massachusetts; 2018. https://www.uptodate.com/contents/clinical-manifestations-diagnosis-and-prognosis-of-primary-biliary-cholangitis-primary-biliary-cirrhosis.

61. Nardi N, Brito-Zeron P, Ramos-Casals M, et al. Circulating auto-antibodies against nuclear and non-nuclear antigens in primary Sjögren's syndrome: prevalence and clinical significance in 335 patients. *Clin Rheumatol.* 2006;25(3):341−346.

62. Gershwin M, Selmi C, Worman H, Gold E, Watnik M, Utts J, Lindor K, Kaplan M, Vierling J, USA PBC Epidemiology Group. Risk factors and comorbidities in primary biliary cirrhosis: a controlled interview-based study of 1032 patients. *Hepatology.* 2005;42(5):1194−1202.

63. Wang L, Zhang F, Chen H, Zhang X, Xu D, Li Y, Wang Q, Gao L, Yang Y, Kong F, Wang K. Connective tissue diseases in primary biliary cirrhosis: a population-based cohort study. *World J Gastroenterol.* 2013;19(31):5131−5137.

64. Selmi C, Generali E, Gershwin ME. Rheumatic manifestations in autoimmune liver disease. *Rheum Dis Clin N Am.* 2018;44:65−87.

65. Baimpa E, Dahabreh IJ, Voulgarelis M, Moutsopoulos HM. Hematologic manifestations and predictors of lymphoma development in primary Sjögren syndrome: clinical and pathophysiologic aspects. *Medicine.* 2009;88(5):284−293.

66. Ramos-Casals M, Font J, Garcia-Carrasco M, Brito M, Rosas J, Calvo-Alen J, Pallares L, Cervera R, Ingelmo M. Primary Sjögren's syndrome: Hematologic patterns of disease expression. *Medicine.* 2002;81(4):281−292.

67. Brito-Zeron P, Soria N, Muñoz S, Bové A, Akasbi M, Belenguer R, Sisó A, Ramos-Casals M. Prevalence and clinical relevance of autoimmune neutropenia in patients with primary Sjögren's syndrome. *Semin Arthritis Rheum.* 2009;38(5):389−395.

68. Manganelli P, Fietta P, Quiani F. Hematologic manifestations of primary Sjögren's syndrome. *Clin Exp Rheumatol.* 2006;24(4):438−448.

69. Brito-Zeron P, Ramos-Casals M, Nardi N, Cervera R, Yagüe J, Ingelmo M, Font J. Circulating monoclonal immunoglobulins in Sjögren's syndrome: prevalence and clinical significance in 237 patients. *Medicine.* 2005;84(2):90−97.

70. Tzioufas A, Boumba D, Skopouli F, Moutsopoulos H. Mixed monoclonal cryoglobulinemia and monoclonal rheumatoid factor cross-reactive idiotypes as predictive factors for the development of lymphoma in primary Sjögren's syndrome. *Arthritis Rheum.* 1996; 39(5):767−772.

71. Ramos-Casals M, Cervera R, Yague J, García-Carrasco M, Trejo O, Jiménez S, Morlà R, Font J, Ingelmo M. Cryoglobulinemia in primary Sjögren's syndrome: prevalence and clinical characteristics in a series of 115 patients. *Semin Arthritis Rheum.* 1998;28(3): 200−205.

72. Nishinshinya MB, Pereda CA, Munoz-Fernandez S, Pego-Reigosa JM, Rua-Figueroa I, Andreu JL, Fernandez-Castro M, Rosas J, Santamaria EL. Identification of lymphoma predictors in patients with primary Sjögren's syndrome: a systemic literature review and meta-analysis. *Rheumatol Int.* 2015;35:17−26.

73. Jhorar P, Torre K, Lu J. Cutaneous features and diagnosis of primary Sjögren syndrome: an update and review. *J Am Acad Dermatol.* 2018;79(4):736−745.

74. Dipalma J. Tartrazine sensitivity. *Am Fam Physician.* 1990;42(5):1347−1350.

75. Stenius B, Lemola M. Hypersensitivity to acetylsalicylic acid (ASA) and tartrazine in patients with asthma. *Clin Allergy.* 1976;6(20):119−129.

76. Bournia V-K, Diamanti K, Vlachoyiannopoulos P, Moutsopoulos H. Anticentromere antibody positive Sjögren's Syndrome: a retrospective descriptive analysis. *Arthritis Res Ther.* 2010;12(2):R47.

77. Brito-Zerón P, Retamozo S, Akasbi M, Gandía M, Perez-De-Lis M, Soto-Cardenas MJ, Diaz-Lagares C, Kostov B, Bove A, Bosch X, Perez-Alvarez R, Siso A, Ramos-Casals M. Annular erythema in primary Sjögren's syndrome: description of 43 non-Asian cases. *Lupus*. 2014;23(2):166–175.

78. Molina R, Provost T, Alexander E. Two types of inflammatory vascular disease in Sjögren's syndrome. *Arthritis Rheum*. 1985;28:1251–1258.

79. Retamozo S, Gheitasi H, Quartuccio L, Kostov B, Corazza L, Bove A, Siso-Almirall A, Gandia M, Ramos-Casals M, De Vita S, Brito-Zeron P. Cryoglobulinemic vasculitis at diagnosis predicts mortality in primary Sjögren's syndrome: analysis of 515 patients. *Rheumatology*. 2016;55:1443–1451.

80. Cha SI, Fessler MB, Cool CD, Schwarz MI, Brown KK. Lymphoid interstitial pneumonia: clinical features, associations and prognosis. *Eur Respir J*. 2006;28:364–369.

81. Pokorny G, Karácsony G, Lonovics J, Hudák J, Németh J, Varró V. Types of atrophic gastritis in patients with primary Sjögren's syndrome. *Ann Rheum Dis*. 1991;50(2): 97–100.

82. Krogh K, Asmussen K, Stengaard-Pedersen K, Laurberg S, Deleuran BW. Bowel symptoms in patients with primary Sjögren's syndrome. *Scand J Rheumatol*. 2009;36(5): 407–409.

83. Coll J, Navarro S, Tomas R, Elena M, Martinez E. Exocrine pancreatic function in Sjögren's syndrome. *Arch Intern Med*. 1989;149(4):848–852.

84. Gobelet C, Gerster J, Rappoport G, Hiroz C, Maeder E. Pancreatic function in Sjögren's syndrome. *Clin Rheumatol*. 1983;2(2):139–143.

85. Montefusco P, Geiss A, Bronzo R, Randall S, Kahn E, McKinley M. Sclerosing cholangitis, chronic pancreatitis, and Sjögren's syndrome: a symptom complex. *Am J Surg*. 1984;147:822–826.

86. Kulling D, Tresch S, Renner E. Triad of sclerosing cholangitis, chronic pancreatitis, and Sjögren's syndrome: case report and review. *Gastrointest Endosc*. 2003;57(1):118–120.

87. Nieminen U, Koivisto T, Kahri A, Färkkilä M. Sjögren's syndrome with chronic pancreatitis, sclerosing cholangitis, and pulmonary infiltrations. *Am J Gastroenterol*. 1997; 92(1):139–142.

88. Fukui T, Okazaki K, Yoshizawa H, Ohashi S, Tamaki H, Kawasaki K, Matsuura M, Asada M, Nakase H, Nakashima Y, Nishio A, Chiba T. A case of autoimmune pancreatitis associated with sclerosing cholangitis, retroperitoneal fibrosis and Sjögren's syndrome. *Pancreatology*. 2005;5(1):86–91.

89. Pickartz T1, Pickartz H, Lochs H, Ockenga J. Overlap syndrome of autoimmune pancreatitis and cholangitis associated with secondary Sjögren's syndrome. *Eur J Gastroenterol Hepatol*. 2004;16(12):1295–1299.

90. Meijer J, Schonland S, Palladini G, Merlini G, Hegenbart U, Ciocca O, Perfetti V, Leijsma M, Bootsma H, Hazenberg B. Sjögren's syndrome and localized nodular cutaneous amyloidosis: coincidence or a distinct clinical entity? *Arthritis Rheum*. 2008; 58(7):1992–1999.

Vasculitis in Sjögren's syndrome

Ghaith Noaiseh, MD

*Associate Professor of Medicine, Division of Allergy, Clinical Immunology and Rheumatology,
University of Kansas, Kansas City, KS, United States*

Definition and classification

Vasculitis is characterized by inflammation and/or destruction of blood vessel walls.[1] It comprises a heterogeneous group of disorders that are commonly classified based on the size of the blood vessels affected. According to the Chapel Hill Consensus Conference Nomenclature, small vessel vasculitis involves intraparenchymal arteries, arterioles, capillaries, and postcapillary venules. Medium vessel vasculitis involves muscular arteries, essentially the main visceral arteries and veins, and their initial branches. Large vessel vasculitis affects the aorta; its major branches to the head, neck, and extremities; and the analogous veins.[2] The vasculitides are also classified as primary (idiopathic) and secondary (i.e., caused by another systemic disease).[2] Vasculitic features discussed in this chapter refer to secondary phenomena occurring in the context of primary Sjögren's syndrome (SS).

Clinical manifestations
Cutaneous vasculitis

The clinical expression of vasculitis depends on the size and location of the vessels affected, with the skin being the organ predominantly involved in SS.[3,4] A wide spectrum of cutaneous vasculitic manifestations has been observed in primary SS and summarized in Table 7.1. The prevalence of cutaneous vasculitis was approximately 9% in a large Spanish cohort involving 1010 SS patients[5] and is estimated to range from 9% to 32% based on previous reports.[6] Although palpable purpura is the most frequent cutaneous manifestation of SS vasculitis[7,8] (Fig. 7.1), other common patterns may also include erythematosus macules/papules and urticaria-like lesions.[7,9]

Histologically, small vessel vasculitis accounts for most SS-related vasculitis, including cutaneous vasculitis, with a minority of cases exhibiting involvement of medium vessels, similar to polyarteritis nodosa (PAN).[7,10,11] In a cohort of 558 patients from Spain with primary SS,[7] 89 (16%) had skin manifestations, of whom, 52

Table 7.1 Cutaneous manifestations of vasculitis in primary Sjögren's syndrome.

Common
Palpable purpura
Erythematous macules/papules
Urticaria-like lesions

Uncommon
Nodules
Vesicles
Ulcers
Pustules
Bullae
Livedo reticularis
Ischemic lesions

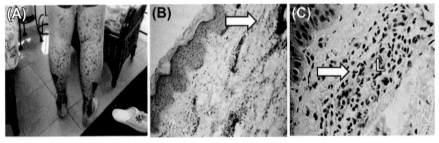

FIGURE 7.1

(A) Cutaneous purpura in a Sjögren's syndrome patient caused by (B) leukocytoclastic vasculitis (*arrows*). (C) Higher magnification view shows neutrophil infiltration with leukocytoclasis around vessel lumen.

were diagnosed with cutaneous vasculitis based on a clinical evaluation by an expert dermatologist.[7] Among 38 patients who underwent a skin biopsy, the main histologic pattern observed was leukocytoclastic vasculitis (LCV) ($n = 36$); 1 had lymphocytic vasculitis and 2 had medium vessel vasculitis with 1 overlapping with LCV. Hepatitis C was ruled out in all patients. Observations in this report emphasized the overwhelming predominance of neutrophilic vascular inflammation and contrasted sharply with the higher frequency of mononuclear cell—predominant infiltration documented in an earlier report.[8] It was postulated that early skin biopsies performed within 24—48 hours of symptom onset would be more likely to demonstrate LCV than mononuclear cell vasculitis, which is considered a later finding in the evolution of neutrophilic vasculitis.[12] Additionally, the high prevalence of cryoglobulinemia in the Spanish cohort may also explain the higher percentage of leukocytoclastic versus mononuclear vasculitis that was observed.[7]

Notably, cutaneous vasculitis can sometimes be the presenting manifestation of SS.[13,14] In the Spanish cohort, 48 patients (92%) had lower limb involvement and the upper extremities (25%), trunk (10%), and face (6%) were less commonly affected. In 48% the cutaneous vasculitis was monophasic, whereas the remaining patients experienced recurrent episodes.

Cutaneous vasculitis as a prognostic indicator

Of the 52 patients with cutaneous vasculitis in the Spanish cohort, 23 patients (44%) had vasculitic involvement beyond the skin suggesting the presence of systemic vasculitis including peripheral neuropathy in 16, pulmonary involvement in 7, glomerulonephritis (GN) in 5, mesenteric vasculitis in 2, and pancreatic vasculitis in 1. Thus in nearly half of the patients, cutaneous vasculitis was a marker for more serious systemic vasculitic involvement.[7]

Additionally, the presence of cutaneous vasculitis has been associated with a more severe clinical phenotype and more robust serologic expression than in patients without cutaneous vasculitis, including more frequent arthritic, neuropathic, and renal involvement; Raynaud phenomenon; hospitalization; and seropositivity for SS antibodies A and B (SSA and SSB), rheumatoid factor, and antinuclear antibodies.[7]

In another study, it was reported that cutaneous vasculitis was the most powerful predictor of mortality in SS when this group was compared to patient controls without this complication.[15] A retrospective study of 163 patients in the United States also found a significant association between vasculitis and severe (i.e., vision threatening) ocular complications of SS.[16] Analysis of 266 patients from Spain observed that vasculitis (including cutaneous vasculitis) when present at the time of diagnosis was an independent predictor of death.[11]

Cutaneous vasculitis patient subsets

Further work was done to classify cutaneous small vessel vasculitis in SS using laboratory markers and revealed at least two distinct clinical subsets with different prognoses: (1) cryoglobulinemic vasculitis (CV) and (2) noncryoglobulinemic vasculitis (NCV).[7,17] CV accounts for roughly 30% of cutaneous vasculitis cases in SS and typically presents with palpable purpura and mixed monoclonal and polyclonal cryoglobulins (type II) in the blood; infrequently, it may also cause digital ischemia and/or ulcers. In contrast, NCV may present with purpura, urticaria, or other lesions and is almost universally associated with hypergammaglobulinemia but not cryoglobulins. For this reason, the latter group has sometimes been labeled with the term "hypergammaglobulinemic vasculitis" or HGV.[17] However, it must be remembered that hypergammaglobulinemia occurs in up to 50% of patients with SS but only a very small subset actually develop NCV. Thus hypergammaglobulinemia serves as a better marker for polyclonal B-cell activation and disease activity than vasculitis.

To more precisely determine the clinical and laboratory differences between CV and NCV, which have long been viewed as distinct patterns of cutaneous vasculitis in SS,[7,18–20] a large multicenter database from five Italian referral centers was analyzed.[17] A total of 652 subjects were included, and 63 developed purpura, of whom, positive results for serum cryoglobulins were present in 23 (36%) and elevated serum gamma globulin levels were present in 40 (but repeatedly negative result for serum cryoglobulins). A total of 589 patients served as controls and had no purpura, negative result for serum cryoglobulins, and no hypergammaglobulinemia. Associations with different phenotypical as well as serologic features were evaluated.[17]

Peripheral neuropathy, low complement C4 levels, monoclonal gammopathy, leukopenia, anti-SSB/La antibodies, and lymphoma were all strongly associated with CV versus controls, whereas rheumatoid factor, monoclonal gammopathy, leukopenia, and anti-SSA/Ro antibodies were associated with HGV. The authors concluded that CV and HGV represented two distinct subsets of vasculitis patients with different clinical and serologic associations. CV is a systemic immunocomplex-mediated vasculitis with complement consumption, increased risk of lymphoma development, and systemic complications, whereas HGV, or NCV, represents an isolated cutaneous vasculitis related to benign B-cell proliferation.[17]

In the aforementioned Spanish study,[7] the long-term outcomes of the 52 patients with cutaneous vasculitis were described. Six patients died (mortality rate, 12%) from 1 to 11 years following the diagnosis of vasculitis. All six patients had severe, systemic CV with more than one organ involved: neuropathic ($n = 5$), renal ($n = 4$), pulmonary ($n = 3$), mesenteric ($n = 2$), and pancreatic ($n = 1$). This experience further exemplifies the bad prognosis associated with SS-related CV compared to NCV.

Given the importance of serum cryoglobulins as a prognostic marker in SS and the difficulty with accurately performing the assay, repeat testing for serum cryoglobulins may be warranted when the initial assay result is negative or a new problem occurs.

In summary, several important clinical pearls should be emphasized regarding the features of cutaneous vasculitis in SS patients (Table 7.2).

Peripheral nervous system involvement

A wide variety of peripheral neuropathies have been described in patients with SS.[21] Mononeuropathy and multiple mononeuropathy, although uncommon in SS,[22,23]

Table 7.2 Important features of cutaneous vasculitis in Sjögren's syndrome.

Usually leukocytoclastic vasculitis
Cryoglobulinemic and noncryoglobulinemic subsets
Typically affects lower extremities
Monophasic in half of the cases
Associated with systemic vasculitis in half the cases
Cryoglobulinemic vasculitis associated with more severe phenotype, increased mortality, and lymphomas

seem to correlate well with the presence of vasculitis.[22–24] In SS patients presenting with neuropathy and vasculitic features, a causative relationship may be inferred.[22,25,26] Compared with SS patients without cutaneous vasculitis,[7] patients with cutaneous vasculitis had a significantly higher frequency of peripheral neuropathy, and approximately one-third of patients (5 of 16) with peripheral neuropathy died from severe multisystemic CV.[7]

In another study, 40 SS patients with neuropathy underwent a nerve and/or muscle biopsy.[24] Of the 14 patients with histologic pattern of necrotizing vasculitis, 64% had skin involvement suggestive of cutaneous vasculitis. Importantly, none of the cases affected the kidney, gastrointestinal tract, or central nervous system (CNS), as assessed by clinical and biologic evaluation.[24] Therefore despite the absence of life-threatening organ involvement, necrotizing vasculitis should be considered as an underlying cause in patients with concurrent peripheral neuropathy and vasculitic skin involvement.[24]

The clinical presentation of vasculitic neuropathy includes sensory and/or motor deficits involving a territory innervated by individual nerves. Pain is common with acute or subacute presentation. Systemic presentation including constitutional symptoms and palpable purpura may, be present, suggesting the presence of systemic vasculitis. Inflammatory marker levels are usually elevated.[22] Compared with nonvasculitic neuropathies, patients with biopsy-proven neuropathic vasculitis (necrotizing or lymphocytic) were more likely to have acute onset of neuropathy, multiple mononeuropathy and clinical sensorimotor involvement, constitutional symptoms, vascular purpura, increased C-reactive protein levels, hypocomplementemia, monoclonal gammopathy, and rheumatoid factor positivity.[22] Therefore these clinical and biologic variables may be helpful in distinguishing patients with and without vasculitic neuropathies.[22]

Electrophysiologic findings include an axonal pattern of dysfunction and "pseudoblocks" at affected areas.[22]

Nerve biopsy may reveal varying degrees of vessel wall damage, fibrinoid necrosis, and mononuclear vascular or perivascular infiltrates.[23,27] The sural nerve is usually sampled, alone[23,28] or with concomitant muscle biopsy.[24] Alternatively, a superficial peroneal nerve/peroneus brevis muscle biopsy can also be utilized for histologic assessment of vasculitis.[29] Obtaining a combined nerve and muscle biopsy may increase the diagnostic sensitivity compared with nerve biopsy alone.[29]

Central nervous system involvement

Difficulty in obtaining brain and spinal cord tissue of patients with SS with active CNS manifestations has made ascertainment of the exact pathogenesis of CNS involvement very challenging.[8] Generally, in patients with nervous system disease not attributable to other causes, the strategy to diagnose probable SS-related CNS vasculitis is to document histologic evidence of vasculitis somewhere else, usually in the skin.[8]

One study reported that CNS SS was caused by a mononuclear inflammatory ischemic cerebral vasculopathy of small vessels, with some patients who were SSA positive exhibiting frank angiitis.[25] Cerebral angiography was performed to exclude other causes of CNS disease and to potentially establish the diagnosis of CNS vasculitis. Abnormalities of small cerebral arteries consistent with but not diagnostic of angiitis have been reported in up to 20% of highly selected cases[25] and include one or more focal areas of narrowing, delayed emptying of vessels, vascular occlusion, and poststenotic dilatation. In cases with a high suspicion of CNS vasculitis based on symptoms, angiographic abnormalities, other imaging abnormalities, and lack of alternative explanation, treatment with high-dose corticosteroids and immunosuppressive therapy is usually instituted.[30,31]

Renal involvement

Circulating cryoglobulins can trigger immunocomplex deposition in the kidneys with binding to endothelial cells, leading to complement activation, recruitment of inflammatory cells, and the development of small vessel vasculitis. Most cases of SS-related glomerular disease are immunocomplex mediated, and a renal biopsy will typically show membranoproliferative GN; this may occur as an isolated phenomenon or as part of a systemic vasculitis.[32,33]

The clinical presentation includes hematuria, proteinuria, hypertension, acute kidney injury, and nephrotic syndrome. In a series of 715 SS patients from Greece, 35 patients (4.9%) had clinically significant renal involvement. Among them, 17 patients had GN alone and 5 patients had GN in combination with interstitial nephritis. Of the GN cases, 64% were associated with cryoglobulinemia.[33] Importantly, GN was also associated with the development of lymphomas and poor survival.[33] Another retrospective, multicenter French study[34] examined 95 patients with biopsy-proven renal involvement and found glomerular lesions in 22 patients (23.2%), mainly related to cryoglobulinemia.

Other organs

The parotid glands, lungs, gastrointestinal tract, pancreas, gallbladder, spleen,[7,10] skeletal muscles, and probably the heart[35] can also be involved and, this usually occurs, as part of a systemic vasculitic process.

Although rare, a PAN-like presentation has long been recognized to occur in SS.[10,36−39] The first case of PAN-like presentation in the Spanish cohort[7] involved skin and muscles and another case had pancreatic and mesenteric involvement. The author identified 19 more reports in the literature of SS patients with a PAN-like presentation, and the frequency of organs involved is as follows: muscle ($n = 10$), gastrointestinal tract ($n = 7$), peripheral nerves ($n = 4$), kidney ($n = 3$), brain ($n = 2$), and one case, respectively, in the parotid glands, pancreas, gallbladder, spleen, and spinal cord. Among the 19 cases, 5 had associated cryoglobulinemia. Among selected cases, no evidence of aneurysmal formation has been documented by visceral angiogram thus far.[10]

Additionally, the interpretation of this literature remains very challenging because reports before 1990[10,37,39] could not rule out hepatitis C, because of the lack of available testing, while the value of other reports[40] was limited by including patients with secondary SS.

Antineutrophil cytoplasmic antibody-associated vasculitis and Sjögren syndrome overlap

A case series of seven patients described an overlap of antineutrophil cytoplasmic antibody (ANCA) vasculitis (AAV) in primary SS and identified 15 more cases in the literature. Of the 22 subjects studied, 76% were perinuclear ANCA positive with myeloperoxidase specificity. In all subjects, diagnosis of SS preceded the diagnosis of AAV, and AAV correlated with extraglandular manifestations of SS.[41] Many of these patients presented with pulmonary hemorrhage or acute kidney injury with a biopsy suggestive of AAV. It remains unclear whether these patients had SS with granulomatous vasculitis, AAV with salivary involvement, or both diseases independently. Determining how these conditions are interrelated is difficult, given the rarity of such patients.[36]

A few publications have also reported an association between SS syndrome and biopsy-proven IgA vasculitis.[42,43] Confirmation of this association by other investigators at other centers is also needed.

European Sjögren's syndrome disease activity index score and vasculitis

Vasculitis as a marker of systemic disease activity is prominently featured in the European Sjögren's Syndrome Disease Activity Index (ESSDAI) that was developed by the European League Against Rheumatism SS task force to assess activity and response to therapy in both clinical trials and in clinical practice settings.[44] ESSDAI is composed of 12 weighted domains that capture disease activity in different body organs. In the cutaneous domain, ESSDAI classifies cutaneous vasculitic activity as moderate or high according to the extent of skin involvement (<18% or >18% of body surface area involved, respectively) and the presence or absence of ulcers (high activity). Interestingly, a clinical diagnosis of cutaneous vasculitis without histologic proof was permissible. Extracutaneous vasculitis, including renal and neuropathic cryoglobulinemic involvement, was included in the corresponding renal and peripheral nervous system ESSDAI domains.[4]

Treatment

Currently, no randomized clinical trials are available to assess the efficacy of therapeutic interventions in SS patients with vasculitic syndromes. Therefore treatment algorithms are based on small uncontrolled studies, case series/reports, and expert opinion derived from the experience with treating similar manifestations in closely related disorders such as systemic lupus and rheumatoid arthritis. The choice of therapy is also influenced by the organs involved and the overall disease severity.

In the Spanish series of 52 patients with cutaneous vasculitis (mostly LCV),[7] the majority of patients were treated with systemic glucocorticoids (73%), of whom, about 20% required high doses (>30 mg/day). Seven patients (13%) received immunosuppressive agents (cyclophosphamide, $n = 4$; azathioprine, $n = 3$), and two received plasmapheresis. Ten patients were treated with nonsteroidal antiinflammatory drugs, five with antihistamines, four with chloroquine, and one with dapsone. Nine patients were not treated.[7] There was no mention of outcome or disease course following therapy. In the United states, low-dose colchicine is also sometimes used for prophylaxis of recurrent attacks of LCV.

In a phase II pilot study involving 15 patients with primary SS who had early and active disease, patients received leflunomide 20 mg once daily for 24 weeks[45]; 3 cases (20%) had biopsy-proven LCV and all experienced resolution of their skin rash with this therapy. The results of this trial, however, were otherwise disappointing.[45]

In a French series of 40 patients with biopsy-confirmed vasculitic neuropathy,[24] the majority of patients received systemic corticosteroids (95%), including high-dose intravenous methylprednisolone in over half of them. Cyclophosphamide was used in 10 patients (25%), azathioprine alone in 8 (20%), plasmapheresis in 4, hydroxychloroquine in 3, and a few treatment refractory cases were managed with rituximab in combination with one of the following options: cyclophosphamide alone, methotrexate, or CHOP (cyclophosphamide, doxorubicin, vincristine, and prednisone) regimen. Successful outcomes using intravenous rituximab as monotherapy or in combination with other treatments for SS-related vasculitic neuropathies (multiple mononeuropathy, sensorimotor neuropathy) have been reported by other centers as well.[46,47] One group also observed improvement with this therapy in two patients with cryoglobulinemic cerebral vasculitis.[48]

In another series from France, treatment with cyclophosphamide resulted in either partial recovery or stabilization of multiple mononeuropathy in all treated patients ($N = 8$).[49] Several authors have also agreed that the prompt initiation of aggressive immunosuppressive therapy combined with the timely use of corticosteroids is essential in the management of vasculitic neuropathy to prevent permanent axonal degeneration.[22,24,50] Cyclophosphamide therapy was also successfully used to reverse one case of suspected vasculitis-related cardiomyopathy.[35]

Although not commonly used to treat vasculitic neuropathies, intravenous immunoglobulin has been reportedly used in several treatment refractory cases, including patients in whom immunosuppressive therapies either failed or were contraindicated.[24,51]

Conclusions

Several vasculitic features can be seen in SS patients, predominantly affecting the skin and peripheral nervous system. Vasculitis in SS patients correlates with a more severe phenotype and poorer outcome, especially when associated with cryoglobulinemia. Such patients need to be carefully monitored and promptly treated with immunosuppressive therapy to alleviate severe disease manifestations and to prevent permanent end-organ damage.

References

1. Ramos-Casals M, Brito-Zeron P, Siso-Almirall A, Bosch X. Primary Sjögren syndrome. *BMJ*. 2012;344:e3821.
2. Jennette JC, Falk RJ, Bacon PA, Basu N, Cid MC, Ferrario F, Flores-Suarez LF, Gross WL, Guillevin L, Hagen EC, Hoffman GS, Jayne DR, Kallenberg CG, Lamprecht P, Langford CA, Luqmani RA, Mahr AD, Matteson EL, Merkel PA, Ozen S, Pusey CD, Rasmussen N, Rees AJ, Scott DG, Specks U, Stone JH, Takahashi K, Watts RA. 2012 revised International Chapel Hill consensus conference nomenclature of vasculitides. *Arthritis Rheum*. 2013;65(1):1–11.
3. Doyle MK. Vasculitis associated with connective tissue disorders. *Curr Rheumatol Rep*. 2006;8(4):312–316.
4. Ramos-Casals M, Brito-Zerón P, Seror R, Bootsma H, Bowman SJ, Dörner T, Gottenberg JE, Mariette X, Theander E, Bombardieri S, De Vita S, Mandl T, Ng WF, Kruize A, Tzioufas A, Vitali C, EULAR Sjögren Syndrome Task Force. Characterization of systemic disease in primary Sjögren's syndrome: EULAR-SS Task Force recommendations for articular, cutaneous, pulmonary and renal involvements. *Rheumatol*. 2015; 54(12):2230–2238.
5. Ramos-Casals M, Solans R, Rosas J, Camps MT, Gil A, Del Pino-Montes J, Calvo-Alen J, Jiménez-Alonso J, Micó ML, Beltrán J, Belenguer R, Pallarés L, GEMESS Study Group. Primary Sjögren syndrome in Spain: clinical and immunologic expression in 1010 patients. *Medicine (Baltim)*. July 2008;87(4):210–219.
6. Garcia-Carrasco M, Ramos-Casals M, Rosas J, Pallares L, Calvo-Alen J, Cervera R, Font J, Ingelmo M. Primary Sjögren syndrome: clinical and immunologic disease patterns in a cohort of 400 patients. *Medicine (Baltim)*. July 2002;81(4):270–280.
7. Ramos-Casals M, Anaya JM, García-Carrasco M, Rosas J, Bové A, Claver G, Diaz LA, Herrero C, Font J. Cutaneous vasculitis in primary Sjögren syndrome: classification and clinical significance of 52 patients. *Medicine (Baltim)*. March 2004;83(2):96–106.
8. Molina R, Provost TT, Alexander EL. Two histopathologic prototypes of inflammatory vascular disease in Sjögren's syndrome: differential association with seroactivity to rheumatoid factor and antibodies to Ro (SS-A) and with hypocomplementemia. *Arthritis Rheum*. November 1985;28(11):1251–1258.
9. Wisnieski JJ. Urticarial vasculitis. *Curr Opin Rheumatol*. January 2000;12(1):24–31.
10. Tsokos M, Lazarou SA, Moutsopoulos HM. Vasculitis in primary Sjögren's syndrome. Histologic classification and clinical presentation. *Am J Clin Pathol*. July 1987;88(1): 26–31.
11. Brito-Zerón P, Ramos-Casals M, Bove A, Sentis J, Font J. Predicting adverse outcomes in primary Sjögren's syndrome: identification of prognostic factors. *Rheumatol*. August 2007;46(8):1359–1362.
12. Gower RG, Sams Jr WM, Thorne EG, Kohler PF, Claman HN. Leukocytoclastic vasculitis: Sequential appearance of immunoreactants and cellular changes in serial biopsies. *J Investig Dermatol*. November 1977;69(5):477–484.

13. Markusse HM, Schoonbrood M, Oudkerk M, Henzen-Logmans SC. Leucocytoclastic vasculitis as presenting feature of primary Sjögren's syndrome. *Clin Rheumatol.* June 1994;13(2):269−272.

14. Cardoso R, Goncalo M, Tellechea O, Maia R, Borges C, Silva JA, Figueiredo A. Livedoid vasculopathy and hypercoagulability in a patient with primary Sjögren's syndrome. *Int J Dermatol.* April 2007;46(4):431−434.

15. Horvath IF, Szanto A, Papp G, Zeher M. Clinical course, prognosis, and cause of death in primary Sjögren's syndrome. *J Immunol Res.* 2014;2014:647507.

16. Akpek EK, Mathews P, Hahn S, Hessen M, Kim J, Grader-Beck T, Birnbaum J, Baer AN. Ocular and systemic morbidity in a longitudinal cohort of Sjögren's syndrome. *Ophthalmology.* January 2015;122(1):56−61.

17. Quartuccio L, Isola M, Baldini C, Priori R, Bartoloni E, Carubbi F, Gregoraci G, Gandolfo S, Salvin S, Luciano N, Minniti A, Alunno A, Giacomelli R, Gerli R, Valesini G, Bombardieri S, De Vita S. Clinical and biological differences between cryoglobulinaemic and hypergammaglobulinaemic purpura in primary Sjögren's syndrome: results of a large multicenter study. *Scand J Rheumatol.* 2015;44(1):36−41.

18. Sugai S, Shimizu S, Tachibana J, Sawada M, Yoshioka R, Hirose Y, Takiguchi T, Konda S, Murayama T. Hypergammaglobulinemic purpura in patients with Sjögren's syndrome: a report of nine cases and a review of the Japanese literature. *Jpn J Med.* 1989;28(2):148−155.

19. Alexander E, Provost TT. Sjögren's syndrome. Association of cutaneous vasculitis with central nervous system disease. *Arch Dermatol.* June 1987;123(6):801−810.

20. Quartuccio L, Isola M, Corazza L, Maset M, Monti G, Gabrielli A, Tzioufas AG, Ferri C, Ferraccioli G, Ramos-Casals M, Voulgarelis M, Lenzi M, Mascia MT, Sansonno D, Cacoub P, Tomsic M, Tavoni A, Pietrogrande M, Zignego AL, Scarpato S, Pioltelli P, Steinfeld S, Lamprecht P, Galli M, Bombardieri S, De Vita S. Performance of the preliminary classification criteria for cryoglobulinaemic vasculitis and clinical manifestations in hepatitis C virus-unrelated cryoglobulinaemic vasculitis. *Clin Exp Rheumatol.* 2012;30(1 Suppl. 70):S48−S52.

21. Pavlakis PP, Alexopoulos H, Kosmidis ML, Stamboulis E, Routsias JG, Tzartos SJ, Tzioufas AG, Moutsopoulos HM, Dalakas MC. Peripheral neuropathies in Sjögren syndrome: a new reappraisal. *J Neurol Neurosurg Psychiatry.* July 2011;82(7):798−802.

22. Pavlakis PP, Alexopoulos H, Kosmidis ML, Mamali I, Moutsopoulos HM, Tzioufas AG, Dalakas MC. Peripheral neuropathies in Sjögren's syndrome: a critical update on clinical features and pathogenetic mechanisms. *J Autoimmun.* August 2012;39(1−2):27−33.

23. Grant IA, Hunder GG, Homburger HA, Dyck PJ. Peripheral neuropathy associated with sicca complex. *Neurology.* April 1997;48(4):855−862.

24. Terrier B, Lacroix C, Guillevin L, Hatron PY, Dhote R, Maillot F, Diot E, Sarrot-Reynauld F, Sordet C, Dubourg O, Meyer L, Mariette X, Gottenberg JE, Club Rhumatismes et Inflammation. Diagnostic and prognostic relevance of neuromuscular biopsy in primary Sjögren's syndrome-related neuropathy. *Arthritis Rheum.* December 15, 2007;57(8):1520−1529.

25. Alexander EL. Neurologic disease in Sjögren's syndrome: mononuclear inflammatory vasculopathy affecting central/peripheral nervous system and muscle. A clinical review and update of immunopathogenesis. *Rheum Dis Clin N Am.* November 1993;19(4):869−908.

26. Alexander EL, Provost TT, Stevens MB, Alexander GE. Neurologic complications of primary Sjögren's syndrome. *Medicine (Baltim).* July 1982;61(4):247−257.

27. Mori K, Iijima M, Koike H, Hattori N, Tanaka F, Watanabe H, Katsuno M, Fujita A, Aiba I, Ogata A, Saito T, Asakura K, Yoshida M, Hirayama M, Sobue G. The wide spectrum of clinical manifestations in Sjögren's syndrome-associated neuropathy. *Brain*. November 2005;128(Pt 11):2518−2534.

28. Mellgren SI, Conn DL, Stevens JC, Dyck PJ. Peripheral neuropathy in primary Sjögren's syndrome. *Neurol*. March 1989;39(3):390−394.

29. Collins MP, Mendell JR, Periquet MI, Sahenk Z, Amato AA, Gronseth GS, Barohn RJ, Jackson CE, Kissel JT. Superficial peroneal nerve/peroneus brevis muscle biopsy in vasculitic neuropathy. *Neurol*. September 12, 2000;55(5):636−643.

30. Hasiloglu ZI, Albayram S, Tasmali K, Erer B, Selcuk H, Islak C. A case of primary Sjögren's syndrome presenting primarily with central nervous system vasculitic involvement. *Rheumatol Int*. March 2012;32(3):805−807.

31. Berman JL, Kashii S, Trachtman MS, Burde RM. Optic neuropathy and central nervous system disease secondary to Sjögren's syndrome in a child. *Ophthalmol*. December 1990;97(12):1606−1609.

32. François H, Mariette X. Renal involvement in primary Sjögren's syndrome. *Nat Rev Nephrol*. February 2016;12(2):82−93.

33. Goules AV, Tatouli IP, Moutsopoulos HM, Tzioufas AG. Clinically significant renal involvement in primary Sjögren's syndrome: clinical presentation and outcome. *Arthritis Rheum*. November 2013;65(11):2945−2953.

34. Jasiek M, Karras A, Le Guern V, Krastinova E, Mesbah R, Faguer S, Jourde-Chiche N, Fauchais AL, Chiche L, Dernis E, Moulis G, Fraison JB, Lazaro E, Jullien P, Hachulla E, Le Quellec A, Rémy P, Hummel A, Costedoat-Chalumeau N, Ronco P, Vanhille P, Meas-Yedid V, Cordonnier C, Ferlicot S, Daniel L, Seror R, Mariette X, Thervet E, François H, Terrier B. A multicentre study of 95 biopsy-proven cases of renal disease in primary Sjögren's syndrome. *Rheumatol*. March, 2017;56(3):362−370.

35. Golan TD, Keren D, Elias N, Naschitz JE, Toubi E, Misselevich I, Yeshurun D. Severe reversible cardiomyopathy associated with systemic vasculitis in primary Sjögren's syndrome. *Lupus*. 1997;6(6):505−508.

36. Scofield RH. Vasculitis in Sjögren's syndrome. *Curr Rheumatol Rep*. December 2011; 13(6):482−488.

37. Alexander EL, Craft C, Dorsch C, Moser RL, Provost TT, Alexander GE. Necrotizing arteritis and spinal subarachnoid hemorrhage in Sjögren's syndrome. *Ann Neurol*. June 1982;11(6):632−635.

38. Lahoz Rallo C, Arribas Lopez JR, Arnalich Fernandez F, Monereo Alonso A, Llanos Chavarri MC, Camacho Siles J. Necrotizing vasculitis of the panarteritis nodosa type in a long-course primary Sjögren's syndrome. *An Med Interna*. October 1990;7(10): 528−530 [Article in Spanish)].

39. Sato K, Miyasaka N, Nishioka K, Yamaoka K, Okuda M, Nishido T, Uchima H. Primary Sjögren's syndrome associated with systemic necrotizing vasculitis: a fatal case [letter]. *Arthritis Rheum*. June 1987;30(6):717−718.

40. Alexander EL, Arnett FC, Provost TT, Stevens MB. Sjögren's syndrome: association of anti-Ro(SS-A) antibodies with vasculitis, hematologic abnormalities, and serologic hyperreactivity. *Ann Intern Med*. February 1983;98(2):155−159.

41. Guellec D, Cornec-Le Gall E, Groh M, Hachulla E, Karras A, Charles P, Dunogué B, Abad S, Alvarez F, Gérard F, Devauchelle-Pensec V, Pers JO10, Puéchal X, Guillevin L, Saraux A, Cornec D. CRI (Club Rhumatismes et Inflammation) and the French Vasculitis Study Group. ANCA-associated vasculitis in patients with primary

Sjögren's syndrome: detailed analysis of 7 new cases and systematic literature review. *Autoimmun Rev.* August 2015;14(8):742–750.

42. Magro CM, Crowson AN. A clinical and histologic study of 37 cases of immunoglobulin A-associated vasculitis. *Am J Dermatopathol.* June 1999;21(3):234–240.

43. Tsai TC, Chen CY, Lin WT, Lee WJ. Chen HC Sjögren's syndrome complicated with IgA nephropathy and leukocytoclastic vasculitis. *Ren Fail.* 2008;30(7):755–758.

44. Seror R, Ravaud P, Bowman SJ, Baron G, Tzioufas A, Theander E, Gottenberg JE, Bootsma H, Mariette X, Vitali C, EULAR Sjögren's Task Force. EULAR Sjögren's syndrome disease activity index: development of a consensus systemic disease activity index for primary Sjögren's syndrome. *Ann Rheum Dis.* June 2010;69(6):1103–1109.

45. Van Woerkom JM, Kruize AA, Geenen R, van Roon EN, Goldschmeding R, Verstappen SM, van Roon JA, Bijlsma JW. Safety and efficacy of leflunomide in primary Sjögren's syndrome: a phase II pilot study. *Ann Rheum Dis.* August 2007;66(8):1026–1032.

46. Voulgarelis M, Giannouli S, Tzioufas AG, Moutsopoulos HM. Long term remission of Sjögren's syndrome associated aggressive B cell non-Hodgkin's lymphomas following combined B cell depletion therapy and CHOP (cyclophosphamide, doxorubicin, vincristine, prednisone). *Ann Rheum Dis.* August 2006;65(8):1033–1037.

47. Mekinian A, Ravaud P, Hatron PY, Larroche C, Leone J, Gombert B, Hamidou M, Cantagrel A, Marcelli C, Rist S, Breban M, Launay D, Fain O, Gottenberg JE, Mariette X. Efficacy of rituximab in primary Sjögren's syndrome with peripheral nervous system involvement: results from the AIR registry. *Ann Rheum Dis.* January 2012;71(1):84–87.

48. Lioger B, Ferreira-Maldent N, Cottier JP, Debiais S, Gyan E, Maillot F. Rituximab for Sjögren syndrome-associated type II mixed cryoglobulinemic cerebral vasculitis. *Neurol Neuroimmunol Neuroinflamm.* July, 2016;3(4):e253.

49. Delalande S, de Seze J, Fauchais AL, Hachulla E, Stojkovic T, Ferriby D, Dubucquoi S, Pruvo JP, Vermersch P, Hatron PY. Neurologic manifestations in primary Sjögren syndrome: a study of 82 patients. *Medicine (Baltim).* September 2004;83(5):280–291.

50. Schaublin GA, Michet Jr CJ, Dyck PJ, Burns TM. An update on the classification and treatment of vasculitic neuropathy. *Lancet Neurol.* December 2005;4(12):853–865.

51. Levy Y, Uziel Y, Zandman GG, Amital H, Sherer Y, Langevitz P, Goldman B, Shoenfeld Y. Intravenous immunoglobulins in peripheral neuropathy associated with vasculitis. *Ann Rheum Dis.* December 2003;62(12):1221–1223.

Lymphoproliferative disease in Sjögren's syndrome

Alan N. Baer, MD[1], Richard F. Ambinder, MD, PhD[2]

[1]*Professor of Medicine, Division of Rheumatology, Department of Medicine, Johns Hopkins University School of Medicine, Baltimore, MD, United States;* [2]*Professor of Oncology, Department of Oncology, Johns Hopkins University School of Medicine, Baltimore, MD, United States*

Introduction

An association between lymphoma and Sjögren's syndrome (SS) was first recognized in 1964, when Talal and Bunim[1] described its occurrence among 4 of 58 SS patients in a study at the National Institutes of Health. An increased risk of lymphoma in SS has since been a consistent observation in multiple studies, and the risk is higher in SS than in any other autoimmune disease. An increased risk of multiple myeloma in SS has also been documented. The development of lymphoma in SS serves as a prime model of malignant transformation following sustained lymphoproliferation in an autoimmune disease. In this chapter the epidemiology, pathogenesis, risk factors, and management of lymphoma in SS are reviewed, with an emphasis on indolent lymphoma of the salivary glands.

Epidemiology

The risk of lymphoma was first estimated to be 44-fold higher in SS patients than in the general population in 136 women studied at the National Institutes of Health.[2] Subsequent hospital- and population-based studies have reestimated this risk with less biased cohorts, although the focus has been on non-Hodgkin lymphoma (NHL). In hospital-based cohorts, the standardized incidence ratios (SIRs) for NHL have ranged from 13.0 to 44.4.[2–6] A pooled estimate of this risk in a 2014 meta-analysis was 18.9 (95% confidence interval [CI], 11.68–26.12).[7] The risk in population-based studies has been lower, with an SIR range of 7.08–48.10[8–12] and a 2014 pooled estimate of 9.68 (95% CI, 4.98–14.38).[7]

Among 13 hospital-based SS patient cohorts, the median prevalence of NHL was 4.5% (range, 2.2%–11.0%).[4–6,11,13–21] The risk and prevalence of NHL increase progressively with disease duration.[11,17,22] In a 2015 systematic review of seven studies, the prevalence of lymphoproliferative disease following diagnosis was 4% during the first 5 years, 10% at 15 years, and 18% at 20 years.[23]

Sjögren's Syndrome. https://doi.org/10.1016/B978-0-323-67534-5.00008-9

SS is the autoimmune disease with the highest risk of lymphoma. Certain other autoimmune diseases, including systemic lupus erythematosus (SLE), rheumatoid arthritis (RA), and celiac disease, also have an increased risk, but substantially less than is true for SS.[24] In a meta-analysis, the NHL SIR was 18.8 (95% CI, 9.5–37.3) for SS, 7.4 (95% CI, 3.3–17.0) for SLE, and 3.9 (95% CI, 2.5–5.9) for RA.[25] Similarly, the risk of NHL for 16 self-reported autoimmune conditions was determined by Ekstrom Smedby et al.[26] in an analysis of 12 case-control studies with a total of 29,423 participants. The pooled relative risk was highest for SS (6.56; 95% CI, 3.10–13.9) but was also significant for hemolytic anemia (2.57; 95% CI, 1.27–5.21) and SLE (2.69; 95% CI, 1.68–4.30).

Lymphoma in secondary Sjögren's syndrome

The risk of lymphoma in secondary SS (i.e., occurring in association with another systemic rheumatic disease, such as RA, SLE, scleroderma, or myositis) is also increased relative to the general population, but not clearly different than that for primary SS. In their pooled analysis, Ekstrom Smedby et al.[26] noted a higher pooled relative risk of NHL among patients with secondary SS (9.56; 95% CI, 2.90–31.6) than those with primary SS (4.75; 95% CI, 1.79–12.60). However, the risk in secondary SS, relative to primary SS, was lower in two other population-based case-control studies.[12,27]

Lymphoma subtypes

The increased risk of NHL in SS is most pronounced for marginal zone B-cell lymphoma and diffuse large B-cell lymphoma (DLBCL). In the study of Ekstrom Smedby et al.,[26] SS was associated with a 31-fold increased risk of marginal zone B-cell lymphoma and 8.9-fold increased risk of DLBCL. Most striking was the 996-fold increased risk of parotid gland marginal zone lymphoma in SS patients. Similar findings were observed in a population-based case-control study of hematopoietic malignancies using SEER-Medicare data, in which the risk of salivary gland marginal zone lymphoma among SS patients was increased 71-fold.[28] The unique link between SS and salivary gland marginal zone B-cell lymphoma, observed in these studies and in most academic cohorts, supports a role for chronic inflammation and/or antigenic stimulation as the important predisposing factors for lymphomagenesis in SS.[24]

Marginal zone lymphoma, both extranodal involving mucosa-associated lymphoid tissue (MALT) and nodal forms, predominates in most, but not all, cohorts of SS-associated lymphomas.[13–15,22,29,30] The preponderance of DLBCL in some cohorts could relate to the fact that it is the most prevalent form of lymphoma and may arise from transformation of MALT lymphoma.[11,18,25]

SS patients with lymphoma have a higher rate of mortality than those without it[17,22] but this has not generally translated to an overall increase in SS mortality rates.[31–33]

Thus lymphomagenesis in SS is a potentially lethal complication; early identification of more aggressive forms of lymphoma in SS may serve to improve patient outcomes.

Multiple myeloma

Monoclonal proteins have a higher prevalence in SS patients than in the general population,[34] and thus an increased risk of multiple myeloma and Waldenström macroglobulinemia might also be expected. In a study of a large health insurance database, the SIR of multiple myeloma among Taiwanese SS patients was 6.1 (95% CI, 2.0−14.2), which is equivalent to the SIR of 7.1 (95% CI, 4.3−10.3) for NHL.[9] Similarly, an increased risk of myeloma was observed in a study of a tertiary-care-center cohort in China (SIR 37.9; 95% CI, 4.6−136.7)[8] and in a study of 1300 consecutive Spanish SS patients in the GEAS-SS study group (SIR 36.17; 95% CI, 25.44−51.43).[13] Among 352 SS patients, 26 patients with monoclonal gammopathy had an increased risk (odds ratio, 7.5) of malignant hematologic disease, including 4 patients who developed lymphoma and 6 patients who developed myeloma, after a median follow-up of 6.3 years.[34]

Risk factors and prediction models

A number of clinical, laboratory, imaging, and pathologic features have been identified as risk factors for lymphoma development among SS patients (Table 8.1).[23] Some are present at the time of disease diagnosis or cohort entry, whereas others may appear during longitudinal follow-up. The most robust are those that relate to salivary glandular lymphoproliferation (persistent salivary gland enlargement, high focus score), extraglandular lymphoproliferation (splenomegaly, lymphadenopathy), clonal B-cell expansion (monoclonal proteins), and cryoglobulinemic vasculitis (palpable purpura, leg ulcers, serum cryoglobulins, low C4 levels). The presence of an IgM-κ monoclonal protein has a particularly strong association with lymphoma.[15,22,35] These observations have informed our knowledge relating to the pathogenesis of lymphoma in SS, as detailed below.

The 2011 report by Theander et al. that the presence of germinal center−like structures in diagnostic minor salivary gland biopsies predicted lymphoma development sparked a reconsideration of the potential indications for the performance of these biopsies.[36,37] However, this finding has not been universally confirmed and thus may not be sufficient to justify a labial minor salivary gland in every patient being evaluated for SS.[38]

The risk of NHL increases in proportion to the number of risk factors.[17,39,40] Clinical prediction models have been described by Baldini et al.[14] (combining salivary gland enlargement, low C4 levels, and disease duration) and Fragkioudaki et al.[41] (combining Raynaud phenomenon, lymphadenopathy, monoclonal gammopathy, rheumatoid factor positivity, C4 hypocomplementemia, and anti-SSA/SSB positivity).

Table 8.1 Risk factors for lymphoma in Sjögren's syndrome.

Clinical	Laboratory	Radiologic	Pathologic	Novel biomarkers
Parotid swelling[2,14,17,29,33,41,103]	Low C4 levels[11,13,14,17,21,29,33,39,41]	Abnormal salivary gland scintigraphy[104]	High focus score (>1.6–3.0) in labial gland biopsy[41,105]	Fms-like tyrosine kinase 3 ligand[106]
Palpable purpura[11,17,21,29,33,41]	Low C3 levels[11,13,14,17]		Germinal center–like structures in diagnostic biopsies[36,38,107]	CXCL13 and CCL11 serum levels[108]
Lymphadenopathy[2,40,41,103]	Cryoglobulins[13,19–21,29,35,39–41]			Low miR200b-5p levels in minor salivary glands[109]
Splenomegaly[2,29,40]	Lymphocytopenia[17,29]			TNFAIP3 mutation[60]
Radiation treatment for parotid swelling[2]	CD4 lymphocytopenia[11]			
Higher ESSDAI score[13,29]	Leukopenia[17]			
Peripheral neuropathy[41]	Neutropenia[40]			
Skin ulcers[20,103]	Rheumatoid factor[29,41]			
Younger onset SS[2,12]	IgM-κ monoclonal protein[35,110]			
Disease duration[14]	Monoclonal gammopathy[13,29,41,110]			
Raynaud phenomenon[41]	Hypergammaglobulinemia[17]			
	Anti-SSA and/or SSB antibodies[29,39,41]			
	Centromere antibodies[43,44]			
	Anemia[13,17]			
	β_2-Microglobulin[6]			

ESSDAI, *European League Against Rheumatism Sjögren's Syndrome Disease Activity Index*; SS, *Sjögren's syndrome.*

Lymphoma is not restricted to SS patients with anti-SSA/Ro antibodies, although these antibodies do confer increased risk.[23,29,39,41,42] Importantly, SS patients with anti-centromere antibodies, approximately half of whom also have anti-SSA/Ro antibodies, have an increased lymphoma risk as well.[43—45]

Prior treatments for SS, including radiation treatment and chemotherapy, may also impact lymphoma risk, but analysis of this is confounded by indication. Kassan et al.[2] observed an increased risk of NHL among those who received radiation treatment for persistent parotid gland enlargement, but these patients might have already had indolent lymphoma as the cause. These investigators also noted an effect of prior drug treatment, but their study was conducted in an era when cytotoxic agents were used more commonly.[2] This effect was not observed in a more modern SS cohort,[29] but has been observed for RA cohorts.[25]

Pathology and pathogenesis

The evolution of salivary gland lymphoproliferation to MALT lymphoma has been described in pathologic studies.[46—48] The classic pathologic lesion in the SS major salivary gland is lymphoepithelial sialadenitis (LESA), also known as benign lymphoepithelial lesion or myoepithelial sialadenitis; it is characterized by a dense periductal lymphoid infiltrate with histologic and functional features of secondary lymphoid organs (Fig. 8.1). Centrally located and crescent-shaped follicles are surrounded by a broad zone of lymphocytes, the outer edge constituting the marginal zone. The lymphocytes within the marginal zone are monocytoid B cells, characterized as "centrocyte-like" because of their resemblance to follicular center cells. Typically, they are small- to medium-sized lymphocytes with a pale, irregular, centrally located nucleus and abundant clear cytoplasm.[48] These marginal zone lymphocytes focally invade the ductal epithelium, resulting in epithelial hyperplasia and disorganization. The ductal structure may be obliterated, leaving an "island" of epithelial cells in the dense lymphoid infiltrate (the so-called epimyoepithelial island). In more advanced cases of LESA, there is effacement of the salivary gland architecture by a dense lymphoid infiltrate containing myoepithelial islands infiltrated by lymphocytes. Immunohistochemical staining demonstrates a polytypic infiltrate with a predominance of B cells. With evolution to MALT lymphoma, there is expansion of the marginal zone centrocyte-like B-cell population, leading to halos around epimyoepithelial islands and linkage of adjacent islands by broad interconnecting strands. There may be displacement of adjacent follicles and infiltration of the follicle by a centrocyte-like cell infiltrate ("follicular colonization"). The centrocyte-like B-cell population shows light-chain restriction, indicative of monoclonal cell expansion, in contrast to the polytypic follicular centers and mantle zone. With the development of high-grade MALT lymphoma, the salivary gland is effaced by an infiltrate of monomorphic malignant B cells, with blastlike features.

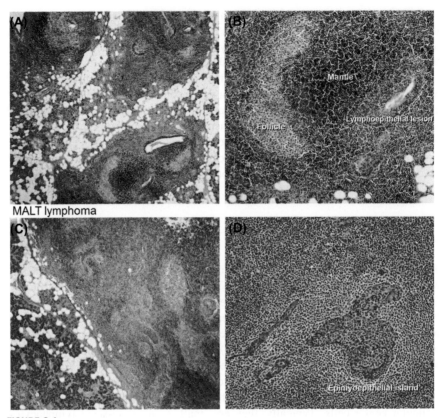

FIGURE 8.1

Lymphoepithelial sialadenitis (LESA) and mucosa-associated lymphoid tissue (MALT) lymphoma of the parotid gland. Parotid gland tissue (A,B) from a Sjögren's syndrome patient with LESA and (C,D) from a different patient with a marginal zone B-cell lymphoma (MALT subtype). In (A) (LESA), there are multiple discrete periductal lymphoid infiltrates with structural features akin to secondary lymphoid organs. A high-power image of one such infiltrate in (B) shows a crescent-shaped lymphoid follicle surrounded by a mantle zone. An early lymphoepithelial lesion is present, arising from the outer margin of the mantle (marginal zone). There is extensive lymphocytic infiltration of the ductal epithelium, associated with ductal epithelial hyperplasia and near occlusion of the ductal lumen. In (C) (MALT lymphoma), there is effacement of the glandular architecture by a dense lymphoid infiltrate. (D) Halos of lighter staining lymphocytes surround epimyoepithelial islands, and these form broad interconnecting strands.

Monoclonality of the B-cell infiltrate does not by itself define the presence of MALT lymphoma.[47,49] The differentiation of a low-grade MALT lymphoma from LESA rests on a number of histopathologic and immunohistochemical findings. Features pointing to lymphoma include soft tissue and perineural invasion, sheets of plasma cells with or without Dutcher bodies, lymph node involvement, and aberrant expression of CD43 by the monoclonal B-cell population.

Current concepts regarding the molecular pathogenesis of lymphoma in SS have been reviewed elsewhere.[24,50,51] These have largely evolved from the study of MALT lymphoma, given the predilection of this neoplasm to arise in the salivary glands of SS patients where there is a persistent lymphocytic infiltration driven by chronic antigenic stimulation. This extranodal lymphoproliferation is characterized by the mono- or oligoclonal expansion of highly selected B-cell populations with receptors exhibiting strong rheumatoid factor activity,[52] indicative of their need for continued antigenic stimulation to proliferate. These B-cell clones may disseminate to distant nodal and extranodal sites of lymphoproliferation or new ones may emerge, depending on the local antigenic milieu.[52–54] With time, accrual of oncogenic events ultimately results in the emergence of one dominant, malignant clone that proliferates without the need for antigenic stimulation.

As noted earlier, the antigen receptor of the malignant B cell in SS-related MALT lymphoma is distinguished by its ability to bind IgG with high affinity (i.e., rheumatoid factor activity).[55,56] This is a feature not shared typically by other forms of lymphoma. These B cells with rheumatoid factor B-cell receptors and toll-like receptors (TLR)-7 are particularly suited for dual-ligand stimulation by immune complexes derived from locally produced IgG autoantibodies directed against RNA-associated autoantigens, such as SSA/Ro52, SSA/Ro60, and SSB/La.[57] Serum levels of B-cell activating factor (BAFF) correlate with SS disease activity and are higher in SS patients with lymphoma; this cytokine is thus thought to drive the proliferation of the autoreactive B cells in the salivary glands.[58]

In the context of chronic antigenic stimulation, autoreactive B cells at the disease site may be prone to malignant transformation by specific oncogenic mutations. In general, translocations involving the *MALT1* gene are involved in the pathogenesis of MALT lymphoma; in SS, they are increased in frequency in those patients with gastric MALT but not MALT involving other extranodal sites, including the salivary glands.[51,59] The A20 protein, encoded by the gene *TNFAIP3*, suppresses nuclear factor (NF)-κB activation but is dysfunctional in the majority of SS patients with lymphoma as a result of germline and somatic mutations; this genetic variation may predispose to lymphomagenesis, given the established role of excessive NF-κB activation in this process.[60]

The pathogenesis of DLBCL in SS is less well studied. Some cases may represent transformation from indolent lymphomas. However, DLBCL is the most common lymphoma subtype in patients with RA,[61] and pathogenetic pathways unique to this lymphoma subtype could also apply to a subset of SS patients.

Clinical presentation

In the majority of patients, lymphoma develops months to years after the diagnosis of SS, the duration reaching as long as 30 years.[22] However, lymphoma can precede the diagnosis of SS in up to 24% of subjects[15,29] and salivary gland lymphoma may provide the first clue of underlying SS.[18,30] Similarly, "occult" MALT lymphoma can be first recognized at the time of initial diagnostic evaluation for SS, in either the minor salivary biopsy[62] or the parotid gland biopsy.[63] The median age of lymphoma diagnosis ranges from 51 to 63 years.[14–17,29,30] The majority of affected patients are women, as is true for SS in general. SS patients with MALT lymphoma present at a significantly younger age than those with DLBCL.[16]

The evolution of certain systemic and glandular manifestations should prompt concern for the presence of an underlying lymphoma, including recurrent fever, purpura, sensorimotor peripheral neuropathy, glomerulonephritis, lymphadenopathy, nodular pulmonary infiltrates, asymmetric glandular enlargement, and intraglandular palpable mass.[15–17,64,65] At the time of lymphoma diagnosis, SS patients more commonly have low C4 levels, serum cryoglobulins, IgM-κ monoclonal proteins, high rheumatoid factor activity, and lymphopenia.[15,22] Anderson and Talal[64] described relatively rapid declines in serum IgM and rheumatoid factor concentrations as markers of imminent or underlying lymphoma, but this was likely a paraneoplastic manifestation and not confirmed in subsequent studies.[66]

Most lymphomas in SS originate in the head and neck and thus present as one or more glandular masses and/or cervical lymphadenopathy.[18] However, they may arise in any lymph node group, within the lacrimal and salivary glands, and at any other extranodal site, including the stomach, nasopharynx, skin, spleen, and lung. The vast majority of patients have excellent functional capacity (as measured by standard oncology performance status) at the time of NHL diagnosis.[16,22] The clinical presentation of lymphoma depends on its subtype and primary location. Those with DLBCL and other aggressive forms present as they would in patients unaffected by SS with a rapidly expanding mass (including in the parotid gland), lymphadenopathy, fever, weight loss, and night sweats.[11,15,17] Patients with MALT lymphoma typically lack B symptoms and have normal serum lactate dehydrogenase and β_2-microglobulin levels. Indolent lymphoma of the salivary glands, usually MALT in subtype, typically presents with a unilateral intraglandular mass, usually of the parotid gland or diffuse glandular swelling. Bilateral glandular swelling can be observed, including patients presenting with diffuse cystic disease of the glands from advanced sialadenitis (Fig. 8.2).[67] The majority have localized (stage IE) or regional disease (stage IIE, with involvement of regional nodes) (Table 8.2).[16,22] There may be synchronous or metachronous involvement of multiple mucosal sites or nonmucosal sites, such as bone marrow, spleen, or liver.[16,22,68,69] DLBCL may arise in the context of a preexisting indolent lymphoma.[22]

Imaging

Computed tomography (CT) and magnetic resonance (MR) imaging of salivary glands affected by lymphoma shows single or multiple soft tissue nodules, generally

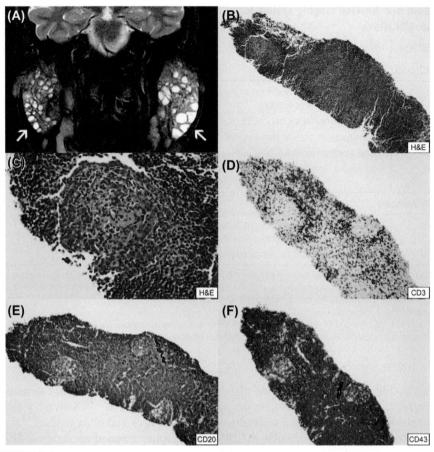

FIGURE 8.2

Diagnosis of mucosa-associated lymphoid tissue lymphoma of parotid glands using core needle biopsy. (A, magnetic resonance T2-fat-suppressed image, coronal view) This patient with Sjögren's syndrome had progressive enlargement of both parotid glands, attributed in part to the presence of multiple cysts (*arrows*). Core needle biopsy showed (B) a dense lymphoid infiltrate with loss of the acinar architecture and (C) lymphoepithelial lesions. The lymphoid infiltrate was composed of both T cells (CD3 stain, D) and B cells (CD20 stain, E), but the B cells were clearly predominant. CD43, a cell surface receptor normally present on T cells, was aberrantly expressed by the malignant B-cell clone (CD43 stain, F). Flow cytometry demonstrated the presence of a monoclonal B-cell population. *H&E*, hematoxylin-eosin.

well demarcated, or diffuse enlargement with or without the presence of intratumoral cysts.[18,70,71] Intraglandular masses have low intensity on T1-weighted MR sequences and isointensity or mild hyperintensity on T2-weighted sequences.[71,72] These findings are not specific for lymphoma and can be seen in glands with

Table 8.2 Revised staging system for primary nodal lymphomas (the Lugano classification).

Stage	Involvement
Limited	
I	Involvement of one node or a group of adjacent nodes (including tonsils, Waldeyer ring, and spleen)
IE	Single extranodal lesions without nodal involvement
II	Involvement of two or more nodal groups on the same side of the diaphragm
IIE	Stage I or II by nodal extent with limited contiguous extranodal involvement
II bulky	II as above with "bulky" disease
Advanced	
III	Involvement of nodes on both sides of the diaphragm
	Involvement of nodes above the diaphragm including that of the spleen
IV	Additional noncontiguous extralymphatic involvement

Bulky disease is defined only for Hodgkin lymphoma as a single nodal mass, in contrast to multiple smaller nodes, of 10 cm or one-third or more of the transthoracic diameter at any level of thoracic vertebrae as determined by computed tomography. No definition is provided for non-Hodgkin lymphoma.
Adapted from *Cheson BD, Fisher RI, Barrington SF et al. Recommendations for initial evaluation, staging, and response assessment of Hodgkin and non-Hodgkin lymphoma: The Lugano classification.* J Clin Oncol. *2014; 32:3059–3068.*

localized lymphoid infiltration and glandular atrophy.[72] The presence of calcification or sialoliths does not exclude the presence of lymphoma.[71,73] Salivary gland lymphoma may be associated with adenopathy in the neck and other regions.[18]

Ultrasonography of glandular MALT lymphoma has a varied appearance. The glands, in general, show multiple ovoid hypoechoic lesions, typical of the appearance of sialadenitis in SS. The presence of lymphoma may be marked by a dominant hypoechoic mass (sometimes palpable), with cystic and solid components and internal septation.[74,75] There may be multiple hypoechoic nodules with increased vascularity by Doppler.[76] In other patients, an intraparotid lymph node may appear pathologic, with peripheral vascularity and loss of the fatty hilum.

[18]F-fluorodeoxyglucose (FDG) positron emission tomography (PET)/CT scanning does not have an established role in the evaluation of suspected MALT or other indolent lymphomas in SS. This technique is known to be less sensitive for the detection of indolent than high-grade NHL.[77] However, this is site specific.[78] MALT lymphoma of the head and neck region and lungs is more FDG avid than it is at other sites, such as the stomach or ocular adnexa. In SS patients with high systemic disease activity, PET/CT may show pathologic uptake in multiple sites, including salivary glands, lymph nodes, lungs, and thyroid.[79] In SS the glandular maximum standardized uptake value (SUVmax) may be higher in patients with lymphoma than in those without lymphoma;

however, the overlap of values limits the diagnostic value of the test.[79] In contrast, PET/CT has particular sensitivity for detecting MALT lymphoma of the lung.[77]

Diagnostic evaluation

Algorithms for diagnosis and staging of lymphomas in SS are discussed in the following section and summarized in Fig. 8.3. The diagnosis of lymphoma always requires a tissue biopsy, with sufficient material for histopathologic examination, including

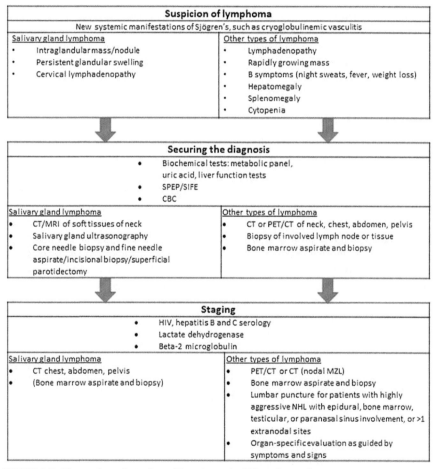

FIGURE 8.3 Diagnosis and staging of lymphoma in Sjögren's syndrome.

CBC, complete blood count; *CT*, computed tomography; *HIV*, human immunodeficiency virus; *MRI*, magnetic resonance imaging; *MZL*, marginal zone lymphoma; *NHL*, non-Hodgkin lymphoma; *PET*, positron emission tomography; *SIFE*, serum immunofixation electrophoresis; *SPEP*, serum protein electrophoresis.

immunohistochemical stains, flow cytometry, and molecular studies. Surgical biopsies remain the gold standard. However, the trend has been to secure pathologic material via needle biopsies, under ultrasound guidance for superficial structures and CT guidance for deeper structures.[80] The choice of technique depends on the resources available to the clinician and local expertise. For evaluation of salivary gland masses or diffuse enlargement, the authors have referred SS patients for ultrasound-guided core needle biopsy.[81,82] Typically, two or more core needle biopsies are obtained from suspicious masses, with one core for histopathologic examination and one for flow cytometry. Cellular material, obtained via fine-needle aspiration, is sent for cytology and also included in the flow cytometry sample. The difficulty in diagnosing marginal zone lymphoma with small tissue samples is a potential drawback.[80]

The finding of a monoclonal B-cell population on flow cytometry or molecular studies is not sufficient to establish a diagnosis of lymphoma, as such monoclonal populations are often seen in LESA.[49]

Lymphoma staging

The benefits of staging are dependent on lymphoma subtype, being much more relevant to high-grade forms. PET/CT imaging is used to stage FDG-avid nodal lymphomas but is generally not recommended for more indolent forms, which are not FDG avid, such as marginal zone lymphoma, lymphoplasmacytic lymphoma (Waldenström macroglobulinemia), and small lymphocytic lymphoma (chronic lymphocytic leukemia). Bone marrow aspiration and biopsy is also an essential component of staging, with the exception of patients with indolent MALT lymphoma (vide infra) and DLBCL (i.e., those with bone marrow involvement evident on PET/CT imaging).

Staging of extranodal MALT lymphoma can be challenging, as CT scans are not optimal for the detection of occult extranodal disease and the tumor may not be FDG avid at certain sites (see earlier discussion). Given that extranodal marginal zone lymphoma of MALT type can be disseminated at initial presentation,[69,83,84] staging generally involves CT imaging of the neck, chest, abdomen, and pelvis. Some authors also recommend a bone marrow aspiration and biopsy,[85,86] but the value of this is questionable because the detection of bone marrow involvement does not influence prognosis. For MALT lymphoma, some authors recommend esophagoduodenoscopy to evaluate for concomitant gastric involvement; if present, this might prompt treatment with antibiotics for *Helicobacter pylori* gastritis. However, this is uncommon, being found in only 1 of 18 patients with salivary gland MALT reported by Ambrosetti et al.[87] The benefits of extensive staging for MALT lymphoma (including upper gastrointestinal endoscopy and colonoscopy in all patients) have been challenged by the observation that there is no difference in progression-free survival or overall survival (OS) between patients with localized disease and those with disseminated disease.[84] In addition, the current availability of several active therapeutic agents for this lymphoma makes staging less important.

Application of the Ann Arbor staging scheme to MALT lymphoma is problematic. Originally developed for Hodgkin lymphoma, the Ann Arbor staging system was modified for NHL (the Lugano classification) and focuses on the number of tumor sites (nodal and extranodal) and their location (Table 8.2).[88] This staging system is ambiguous as to whether lymphomatous involvement of multiple salivary glands should be graded as stage IE or stage IV. There is thus a lack of consistency in the application of this staging system to MALT lymphoma,[63,89–91] making it difficult to compare study results.

Treatment of lymphoma

Treatment approaches are not only dictated by the lymphoma subtype but also influenced by considerations specific to the underlying SS, including systemic disease activity and potential morbidity of certain treatment approaches. Algorithms for the initial treatment of the three major lymphoma subtypes in SS are shown in Fig. 8.4 and discussed below.

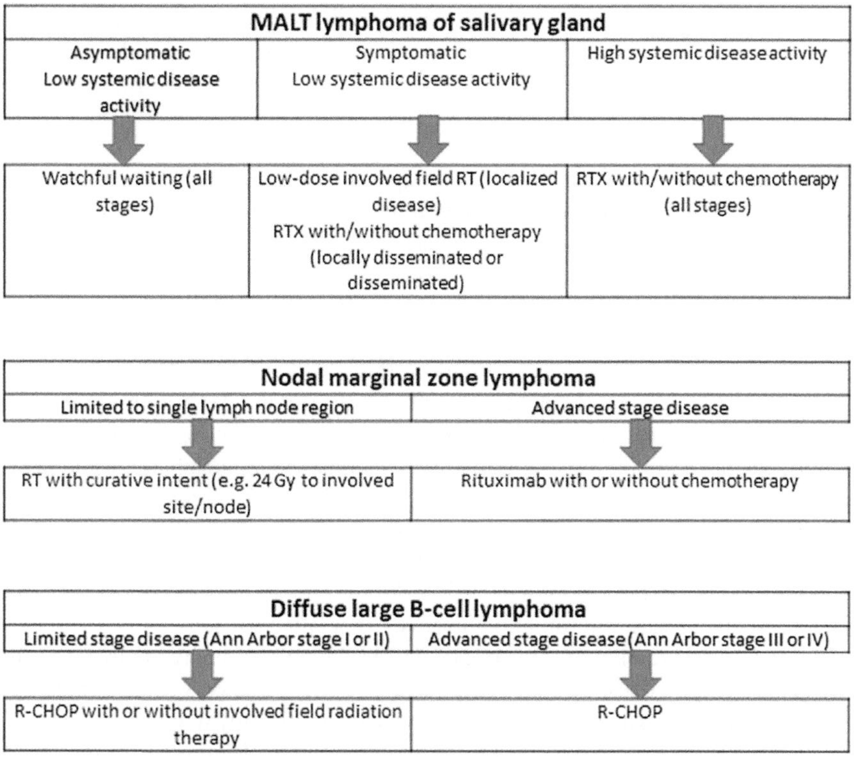

MALT lymphoma of salivary gland		
Asymptomatic Low systemic disease activity	Symptomatic Low systemic disease activity	High systemic disease activity
Watchful waiting (all stages)	Low-dose involved field RT (localized disease) RTX with/without chemotherapy (locally disseminated or disseminated)	RTX with/without chemotherapy (all stages)

Nodal marginal zone lymphoma	
Limited to single lymph node region	Advanced stage disease
RT with curative intent (e.g. 24 Gy to involved site/node)	Rituximab with or without chemotherapy

Diffuse large B-cell lymphoma	
Limited stage disease (Ann Arbor stage I or II)	Advanced stage disease (Ann Arbor stage III or IV)
R-CHOP with or without involved field radiation therapy	R-CHOP

FIGURE 8.4 Initial treatment for three most common lymphoma subtypes in Sjögren's syndrome.

MALT, mucosa-associated lymphoid tissue; *R-CHOP,* Rituxan-cyclophosphamide, doxorubicin, vincristine, and prednisone; *RT,* radiation therapy; *RTX,* rituximab.

For MALT lymphoma localized to one or more salivary glands, watchful waiting is an option if the tumor is asymptomatic or if the patient does not have active systemic disease. In two case series of MALT lymphoma occurring in SS, this approach was applied to 19 of 66 patients. In a study of 35 SS patients with MALT lymphoma, Pollard et al.[63] observed progression or recurrence of lymphoma to be significantly more frequent in those patients with high SS disease activity than in those with low disease activity at the time of lymphoma diagnosis. Features of high systemic disease activity included the presence of monoclonal gammopathy, cryoglobulins, increased rheumatoid factor, and severe extraglandular manifestations, such as arthritis, vasculitis, or internal organ involvement. Watchful waiting is also an option for those patients with severe comorbidity, of advanced age, or in whom the tumor has been surgically resected as part of the initial diagnostic evaluation (e.g., superficial parotidectomy for a salivary gland mass).

For patients with symptomatic MALT lymphoma of the salivary glands, treatment options include low-dose radiotherapy and systemic regimens. Surgical resection of lymphoma is not recommended as a standard treatment option. The use of low-dose involved-field radiotherapy (two doses of 2 Gy on consecutive days) is an option, particularly for a tumor that is <5 cm in size.[63,92,93] However, experience with this therapy is limited in SS and the risk of worsening xerostomia as a side effect has not been defined, although expected to be lower than that of standard radiotherapy.

Rituximab is a key component of systemic treatment protocols for both localized and disseminated MALT lymphoma.[22,63,94] A single cycle of rituximab (375 mg/m^2 weekly for four doses) is an appropriate initial treatment for newly diagnosed MALT lymphoma that is symptomatic, regardless of the stage.[22] There is no known survival advantage with the use of maintenance rituximab therapy, but it is recommended by some authors.[22] Rituximab maintenance therapy would be particularly appropriate if the patient had an early relapse after one initial cycle of rituximab treatment. Initial treatment with rituximab in combination with chemotherapy may be more appropriate for those with severe extraglandular disease, advanced stage involvement, or localized disease in whom a rapid response is needed (e.g., extensive pulmonary lymphoma).[22,63,91] The options for chemotherapy, each in combination with rituximab, include cyclophosphamide and prednisone; cyclophosphamide, doxorubicin, vincristine, and prednisone (CHOP); fludarabine alone or with cyclophosphamide; and chlorambucil. Clinical trials have assessed the benefits of combining rituximab with bendamustine or chlorambucil for treating MALT lymphoma.[91,95,96] Antibiotics are the initial treatment for MALT associated with microbial pathogens, especially gastric.

Relapse or progression of salivary gland MALT lymphoma may involve the salivary gland, lymph nodes, or extranodal sites.[63,87,89] It is treated with systemic regimens, generally, rituximab in combination with chemotherapy (e.g., bendamustine) or with ibrutinib (a Bruton tyrosine kinase inhibitor) alone. Ibrutinib is the only therapeutic agent specifically approved by the FDA for relapsed/refractory marginal zone lymphoma, including MALT lymphoma.[97] It is taken orally once daily and has minimal side effects in most patients.

The treatment of nodal marginal zone lymphoma typically involves chemotherapy, sometimes in combination with rituximab.[22]

Treatment of DLBCL is based on the disease stage and molecular subtype and usually involves systemic chemotherapy (usually CHOP) plus rituximab.

Prognosis

The prognosis of NHL in SS is generally favorable. In a cohort of 77 SS patients with NHL from the University of Athens (1993−2013), the overall survival (OS) and event-free survival for the entire cohort were 91% and 78%, respectively.[16] Actuarial 5-year OS for SS patients was 94% for those with MALT lymphoma, 88% for those with nodal marginal zone lymphoma, and 75% for those with DLBCL. Prognosis was worse for those with high systemic disease activity, bone marrow involvement, and unfavorable international prognostic index score.

These results, specific to patients with SS, correspond well to studies of these lymphoma subtypes in broader patient populations.[69,83,98] Interestingly, the coexistence of SS was associated with improved OS in a multicenter international study of 247 patients with salivary gland MALT lymphoma, including 84 with SS.[89]

In two series of patients with MALT lymphoma of the salivary glands, with a combined 310 patients (including 33%−35% with SS or antecedent sialadenitis), relapse or progression of disease occurred in 31%−37% but did not impact OS.[89,90] Progression/relapse occurred in 29% of the 35 SS patients with MALT lymphoma of the salivary gland in the series of Pollard et al.[63]

Histologic transformation of salivary gland MALT lymphoma to DLBCL occurred in 12% of patients, 35−110 months after diagnosis, in a series reported by Ambrosetti et al.[87]; this frequency corresponds to the frequency for all forms of MALT lymphoma.[99] Risk factors include age >60 years and lymph node involvement at presentation.[87] Transformation occurs independent of dissemination.[83,100]

Screening protocol for lymphoma

There are no established guidelines for screening SS patients for the development of lymphoma.[101,102] As early identification of an indolent lymphoma in SS patients does not affect outcome, screening does not need to go beyond what is routine during the course of longitudinal care of SS patients, with follow-up visits every 6−12 months. This would include history and physical examination (looking for a salivary gland nodule, lymphadenopathy, B symptoms, signs of vasculitis, etc.) and basic laboratory studies (e.g., complete blood count, chemistry panel, urinalysis). For those at high risk of lymphoma (as detailed earlier and in Table 8.1), there is potential value in monitoring complement and immunoglobulin levels and performing serum immunofixation electrophoresis and tests for serum cryoglobulins[33] once yearly. The results of these tests may serve to identify systemic disease that requires treatment in its own right or mandates closer monitoring for end-organ involvement. Similarly, the decision to perform biopsy of the salivary glands of an SS patient with long-standing persistent bilateral glandular enlargement needs to be individualized; it may not influence treatment if the glandular enlargement is not symptomatic and the systemic disease is mild or stable.

Conclusions

The substantial risk of lymphoma in SS is a distinctive feature, setting it apart from other systemic autoimmune rheumatic diseases. The majority are indolent lymphomas of the MALT type with preferential involvement of the salivary gland and excellent survival rates. However, DLBCL and other more aggressive lymphomas constitute a substantial minority of affected SS patients and have less favorable survival rates. The risk factors for development of lymphoma are primarily clinical and laboratory markers of lympho-proliferation, especially persistent glandular enlargement, low C4 levels, and cryoglo-bulinemia. It remains to be determined whether disease-modifying therapy, not yet available for SS, will diminish the risk of lymphoma and whether therapies for indolent lymphoma, such as ibrutinib, may prove effective for the benign lymphoproliferation of SS. Management of lymphoma in SS is dictated by its subtype and histologic grade, associated symptoms, and associated SS disease activity.

References

1. Talal N, Bunim JJ. The development of malignant lymphoma in the course of Sjögren's syndrome. *Am J Med*. 1964;36:529–540.
2. Kassan SS, Thomas TL, Moutsopoulos HM, Hoover R, Kimberly RP, Budman DR, Costa J, Decker JL, Chused TM. Increased risk of lymphoma in sicca syndrome. *Ann Intern Med*. 1978;89:888–892.
3. Davidson BK, Kelly CA, Griffiths ID. Primary Sjögren's syndrome in the North East of England: a long-term follow-up study. *Rheumatology*. 1999;38:245–253.
4. Valesini G, Priori R, Bavoillot D, Osborn J, Danieli MG, Del Papa N, Gerli R, Pietrogrande M, Sabbadini MG, Silvestris F, Valsecchi L. Differential risk of non-Hodgkin's lymphoma in Italian patients with primary Sjögren's syndrome. *J Rheumatol*. 1997;24:2376–2380.
5. Lazarus MN, Robinson D, Mak V, Moller H, Isenberg DA. Incidence of cancer in a cohort of patients with primary Sjögren's syndrome. *Rheumatology*. 2006;45:1012–1015.
6. Pertovaara M, Pukkala E, Laippala P, Miettinen A, Pasternack A. A longitudinal cohort study of Finnish patients with primary Sjögren's syndrome: clinical, immunological, and epidemiological aspects. *Ann Rheum Dis*. 2001;60:467–472.
7. Liang Y, Yang Z, Qin B, Zhong R. Primary Sjögren's syndrome and malignancy risk: a systematic review and meta-analysis. *Ann Rheum Dis*. 2014;73:1151–1156.
8. Zhang W, Feng S, Yan S, Zhao Y, Li M, Sun J, Zhang FC, Cui Q, Dong Y. Incidence of malignancy in primary Sjögren's syndrome in a Chinese cohort. *Rheumatology*. 2010; 49:571–577.

9. Weng MY, Huang YT, Liu MF, Lu TH. Incidence of cancer in a nationwide population cohort of 7852 patients with primary Sjögren's syndrome in Taiwan. *Ann Rheum Dis*. 2012;71:524−527.

10. Johnsen SJ, Brun JG, Goransson LG, Smastuen MC, Johannesen TB, Haldorsen K, Harboe E, Jonsson R, Meyer PA, Omdal R. Risk of non-Hodgkin's lymphoma in primary Sjögren's syndrome: a population-based study. *Arthritis Care Res*. 2013;65: 816−821.

11. Theander E, Henriksson G, Ljungberg O, Mandl T, Manthorpe R, Jacobsson LT. Lymphoma and other malignancies in primary Sjögren's syndrome: a cohort study on cancer incidence and lymphoma predictors. *Ann Rheum Dis*. 2006;65:796−803.

12. Kauppi M, Pukkala E, Isomaki H. Elevated incidence of hematologic malignancies in patients with Sjögren's syndrome compared with patients with rheumatoid arthritis (Finland). *Cancer Causes Control*. 1997;8:201−204.

13. Brito-Zeron P, Kostov B, Fraile G, Caravia-Duran D, Maure B, Rascon FJ, Zamora M, Casanovas A, Lopez-Dupla M, Ripoll M, Pinilla B, Fonseca E, Akasbi M, de la Red G, Duarte-Millan MA, Fanlo P, Guisado-Vasco P, Perez-Alvarez R, Chamorro AJ, Morcillo C, Jimenez-Heredia I, Sanchez-Berna I, Lopez-Guillermo A, Ramos-Casals M, SS Study Group GEAS-SEMI. Characterization and risk estimate of cancer in patients with primary Sjögren syndrome. *J Hematol Oncol*. 2017;10:90.

14. Baldini C, Pepe P, Luciano N, Ferro F, Talarico R, Grossi S, Tavoni A, Bombardieri S. A clinical prediction rule for lymphoma development in primary Sjögren's syndrome. *J Rheumatol*. 2012;39:804−808.

15. Risselada AP, Kruize AA, Bijlsma JW. Clinical features distinguishing lymphoma development in primary Sjögren's Syndrome–a retrospective cohort study. *Semin Arthritis Rheum*. 2013;43:171−177.

16. Papageorgiou A, Ziogas DC, Mavragani CP, Zintzaras E, Tzioufas AG, Moutsopoulos HM, Voulgarelis M. Predicting the outcome of Sjögren's syndrome-associated non-hodgkin's lymphoma patients. *PLoS One*. 2015;10:e0116189.

17. Solans-Laque R, Lopez-Hernandez A, Bosch-Gil JA, Palacios A, Campillo M, Vilardell-Tarres M. Risk, predictors, and clinical characteristics of lymphoma development in primary Sjögren's syndrome. *Semin Arthritis Rheum*. 2011;41:415−423.

18. Tonami H, Matoba M, Kuginuki Y, Yokota H, Higashi K, Yamamoto I, Sugai S. Clinical and imaging findings of lymphoma in patients with Sjögren syndrome. *J Comput Assist Tomogr*. 2003;27:517−524.

19. Kimman J, Bossuyt X, Blockmans D. Prognostic value of cryoglobulins, protein electrophoresis, and serum immunoglobulins for lymphoma development in patients with Sjögren's syndrome. A retrospective cohort study. *Acta Clin Belg*. 2018;73:169−181.

20. Zufferey P, Meyer OC, Grossin M, Kahn MF. Primary Sjögren's syndrome (SS) and malignant lymphoma. A retrospective cohort study of 55 patients with SS. *Scand J Rheumatol*. 1995;24:342−345.

21. Skopouli FN, Dafni U, Ioannidis JP, Moutsopoulos HM. Clinical evolution, and morbidity and mortality of primary Sjögren's syndrome. *Semin Arthritis Rheum*. 2000;29:296−304.

22. Voulgarelis M, Ziakas PD, Papageorgiou A, Baimpa E, Tzioufas AG, Moutsopoulos HM. Prognosis and outcome of non-Hodgkin lymphoma in primary Sjögren syndrome. *Medicine*. 2012;91:1−9.

23. Nishishinya MB, Pereda CA, Munoz-Fernandez S, Pego-Reigosa JM, Rua-Figueroa I, Andreu JL, Fernandez-Castro M, Rosas J, Loza Santamaria E. Identification of

lymphoma predictors in patients with primary Sjögren's syndrome: a systematic literature review and meta-analysis. *Rheumatol Int.* 2015;35:17−26.

24. Baecklund E, Smedby KE, Sutton LA, Askling J, Rosenquist R. Lymphoma development in patients with autoimmune and inflammatory disorders–what are the driving forces? *Semin Cancer Biol.* 2014;24:61−70.

25. Zintzaras E, Voulgarelis M, Moutsopoulos HM. The risk of lymphoma development in autoimmune diseases: a meta-analysis. *Arch Intern Med.* 2005;165:2337−2344.

26. Ekstrom Smedby K, Vajdic CM, Falster M, Engels EA, Martinez-Maza O, Turner J, Hjalgrim H, Vineis P, Seniori Costantini A, Bracci PM, Holly EA, Willett E, Spinelli JJ, La Vecchia C, Zheng T, Becker N, De Sanjose S, Chiu BC, Dal Maso L, Cocco P, Maynadie M, Foretova L, Staines A, Brennan P, Davis S, Severson R, Cerhan JR, Breen EC, Birmann B, Grulich AE, Cozen W. Autoimmune disorders and risk of non-Hodgkin lymphoma subtypes: a pooled analysis within the InterLymph Consortium. *Blood.* 2008;111:4029−4038.

27. Mellemkjaer L, Pfeiffer RM, Engels EA, Gridley G, Wheeler W, Hemminki K, Olsen JH, Dreyer L, Linet MS, Goldin LR, Landgren O. Autoimmune disease in individuals and close family members and susceptibility to non-Hodgkin's lymphoma. *Arthritis Rheum.* 2008;58:657−666.

28. Anderson LA, Gadalla S, Morton LM, Landgren O, Pfeiffer R, Warren JL, Berndt SI, Ricker W, Parsons R, Engels EA. Population-based study of autoimmune conditions and the risk of specific lymphoid malignancies. *Int J Cancer.* 2009;125:398−405.

29. Nocturne G, Virone A, Ng WF, Le Guern V, Hachulla E, Cornec D, Daien C, Vittecoq O, Bienvenu B, Marcelli C, Wendling D, Amoura Z, Dhote R, Lavigne C, Fior R, Gottenberg JE, Seror R, Mariette X. Rheumatoid factor and disease activity are independent predictors of lymphoma in primary Sjögren's syndrome. *Arthritis Rheum.* 2016;68:977−985.

30. Voulgarelis M, Dafni UG, Isenberg DA, Moutsopoulos HM. Malignant lymphoma in primary Sjögren's syndrome: a multicenter, retrospective, clinical study by the European Concerted Action on Sjögren's Syndrome. *Arthritis Rheum.* 1999;42:1765−1772.

31. Theander E, Manthorpe R, Jacobsson LT. Mortality and causes of death in primary Sjögren's syndrome: a prospective cohort study. *Arthritis Rheum.* 2004;50:1262−1269.

32. Maciel G, Crowson CS, Matteson EL, Cornec D. Incidence and mortality of physician-diagnosed primary Sjögren syndrome: time trends over a 40-year period in a population-based US cohort. *Mayo Clin Proc.* 2017;92:734−743.

33. Ioannidis JP, Vassiliou VA, Moutsopoulos HM. Long-term risk of mortality and lymphoproliferative disease and predictive classification of primary Sjögren's syndrome. *Arthritis Rheum.* 2002;46:741−747.

34. Tomi AL, Belkhir R, Nocturne G, Desmoulins F, Berge E, Pavy S, Miceli-Richard C, Mariette X, Seror R. Brief report: monoclonal gammopathy and risk of lymphoma and multiple myeloma in patients with primary Sjögren's syndrome. *Arthritis Rheum.* 2016;68:1245−1250.

35. Tzioufas AG, Boumba DS, Skopouli FN, Moutsopoulos HM. Mixed monoclonal cryoglobulinemia and monoclonal rheumatoid factor cross-reactive idiotypes as predictive factors for the development of lymphoma in primary Sjögren's syndrome. *Arthritis Rheum.* 1996;39:767−772.

36. Theander E, Vasaitis L, Baecklund E, Nordmark G, Warfvinge G, Liedholm R, Brokstad K, Jonsson R, Jonsson MV. Lymphoid organisation in labial salivary gland

biopsies is a possible predictor for the development of malignant lymphoma in primary Sjögren's syndrome. *Ann Rheum Dis.* 2011;70:1363−1368.

37. Fox RI. The importance of minor salivary gland biopsy in prediction of lymphoma in Sjögren's syndrome: should we be obtaining more information about prognosis from minor salivary gland samples? *Ann Rheum Dis.* 2011;70:1351−1353.

38. Haacke EA, van der Vegt B, Vissink A, Spijkervet FKL, Bootsma H, Kroese FGM. Germinal centres in diagnostic labial gland biopsies of patients with primary Sjögren's syndrome are not predictive for parotid MALT lymphoma development. *Ann Rheum Dis.* 2017;76:1781−1784.

39. Quartuccio L, Isola M, Baldini C, Priori R, Bartoloni Bocci E, Carubbi F, Maset M, Gregoraci G, Della Mea V, Salvin S, De Marchi G, Luciano N, Colafrancesco S, Alunno A, Giacomelli R, Gerli R, Valesini G, Bombardieri S, De Vita S. Biomarkers of lymphoma in Sjögren's syndrome and evaluation of the lymphoma risk in prelymphomatous conditions: results of a multicenter study. *J Autoimmun.* 2014;51:75−80.

40. Baimpa E, Dahabreh IJ, Voulgarelis M, Moutsopoulos HM. Hematologic manifestations and predictors of lymphoma development in primary Sjögren syndrome: clinical and pathophysiologic aspects. *Medicine.* 2009;88:284−293.

41. Fragkioudaki S, Mavragani CP, Moutsopoulos HM. Predicting the risk for lymphoma development in Sjögren syndrome: an easy tool for clinical use. *Medicine.* 2016;95: e3766.

42. Quartuccio L, Baldini C, Bartoloni E, Priori R, Carubbi F, Corazza L, Alunno A, Colafrancesco S, Luciano N, Giacomelli R, Gerli R, Valesini G, Bombardieri S, De Vita S. Anti-SSA/SSB-negative Sjögren's syndrome shows a lower prevalence of lymphoproliferative manifestations, and a lower risk of lymphoma evolution. *Autoimmun Rev.* 2015;14:1019−1022.

43. Gulati D, Kushner I, File E, Magrey M. Primary Sjögren's syndrome with anticentromere antibodies–a clinically distinct subset. *Clin Rheumatol.* 2010;29:789−791.

44. Baldini C, Mosca M, Della Rossa A, Pepe P, Notarstefano C, Ferro F, Luciano N, Talarico R, Tani C, Tavoni AG, Bombardieri S. Overlap of ACA-positive systemic sclerosis and Sjögren's syndrome: a distinct clinical entity with mild organ involvement but at high risk of lymphoma. *Clin Exp Rheumatol.* 2013;31:272−280.

45. Baer AN, Medrano L, McAdams-DeMarco M, Gniadek TJ. Anti-centromere antibodies are associated with more severe exocrine glandular dysfunction in Sjögren's syndrome: analysis of the Sjögren's International Collaborative Clinical Alliance cohort. *Arthritis Care Res.* 2016;68:1554−1559.

46. Hyjek E, Smith WJ, Isaacson PG. Primary B-cell lymphoma of salivary glands and its relationship to myoepithelial sialadenitis. *Hum Pathol.* 1988;19:766−776.

47. Quintana PG, Kapadia SB, Bahler DW, Johnson JT, Swerdlow SH. Salivary gland lymphoid infiltrates associated with lymphoepithelial lesions: a clinicopathologic, immunophenotypic, and genotypic study. *Hum Pathol.* 1997;28:850−861.

48. Hsi ED, Zukerberg LR, Schnitzer B, Harris NL. Development of extrasalivary gland lymphoma in myoepithelial sialadenitis. *Mod Pathol.* 1995;8:817−824.

49. Fishleder A, Tubbs R, Hesse B, Levine H. Uniform detection of immunoglobulin-gene rearrangement in benign lymphoepithelial lesions. *N Engl J Med.* 1987;316: 1118−1121.

50. Nocturne G, Mariette X. Sjögren Syndrome-associated lymphomas: an update on pathogenesis and management. *Br J Haematol.* 2015;168:317−327.

51. Kuper-Hommel MJ, van Krieken JH. Molecular pathogenesis and histologic and clinical features of extranodal marginal zone lymphomas of mucosa-associated lymphoid tissue type. *Leuk Lymphoma.* 2012;53:1032–1045.
52. Bahler DW, Swerdlow SH. Clonal salivary gland infiltrates associated with myoepithelial sialadenitis (Sjögren's syndrome) begin as nonmalignant antigen-selected expansions. *Blood.* 1998;91:1864–1872.
53. Gasparotto D, De Vita S, De Re V, Marzotto A, De Marchi G, Scott CA, Gloghini A, Ferraccioli G, Boiocchi M. Extrasalivary lymphoma development in Sjögren's syndrome: clonal evolution from parotid gland lymphoproliferation and role of local triggering. *Arthritis Rheum.* 2003;48:3181–3186.
54. Dong L, Masaki Y, Takegami T, Jin ZX, Huang CR, Fukushima T, Sawaki T, Kawanami T, Saeki T, Kitagawa K, Sugai S, Okazaki T, Hirose Y, Umehara H. Clonality analysis of lymphoproliferative disorders in patients with Sjögren's syndrome. *Clin Exp Immunol.* 2007;150:279–284.
55. Martin T, Weber JC, Levallois H, Labouret N, Soley A, Koenig S, Korganow AS, Pasquali JL. Salivary gland lymphomas in patients with Sjögren's syndrome may frequently develop from rheumatoid factor B cells. *Arthritis Rheum.* 2000;43:908–916.
56. Bende RJ, Aarts WM, Riedl RG, de Jong D, Pals ST, van Noesel CJ. Among B cell non-Hodgkin's lymphomas, MALT lymphomas express a unique antibody repertoire with frequent rheumatoid factor reactivity. *J Exp Med.* 2005;201:1229–1241.
57. Lau CM, Broughton C, Tabor AS, Akira S, Flavell RA, Mamula MJ, Christensen SR, Shlomchik MJ, Viglianti GA, Rifkin IR, Marshak-Rothstein A. RNA-associated autoantigens activate B cells by combined B cell antigen receptor/Toll-like receptor 7 engagement. *J Exp Med.* 2005;202:1171–1177.
58. Quartuccio L, Salvin S, Fabris M, Maset M, Pontarini E, Isola M, De Vita S. BLyS upregulation in Sjögren's syndrome associated with lymphoproliferative disorders, higher ESSDAI score and B-cell clonal expansion in the salivary glands. *Rheumatology.* 2013;52:276–281.
59. Streubel B, Huber D, Wohrer S, Chott A, Raderer M. Frequency of chromosomal aberrations involving MALT1 in mucosa-associated lymphoid tissue lymphoma in patients with Sjögren's syndrome. *Clin Cancer Res.* 2004;10:476–480.
60. Nocturne G, Boudaoud S, Miceli-Richard C, Viengchareun S, Lazure T, Nititham J, Taylor KE, Ma A, Busato F, Melki J, Lessard CJ, Sivils KL, Dubost JJ, Hachulla E, Gottenberg JE, Lombes M, Tost J, Criswell LA, Mariette X. Germline and somatic genetic variations of TNFAIP3 in lymphoma complicating primary Sjögren's syndrome. *Blood.* 2013;122:4068–4076.
61. Baecklund E, Backlin C, Iliadou A, Granath F, Ekbom A, Amini RM, Feltelius N, Enblad G, Sundstrom C, Klareskog L, Askling J, Rosenquist R. Characteristics of diffuse large B cell lymphomas in rheumatoid arthritis. *Arthritis Rheum.* 2006;54: 3774–3781.
62. Van Mello NM, Pillemer SR, Tak PP, Sankar V. B cell MALT lymphoma diagnosed by labial minor salivary gland biopsy in patients screened for Sjögren's syndrome. *Ann Rheum Dis.* 2005;64:471–473.
63. Pollard RP, Pijpe J, Bootsma H, Spijkervet FK, Kluin PM, Roodenburg JL, Kallenberg CG, Vissink A, van Imhoff GW. Treatment of mucosa-associated lymphoid tissue lymphoma in Sjögren's syndrome: a retrospective clinical study. *J Rheumatol.* 2011;38:2198–2208.

64. Anderson LG, Talal N. The spectrum of benign to malignant lymphoproliferation in Sjögren's syndrome. *Clin Exp Immunol*. 1972;10:199—221.
65. Yachoui R, Leon C, Sitwala K, Kreidy M. Pulmonary MALT lymphoma in patients with Sjögren's syndrome. *Clin Med Res*. 2017;15:6—12.
66. McCurley TL, Collins RD, Ball E, Collins RD. Nodal and extranodal lymphoproliferative disorders in Sjögren's syndrome: a clinical and immunopathologic study. *Hum Pathol*. 1990;21:482—492.
67. Stewart A, Blenkinsopp PT, Henry K. Bilateral parotid MALT lymphoma and Sjögren's syndrome. *Br J Oral Maxillofac Surg*. 1994;32:318—322.
68. De Vita S, Boiocchi M, Sorrentino D, Carbone A, Avellini C, Dolcetti R, Marzotto A, Gloghini A, Bartoli E, Beltrami CA, Ferraccioli G. Characterization of prelymphomatous stages of B cell lymphoproliferation in Sjögren's syndrome. *Arthritis Rheum*. 1997; 40:318—331.
69. Thieblemont C, Berger F, Dumontet C, Moullet I, Bouafia F, Felman P, Salles G, Coiffier B. Mucosa-associated lymphoid tissue lymphoma is a disseminated disease in one third of 158 patients analyzed. *Blood*. 2000;95:802—806.
70. Ando M, Matsuzaki M, Murofushi T. Mucosa-associated lymphoid tissue lymphoma presented as diffuse swelling of the parotid gland. *Am J Otolaryngol*. 2005;26:285—288.
71. Kato H, Kanematsu M, Goto H, Mizuta K, Aoki M, Kuze B, Hirose Y. Mucosa-associated lymphoid tissue lymphoma of the salivary glands: MR imaging findings including diffusion-weighted imaging. *Eur J Radiol*. 2012;81:e612—e617.
72. Grevers G, Ihrler S, Vogl TJ, Weiss M. A comparison of clinical, pathological and radiological findings with magnetic resonance imaging studies of lymphomas in patients with Sjögren's syndrome. *Eur Arch Otorhinolaryngol*. 1994;251:214—217.
73. Wickramasinghe A, Howarth A, Drage NA. Multiple bilateral parotid sialoliths in a patient with mucosa-associated lymphoid tissue lymphoma (MALT lymphoma) of the salivary glands. *Oral Surg Oral Med Oral Pathol Oral Radiol Endod*. 2005;99: 496—498.
74. Lewis K, Vandervelde C, Grace R, Ramesar K, Williams M, Howlett DC. Salivary gland mucosa-associated lymphoid tissue lymphoma in 2 patients with Sjögren's syndrome: clinical and sonographic features with pathological correlation. *J Clin Ultrasound*. 2007;35:97—101.
75. Bahn YE, Lee SK, Kwon SY, Kim SP. Sonographic appearances of mucosa-associated lymphoid tissue lymphoma of the submandibular gland confirmed with sonographically guided core needle biopsy. *J Clin Ultrasound*. 2011;39:228—232.
76. Matsushita T, Takashima S, Takayama F, Momose M, Wang J, Ishiyama T. Sonographic detection of secondary MALT lymphoma of the submandibular gland. *J Clin Ultrasound*. 2001;29:462—465.
77. Perry C, Herishanu Y, Metzer U, Bairey O, Ruchlemer R, Trejo L, Naparstek E, Sapir EE, Polliack A. Diagnostic accuracy of PET/CT in patients with extranodal marginal zone MALT lymphoma. *Eur J Haematol*. 2007;79:205—209.
78. Treglia G, Zucca E, Sadeghi R, Cavalli F, Giovanella L, Ceriani L. Detection rate of fluorine-18-fluorodeoxyglucose positron emission tomography in patients with marginal zone lymphoma of MALT type: a meta-analysis. *Hematol Oncol*. 2015;33: 113—124.
79. Cohen C, Mekinian A, Uzunhan Y, Fauchais AL, Dhote R, Pop G, Eder V, Nunes H, Brillet PY, Valeyre D, Fain O, Soussan M. 18F-fluorodeoxyglucose positron emission

tomography/computer tomography as an objective tool for assessing disease activity in Sjögren's syndrome. *Autoimmun Rev.* 2013;12:1109−1114.

80. Farmer PL, Bailey DJ, Burns BF, Day A, LeBrun DP. The reliability of lymphoma diagnosis in small tissue samples is heavily influenced by lymphoma subtype. *Am J Clin Pathol.* 2007;128:474−480.

81. Burke C, Thomas R, Inglis C, Baldwin A, Ramesar K, Grace R, Howlett DC. Ultrasound-guided core biopsy in the diagnosis of lymphoma of the head and neck. A 9 year experience. *Br J Radiol.* 2011;84:727−732.

82. Kim HJ, Kim JS. Ultrasound-guided core needle biopsy in salivary glands: a meta-analysis. *Laryngoscope.* 2018;128:118−125.

83. Zucca E, Conconi A, Pedrinis E, Cortelazzo S, Motta T, Gospodarowicz MK, Patterson BJ, Ferreri AJ, Ponzoni M, Devizzi L, Giardini R, Pinotti G, Capella C, Zinzani PL, Pileri S, Lopez-Guillermo A, Campo E, Ambrosetti A, Baldini L, Cavalli F, International Extranodal Lymphoma Study Group. Nongastric marginal zone B-cell lymphoma of mucosa-associated lymphoid tissue. *Blood.* 2003;101: 2489−2495.

84. Raderer M, Wohrer S, Streubel B, Troch M, Turetschek K, Jager U, Skrabs C, Gaiger A, Drach J, Puespoek A, Formanek M, Hoffmann M, Hauff W, Chott A. Assessment of disease dissemination in gastric compared with extragastric mucosa-associated lymphoid tissue lymphoma using extensive staging: a single-center experience. *J Clin Oncol.* 2006;24:3136−3141.

85. Dreyling M, Thieblemont C, Gallamini A, Arcaini L, Campo E, Hermine O, Kluin-Nelemans JC, Ladetto M, Le Gouill S, Iannitto E, Pileri S, Rodriguez J, Schmitz N, Wotherspoon A, Zinzani P, Zucca E. ESMO Consensus conferences: guidelines on malignant lymphoma. part 2: marginal zone lymphoma, mantle cell lymphoma, peripheral T-cell lymphoma. *Ann Oncol.* 2013;24:857−877.

86. Kahl B, Yang D. Marginal zone lymphomas: management of nodal, splenic, and MALT NHL. *Hematol Am Soc Hematol Educ Program.* 2008;359−364.

87. Ambrosetti A, Zanotti R, Pattaro C, Lenzi L, Chilosi M, Caramaschi P, Arcaini L, Pasini F, Biasi D, Orlandi E, D'Adda M, Lucioni M, Pizzolo G. Most cases of primary salivary mucosa-associated lymphoid tissue lymphoma are associated either with Sjogren syndrome or hepatitis C virus infection. *Br J Haematol.* 2004;126:43−49.

88. Cheson BD, Fisher RI, Barrington SF, Cavalli F, Schwartz LH, Zucca E, Lister TA, Alliance, Australasian Leukaemia and Lymphoma Group, Eastern Cooperative Oncology Group, European Mantle Cell Lymphoma Consortium, Italian Lymphoma Foundation, European Organisation for Research, Treatment of Cancer/Dutch Hemato-Oncology Group, Grupo Espanol de Medula Osea, German High-Grade Lymphoma Study Group, German Hodgkin's Study Group, Japanese Lymphorra Study Group, Lymphoma Study Association, NCIC Clinical Trials Group, Nordic Lymphoma Study Group, Southwest Oncology Group, United Kingdom National Cancer Research Institute. Recommendations for initial evaluation, staging, and response assessment of Hodgkin and non-Hodgkin lymphoma: the Lugano classification. *J Clin Oncol.* 2014;32:3059−3068.

89. Jackson AE, Mian M, Kalpadakis C, Pangalis GA, Stathis A, Porro E, Conconi A, Cortelazzo S, Gaidano G, Lopez Guillermo A, Johnson PW, Martelli M, Martinelli G, Thieblemont C, McPhail ED, Copie-Bergman C, Pileri SA, Jack A, Campo E, Mazzucchelli L, Ristow K, Habermann TM, Cavalli F, Nowakowski GS, Zucca E. Extranodal marginal zone lymphoma of mucosa-associated lymphoid tissue

of the salivary glands: a multicenter, international experience of 248 patients (IELSG 41). *Oncologist.* 2015;20:1149−1153.

90. Anacak Y, Miller RC, Constantinou N, Mamusa AM, Epelbaum R, Li Y, Calduch AL, Kowalczyk A, Weber DC, Kadish SP, Bese N, Poortmans P, Kamer S, Ozsahin M. Primary mucosa-associated lymphoid tissue lymphoma of the salivary glands: a multicenter Rare Cancer Network study. *Int J Radiat Oncol Biol Phys.* 2012;82:315−320.

91. Demaria L, Henry J, Seror R, Frenzel L, Hermine O, Mariette X, Nocturne G. Rituximab-Bendamustine (R-Benda) in MALT lymphoma complicating primary Sjögren syndrome (pSS). *Br J Haematol.* 2018;184:472−475.

92. Luthy SK, Ng AK, Silver B, Degnan KO, Fisher DC, Freedman AS, Mauch PM. Response to low-dose involved-field radiotherapy in patients with non-Hodgkin's lymphoma. *Ann Oncol.* 2008;19:2043−2047.

93. Konig L, Horner-Rieber J, Bernhardt D, Hommertgen A, Rieken S, Debus J, Herfarth K. Response rates and recurrence patterns after low-dose radiotherapy with 4Gy in patients with low-grade lymphomas. *Strahlenther Onkol.* 2018;194:454−461.

94. Conconi A, Martinelli G, Thieblemont C, Ferreri AJ, Devizzi L, Peccatori F, Ponzoni M, Pedrinis E, Dell'Oro S, Pruneri G, Filipazzi V, Dietrich PY, Gianni AM, Coiffier B, Cavalli F, Zucca E. Clinical activity of rituximab in extranodal marginal zone B-cell lymphoma of MALT type. *Blood.* 2003;102:2741−2745.

95. Salar A, Domingo-Domenech E, Panizo C, Nicolas C, Bargay J, Muntanola A, Canales M, Bello JL, Sancho JM, Tomas JF, Rodriguez MJ, Penalver J, Grande C, Sanchez-Blanco JJ, Palomera L, Arranz R, Conde E, Garcia M, Garcia JF, Caballero D, Montalban C. Long-term results of a phase 2 study of rituximab and bendamustine for mucosa-associated lymphoid tissue lymphoma. *Blood.* 2017;130:1772−1774.

96. Zucca E, Conconi A, Martinelli G, Bouabdallah R, Tucci A, Vitolo U, Martelli M, Pettengell R, Salles G, Sebban C, Guillermo AL, Pinotti G, Devizzi L, Morschhauser F, Tilly H, Torri V, Hohaus S, Ferreri AJM, Zachee P, Bosly A, Haioun C, Stelitano C, Bellei M, Ponzoni M, Moreau A, Jack A, Campo E, Mazzucchelli L, Cavalli F, Johnson P, Thieblemont C. Final results of the IELSG-19 randomized trial of mucosa-associated lymphoid tissue lymphoma: improved event-free and progression-free survival with rituximab plus chlorambucil versus either chlorambucil or rituximab monotherapy. *J Clin Oncol.* 2017;35:1905−1912.

97. Noy A, de Vos S, Thieblemont C, Martin P, Flowers CR, Morschhauser F, Collins GP, Ma S, Coleman M, Peles S, Smith S, Barrientos JC, Smith A, Munneke B, Dimery I, Beaupre DM, Chen R. Targeting Bruton tyrosine kinase with ibrutinib in relapsed/refractory marginal zone lymphoma. *Blood.* 2017;129:2224−2232.

98. Ziepert M, Hasenclever D, Kuhnt E, Glass B, Schmitz N, Pfreundschuh M, Loeffler M. Standard International prognostic index remains a valid predictor of outcome for patients with aggressive CD20+ B-cell lymphoma in the rituximab era. *J Clin Oncol.* 2010;28:2373−2380.

99. Zucca E, Bertoni F. The spectrum of MALT lymphoma at different sites: biological and therapeutic relevance. *Blood.* 2016;127:2082−2092.

100. Thieblemont C, Bastion Y, Berger F, Rieux C, Salles G, Dumontet C, Felman P, Coiffier B. Mucosa-associated lymphoid tissue gastrointestinal and nongastrointestinal lymphoma behavior: analysis of 108 patients. *J Clin Oncol.* 1997;15:1624−1630.

101. Routsias JG, Goules JD, Charalampakis G, Tzima S, Papageorgiou A, Voulgarelis M. Malignant lymphoma in primary Sjögren's syndrome: an update on the pathogenesis and treatment. *Semin Arthritis Rheum.* 2013;43:178−186.

102. Jonsson MV, Theander E, Jonsson R. Predictors for the development of non-Hodgkin lymphoma in primary Sjögren's syndrome. *Presse Med.* 2012;41:e511−e516.

103. Sutcliffe N, Inanc M, Speight P, Isenberg D. Predictors of lymphoma development in primary Sjögren's syndrome. *Semin Arthritis Rheum.* 1998;28:80−87.

104. Ramos-Casals M, Brito-Zeron P, Perez-DE-Lis M, Diaz-Lagares C, Bove A, Soto MJ, Jimenez I, Belenguer R, Siso A, Muxi A, Pons F. Clinical and prognostic significance of parotid scintigraphy in 405 patients with primary Sjögren's syndrome. *J Rheumatol.* 2010;37:585−590.

105. Risselada AP, Kruize AA, Goldschmeding R, Lafeber FP, Bijlsma JW, van Roon JA. The prognostic value of routinely performed minor salivary gland assessments in primary Sjögren's syndrome. *Ann Rheum Dis.* 2014;73:1537−1540.

106. Tobon GJ, Saraux A, Gottenberg JE, Quartuccio L, Fabris M, Seror R, Devauchelle-Pensec V, Morel J, Rist S, Mariette X, De Vita S, Youinou P, Pers JO. Role of Fms-like tyrosine kinase 3 ligand as a potential biologic marker of lymphoma in primary Sjögren's syndrome. *Arthritis Rheum.* 2013;65:3218−3227.

107. Sene D, Ismael S, Forien M, Charlotte F, Kaci R, Cacoub P, Diallo A, Dieude P, Liote F. Ectopic germinal center-like structures in minor salivary gland biopsy tissue predict lymphoma occurrence in patients with primary Sjögren's syndrome. *Arthritis Rheum.* 2018;70:1481−1488.

108. Nocturne G, Seror R, Fogel O, Belkhir R, Boudaoud S, Saraux A, Larroche C, Le Guern V, Gottenberg JE, Mariette X. CXCL13 and CCL11 serum levels and lymphoma and disease activity in primary Sjögren's syndrome. *Arthritis Rheumatol.* 2015;67:3226−3233.

109. Kapsogeorgou EK, Papageorgiou A, Protogerou AD, Voulgarelis M, Tzioufas AG. Low miR200b-5p levels in minor salivary glands: a novel molecular marker predicting lymphoma development in patients with Sjögren's syndrome. *Ann Rheum Dis.* 2018;77:1200−1207.

110. Brito-Zeron P, Retamozo S, Gandia M, Akasbi M, Perez-De-Lis M, Diaz-Lagares C, Bosch X, Bove A, Perez-Alvarez R, Soto-Cardenas MJ, Siso A, Ramos-Casals M. Monoclonal gammopathy related to Sjögren syndrome: a key marker of disease prognosis and outcomes. *J Autoimmun.* 2012;39:43−48.

Sjögren's syndrome: peripheral and autonomic nervous system involvement

David S. Younger, MD, MPH, MS

Department of Clinical Medicine, CUNY School of Medicine at City College, Graduate School of Public Health and Health Policy, City University of New York, New York, NY, United States

Epidemiology
Peripheral neuropathy

The initial investigation of the neurologic manifestations in Sjögren's syndrome (SS) dates back to the 1980s,[1] and a recent review found wide variations in the reported overall prevalence appearing to center around 20% of individuals.[2] For example, a retrospective review of 420 SS patients in France who met the 2002 American European Consensus Group criteria (Chapter 2) and were followed for an average of over 7 years reported 95 patients (22%) with neurologic involvement documented by objective findings on physical examination, imaging, and/or other neurodiagnostic studies.[3] Also, 62 patients had peripheral nervous system (PNS) involvement, 41 patients had central nervous system (CNS) involvement, and 10 patients had both. Pure sensory neuropathies occurred mainly in patients without extraglandular manifestations and in individuals who were anti-Ro/SSA antibody negative ($P < .05$). Mononeuritis multiplex (MNM) and axonal sensorimotor polyneuropathies were most frequently associated with active systemic disease (e.g., Raynaud phenomenon, cutaneous vasculitis, renal involvement, and cryoglobulinemia) ($P < .05$).

Neuropathies in SS can be the presenting manifestations of the disease or occur later in the course. Peripheral neuropathies may occur as an isolated problem or in association with CNS disease (Chapter 10) or cranial or autonomic neuropathy (AN). In one study of 82 patients, the neurologic manifestations of SS (CNS > PNS) preceded the onset of sicca symptoms in 47% cases, with a mean delay of 6 years between neurologic onset and the development of sicca. In 19% of cases the diagnosis of SS could not be established at the time of initial presentation.[4] In another series, neurologic manifestations, particularly PNS, preceded sicca symptoms in 40%–93% cases, depending on the institutional referral bias.[5] Thus the exact prevalence of PNS in SS remains challenging to estimate because of the limited size of available cohorts, referral bias, the differences in case definitions, the diagnostic criteria used for SS, and the degree of neurologic assessment.[6]

Autonomic neuropathies

AN is common in SS and characterized by predominant autonomic dysfunction as discussed below in *Autonomic diagnosis*. Autonomic nervous system (ANS) dysfunction may contribute to other key SS symptoms including chronic fatigue. One multicenter, prospective, cross-sectional study of 317 patients in the United Kingdom with well-characterized SS found a significantly higher prevalence of autonomic symptoms in patients than in community controls.[7] Additionally, 55% of SS patients but only 20% controls met the case definition of AN ($P < .0001$) using the Composite Autonomic Symptom Scale (COMPASS), a validated item-weighted symptom questionnaire that correlates well with other instruments and objective measures including the Composite Autonomic Scoring Scale (CASS) used to quantify autonomic deficits.[8] Total COMPASS scores were also independently associated with certain patient-reported outcomes (e.g., ESSPRI [European League Against Rheumatism (EULAR) Sjögren's Syndrome Patient Reported Index]) and disease activity measures [e.g., ESSDAI (EULAR Sjögren's Syndrome Disease Activity Index)], and the authors speculated that dysautonomia may be a key element of the pathologic processes of SS.[7]

When ANS dysfunction is assessed by objective measures the prevalence of autonomic neuropathies in SS is also high but varies according to methods of assessment. Andonopoulos and colleagues[9] studied 32 patients with SS and 22 age- and sex-matched healthy individuals who were asked specific questions about symptoms suggestive of AN and subjected them to a battery of five cardiovascular tests including response of blood pressure (BP) to sustained hand grip or Valsalva maneuver (VM), heart rate (HR) response to deep breathing, and HR and BP response to standing. Sixteen patients (50%) had symptoms of AN when specifically asked versus none of the controls ($P < .0005$). However, objective testing revealed severe cardiovascular AN in 68.8% of patients but in only 12.7% of controls ($P < .0001$), indicating that subclinical cases of AN also exist. Koh and coworkers[10] reported a significantly higher prevalence (36%) of autonomic dysfunction by using a standardized 5-minute, supine, resting HR variability test among 154 Korean patients with SS compared with 154 age- and sex-matched Korean controls. Abnormal results were associated with the fatigue score in ESSPRI but not the total scores of ESSPRI or ESSDAI.

Clinical presentation

Patients with SS develop a variety of peripheral and autonomic neuropathies with a clinical presentation that depends on the type of neuron involved and the caliber of the axon and its location (e.g., large and myelinated or microscopic and intraepidermal). Multiple patterns of peripheral neuropathy have been described in several case series and reviews.[4,11–18] These include small fiber sensory neuropathy (SFN), sensory ataxic neuronopathy/ganglionopathy, axonal sensory or sensorimotor polyneuropathy, cranial neuropathies, mononeuritis multiplex, radiculoneuropathy, chronic inflammatory demyelinating polyneuropathy (CIDP), motor neuron disease, and AN. The neuropathies can be broadly categorized in two major groups. Sensory symptoms without substantial motor involvement is a feature of SFN, sensory ataxic neuronopathy/ganglionopathy, trigeminal neuropathy, and AN, although the affected sensory modalities and distribution pattern vary. In contrast, motor weakness and muscle atrophy were observed in MNM, multiple cranial neuropathy, and radiculoneuropathy. Autonomic symptoms were seen in all forms of sensory neuropathy. Acute and subacute onsets were frequent in MNM and multiple cranial neuropathy, whereas chronic progression was predominant in the other forms. Age at onset and first evaluation, female predominance, and the prevalence of typical sicca symptoms were similar for each neuropathy type. Patterns sometimes overlapped and, in certain instances, more than one neuropathy could be identified in the same individual.[11,15,16]

Small fiber neuropathy

Painful small fiber neuropathy (SFN) is the most common type of neuropathy in autoimmune patients, including in SS. It preferentially damages small-diameter, unmyelinated C-fibers and/or thinly myelinated A-δ pain-sensitive and autonomic fibers that signal pain and tissue damage/inflammation and regulate autonomic function.[19] Sensory symptoms in SFN include spontaneous chronic distal or widespread burning or shooting pain, stimulus-evoked hyperalgesia/allodynia, reduced nociceptive sensation, and neuropathic itching. Examination often shows loss of pinprick and temperature sensation in the distal extremities in a symmetric length-dependent distribution but intact proprioception, sensation to light touch and vibration, strength, and deep tendon reflexes. When SFN occurs in a nonlength-dependent distribution, the face, scalp, trunk, and proximal limbs may also be affected. Symptoms of cardiovascular, gastrointestinal (GI), or microvascular dysfunction and altered sweating reflect concomitant autonomic end-organ involvement. Neurogenic dysregulation of the microvessels causes a wide array of symptoms including postural orthostatic dizziness, tachycardia,[20] and fatigue. In SFN, electromyographic (EMG)/nerve conduction velocity (NCV) study results are typically normal, except in rare instances when another neuropathy also coexists. The course in most patients will be insidious and chronic but acute and subacute progression may occasionally occur.[21]

A 3-mm skin biopsy as described below for epidermal nerve fiber staining is the most reliable means to document the diagnosis and distinguish between a length-dependent and nonlength-dependent SFN. The biopsy sample is taken from the distal and proximal sites of the leg to determine the site of injury of nociceptive pathways from dorsal root ganglia (DRG) sensory neurons peripherally along macroscopic peripheral axons to microscopic nerve terminals in the skin, visualized as intraepidermal nerve fibers (IENFs). The density of IENFs is counted and depletion of IENFs along the distal lateral calf suggests a length-dependent peripheral degenerative process, whereas proximal depletion along the lateral thigh indicates that a nonlength-dependent mechanism is likely due to loss of integrity of the DRG and/or autonomic ganglia.

Small fiber neuropathy is common among patients with autoimmune diseases but it may also occur in other comorbidities some of which (e.g., celiac, vitamin B_{12} deficiency) occur as complications of SS (Table 9.1). This must be considered in the evaluation of the SS patient with neuropathic symptoms and multiple comorbidities. The National Health and Nutrition Examination Survey reported a 14.8% prevalence of SFN among people older than 40 years.[22] Bakkers and colleagues[23] studied 365 patients with SFN from various causes and compiled a detailed survey of SFN symptoms using a Standard Inventory Questionnaire. The study identified four predominant sensory neuropathic symptoms characteristic of SFN, including burning pain, sheet intolerance, restless legs, and skin sensitivity. Prominent symptoms of autonomic involvement included changes in sweating pattern, diarrhea, constipation, bladder disturbance, dizziness on standing, palpitations, hot flashes, dry eyes, and dry mouth. Using a generic Medical Outcomes Study 36-Iitem Short Form Health Survey, the investigators also observed severe reduction in patients' quality of life, with the most significant deficits in Role Functioning-Physical, Body Pain, and Physical Component Summary scores.

Sensory ataxic neuronopathy

Sensory ataxic neuronopathy also known as sensory ganglionopathy or dorsal root ganglionitis, is an uncommon but disabling large fiber sensory neuropathy, predominantly manifesting as impairment of joint-position sense leading to sensory ataxia. Muscle power, muscle volume, and motor nerve function are preserved.[12] Lymphocytic infiltration of the DRG has been described in several cases of sensory ataxic neuronopathy.[24,25]

The symptoms of sensory ganglionopathy depend on the type of neuron targeted. Damage to large myelinated sensory neurons reduces touch, vibration, and proprioception, causing ataxia, athetoid limb movements, positive result in Romberg test, diminished deep tendon reflexes, and difficulty moving, despite preserved strength. There may occasionally be difficulty with fine motor movements. Sensory ganglionopathies typically cause patchy, asymmetric, and often proximal signs and symptoms in a nonlength-dependent distribution, sometimes with rapid onset. The sudden onset of proximal or patchy unexplained neuropathic pain in the hands and feet should raise the possibility of involvement of DRG neurons and their peripheral sensory axons. Trigeminal nerve abnormalities and ANS dysfunction, including abnormal pupils, hypohidrosis/anhidrosis, fixed tachycardia, and orthostatic hypotension, frequently coexist.[25] An EMG/NCV study will typically show

Table 9.1 Differential diagnosis of small fiber peripheral neuropathy.

Amyloid
Familial amyloidosis
Primary systemic amyloidosis
Connective tissue disorders/Autoimmune
Celiac
Sjögren's syndrome
Rheumatoid arthritis
Mixed connective tissue
Sarcoidosis
Systemic lupus erythematosus
Hematologic
Monoclonal gammopathy
Hereditary
Fabry disease
SCN9A mutation 17
SCN10A
Idiopathic
Infections
Hepatitis C
HIV
Lyme disease
Malignancy
Chronic lymphocytic leukemia
Paraneoplastic
Metabolic/Endocrinologic
Diabetes mellitus
Impaired glucose tolerance
Porphyrias
Thyroid dysfunction
Toxins
Alcohol
Chemotherapy
Drugs
Vitamins
Pyridoxine toxicity
Vitamin B_{12} deficiency

a decrease or absence in sensory nerve action potentials in the affected areas, with preserved motor nerve conduction. Abnormal magnetic resonance images (MRI) (e.g., hyperintensity of T_2 signal in the posterior columns) of DRG have also been reported.[26,27]

Axonal sensory and sensorimotor polyneuropathy

Distal axonal sensory neuropathy is common in SS, particularly in patients with active systemic disease, and targets large myelinated nerve fibers of the distal lower extremities in a length-dependent symmetric distribution.[14] It typically presents with the insidious onset of distal paresthesias and tingling followed by balance and gait disturbances. Examination shows vibratory, proprioceptive, and discriminative sensory loss in a stocking/glove distribution, hyporeflexia or areflexia, and trophic skin changes. This type of neuropathy may occasionally coexist with SFN. Mixed sensorimotor polyneuropathy, which involves both the motor and sensory large-caliber myelinated fibers, causes additional complaints of muscle cramps, muscle wasting, weakness, fasciculations, and tremors. Examination will show weakness of the foot and toe extensors. NCV studies show reduced amplitude of the sensory nerve action potential (SNAP) with or without a reduction in the compound muscle action potential (CMAP) in the setting of preserved conduction velocity. A variety of conditions that can mimic or complicate SS should be considered in the differential diagnosis, especially in patients who present with neurologic signs and symptoms (Table 9.2). Patients who present with painful, asymmetric, or rapid-onset axonal neuropathies that exhibit stepwise progression should undergo evaluation for vasculitis.

Cranial neuropathy

Among SS patients with neurologic involvement, the prevalence of cranial neuropathies ranges from 16% to 20%.[4,11] Trigeminal neuropathy most commonly occurs and is defined as a pure sensory neuropathy restricted to the territory of the sensory trigeminal nerves. It causes facial numbness, tingling, and/or burning pain that is typically unilateral but may also occur in a bilateral distribution.[17] Facial dysesthesias may occur spontaneously or after certain activities such as putting on makeup or brushing the teeth.

Other cranial neuropathies in SS may cause recurrent diplopia (cranial nerves [CNs] III and VI), Bell palsy (CN VII), and hearing loss and vestibular symptoms (cochlear nerve).[18] Mori and coworkers[11] also described patients with multiple cranial neuropathies (CNs III, V, VI, VII, VIII, IX, X, and XII) in various combinations.

Mononeuritis multiplex

Mononeuritis multiplex is characterized by multiple mononeuropathies in the arms or legs, involving motor and sensory fibers. Typically, there is simultaneous or consecutive asymmetric damage of at least two nerves in the same limb, which do not form a continuity with one another. It frequently presents with acute or subacute painful dysesthesias in one limb followed by motor involvement. Symptoms often occur in a stepwise fashion. Examination will show patchy sensory loss and motor weakness in a nondermatomal distribution; motor weakness sometimes manifests as wrist drop, or foot drop with gait disturbance. Sensory involvement generally affects both superficial and deep sensation. Electrophysiologic studies

Table 9.2 Differential diagnosis of axonal sensorimotor polyneuropathy.

Amyloid polyneuropathy
Connective tissue disorders/Autoimmune
Cryoglobulinemia
Guillain-Barré syndrome
Mixed connective tissue
Rheumatoid arthritis
Sarcoidosis
Sjögren's syndrome
Systemic lupus erythematosus
Vasculitis
Hematologic
Monoclonal gammopathy
Hereditary
Hereditary sensory neuropathy type IA
Charcot-Marie-tooth disease (type 2)
Idiopathic

Infections
HIV
Leprosy
Lyme disease
Zika virus
Malignancy
Chronic lymphocytic leukemia
Paraneoplastic
Metabolic/Endocrinologic
Diabetes mellitus
Impaired glucose tolerance
Hypothyroidism
Porphyrias
Neurologic
Parkinson disease
Toxins
Alcohol
Chemotherapy
Drugs
Heavy metals
Uremia
Vitamins
Vitamin B_1 deficiency
Vitamin B_6
Vitamin B_{12} deficiency
Vitamin E deficiency

document axonal damage and "pseudoblocks" corresponding to the areas of nerve ischemia. MNM can be associated with trigeminal or multiple cranial neuropathies. When indicated, a cutaenous nerve or simultaneous nerve-muscle biopsy may reveal underlying vasculitis. Vasculitic neuropathies in SS are often associated with cryoglobulinemia, constitutional symptoms, and vasculitis in other organs (Chapter 7).[28]

Other neuropathies in Sjögren's syndrome

Other neuropathies that can occur in SS, albeit rarely, are listed in the following and described in some case series but not others. It remains unclear whether this variance is explained by differences in the genetics of the SS population under study, the clinical interests and evaluation done by the neurologist, or simply reflects the chance occurrence of two unrelated disorders.

Chronic inflammatory demyelinating polyneuropathy

CIDP is rare in SS and characterized by the slow development (>8weeks) of symmetric weakness (both proximal and distal) in all four extremities, sensory abnormalities, and absent deep tendon reflexes.[17] Cerebrospinal fluid (CSF) analysis will usually show high total protein levels. EMG/NCV findings include prolonged distal motor latency with slowed conduction velocity, abnormal temporal dispersion or partial conduction block, and absence of the F-wave or prolongation of its latency.[17]

Radiculoneuropathy

Polyradiculoneuropathy, also known as inflammatory polyradiculoneuropathy, radiculoneuropathy, or chronic sensorimotor polyradiculopathy, is also uncommon in SS[4,5] and manifests as a CIDP-like syndrome caused by lesions restricted to the spinal roots or the very proximal portion of spinal nerves.[11,29] It presents with loss of sensation in the extremities in a stocking-glove distribution, sensory ataxia, and muscle weakness. Levels of CSF protein are usually increased. Electrodiagnostic studies demonstrate normal or near-normal motor and sensory NCVs, F-wave abnormalities, poor occurrence, and prolonged latencies.[11] An MRI of the lumbar spine can show gadolinium enhancement of the dorsal spinal roots and cauda equina. In one series, when sural nerve biopsies were performed, varying degrees of myelinated fiber loss and mild-moderate demyelinating changes were observed in all specimens.

Motor neuron disease

Motor neuron disease of various forms has been described in a handful of patients with SS. Onset may be acute, subacute, or chronic. Most patients lack sicca symptoms at the time of presentation.

An acute motor axonal neuropathy resembling a variant of Guillain-Barré syndrome was described in a young man with no significant medical history or sicca symptoms; this began as distal lower extremity weakness with gait dysfunction that rapidly progressed to cause flaccid quadriparesis with areflexia but no sensory signs or symptoms. An extensive workup revealed positive antinuclear antibodies at 1:2560 (speckled), positive anti-SSA, positive anti-GM1 antibodies, and a positive minor salivary gland biopsy.[30] A similar case without anti-GM1 antibodies and subacute onset was also described in an elderly female with SS.[31]

Anterior horn cell disease of gradual onset also occurs in SS and causes paresis of the limbs affecting the distal extremities first that eventually leads to quadriparesis, muscle atrophy, and fasciculations, without accompanying sphincter dysfunction or upper motor neuron signs.[17,32] NCV studies show normal sensory nerve conduction but reduced compound muscle action potential amplitudes and prolonged distal motor latencies and delayed F-response latencies. EMG will reveal signs of acute denervation and fasciculation potentials. Histopathologic examination from limited autopsy studies has shown mononuclear cell infiltration in the area of motor neurons, axonal degeneration, and motor root atrophy and fibrosis.

Diagnostic evaluation
Nerve conduction studies and electromyography
General considerations

Readers are referred to a standard textbook with chapters on the relevant subjects of neuromuscular[33] and autonomic disorders.[34] Standard NCV studies assess the large myelinated nerve fibers of named sensory, motor, and mixed nerves. The study results should therefore be normal in a patient with SFN. The recorded *sensory nerve action potential* (SNAP) is the summation of many evoked sensory nerve fiber action potentials. The recordings are generally made with surface recording electrodes placed proximal or distal to the stimulating electrodes termed orthodromic or antidromic, respectively.

The pathophysiologic nature of a sudden mononeuropathy such as common fibular neuropathies at the fibular head, radial neuropathy at the spiral groove, and selected ulnar neuropathy at the elbow, presenting respectively in the foot, as wrist drop, and intrinsic hand weakness, is due to loss of excitability of the subserved myofibers. Although demyelinating processes due to the focal demyelinating block of conduction resolve over several weeks, an axonal component due to Wallerian degeneration is the likeliest dominant process if weakness persists longer. Electrodiagnostic studies add precision in monitoring the remyelinating and regenerating process underlying recovery through serial studies that should begin soon after the injury, at 21 days when the demyelinating block should begin to subside, and afterward at several month intervals.

Sensory nerve integrity

The onset and peak latencies, amplitude, duration, and morphology are recorded and the *NCV* is calculated between two sites of stimulation. The *onset latency* reflects the NCV along the fastest conducting fibers, whereas the *peak latency* corresponds to the average velocity of the conducting fibers. Sensory NCV studies can localize lesions involving the sensory system from the DRG to the nerve terminal. Most experts routinely record the median (recording index finger), ulnar (recording fifth finger), radial (recording the thumb base), sural (recording lateral malleolus), and superficial fibular (recording dorsum of ankle) NCVs.

Motor neuron integrity

Orthostatic motor NCV studies are performed using the belly-tendon method wherein the recorded response is a summation of individual muscle fiber *compound muscle action potentials* (CMAPs) generated by the stimulated motor axons. The innervation ratio or the number of muscle fibers innervated per motor axon explains why motor responses measured in millivolts are so much larger than sensory responses measured in microvolts. CMAPs are more resistant to physiologic temporal dispersion, permitting the distance between the stimulating and recording electrodes to be greater and assessment of longer nerve segments compared with sensory NCV studies, thus rendering them useful for the localization of focal demyelinating conduction blocks, a feature of demyelination. *Distal latency* is never used to calculate the motor NCV because in addition to the desired motor NCV time, it incorporates the tissue transit and nerve fiber activation times, neuromuscular junction transmission, and muscle fiber conduction times. The motor NCV between the two sites of stimulation is expressed in milliseconds (ms) and calculated by dividing the distance between the two sites in millimeters by the latency difference in milliseconds. The median, ulnar, fibular, and posterior tibial motor responses are recorded from the abductor pollicis brevis, abductor digiti minimi, extensor digitorum brevis, and abductor hallucis muscles, respectively, and compose the standard motor NCV study. Other additional limb and/or cranial motor nerves may be studied based on the clinical situation.

Nerve injury

The pathologic responses to nerve injury are essentially limited to *axon loss, focal demyelination,* or some combination thereof. Lesions that produce axon disruption or DRG cell loss are identifiable by a loss of the amplitude of the recorded sensory or motor response. Such changes are more noticeable in the sensory nerves, which are more sensitive to a given percentage of axon disruption than the corresponding CMAP amplitude. A loss of approximately 50% of the axons of a mixed nerve leads to comparatively lower amplitudes in the SNAP responses than those of the CMAP, which appears to follow a linear relationship. Distal latency and NCV measurements tend to be normal in partial axon loss lesions, indicating preservation of the fastest conducting fibers rather than the total number of conducting fibers. The observed alterations with demyelinating lesions (e.g., CIDP) depend on the severity with which such processes tend to affect the largest and fastest conducting fibers. Mild demyelinating lesions cause widening of the nodal gap and slowing of the rate of propagation of nerve fiber action potentials, leading to prolongation of distal latencies and decreased NCV, with all the propagating impulses reaching their target organ in a delayed manner. With both axon loss and demyelinating conduction block, the amplitude of the response is the most important parameter measured, with the degree of amplitude reduction dependent on the number of nerve fibers affected. The clinical correlation of the motor axonal pathophysiologic condition is that clinical weakness occurs when the propagating nerve fiber action potentials fail to reach their myofiber target, an outcome that occurs only with axon loss—induced conduction failure or demyelinating conduction block, but not with lesions producing solely demyelinating conduction slowing. Analogously, fixed sensory deficits are expected with dropout of propagating SNAPs, a condition that associates with axon loss—induced conduction failure or demyelinating conduction block. Regardless of the type of nerve fiber lesion, demyelinating conduction slowing has little clinical accompaniment. *F-waves* are elicited by the supramaximal stimulation of a motor nerve to study conduction along the proximal segments of the nerve as far up as the root level. This leads to bidirectional propagating action potentials, with those traveling distally producing the muscular (M) wave and the others traveling proximally reaching the spinal cord. These waveforms are most useful in detecting root lesions or confirming the degree of demyelination along the proximal nerve segments.

Electromyography

Needle EMG is the most sensitive test for detecting motor axon loss lesions and the only portion of the EMG examination capable of identifying disorders involving the upper motor neuron (UMN) system, and, for practical purposes, the muscle fibers themselves. Both concentric and monopole needle electrodes are used. The former are hollow and contain a thin centrally located metal wire that is surrounded by an insulating resin. The tip of the wire is exposed distally and functions as the G1 electrode, whereas the intramuscular portion of the cannula functions as the G2 electrode. Monopole needles are composed of a metal shaft that is coated with Teflon, except at its tip, which functions as the G1 recording electrode. It is used in conjunction with a separate surface electrode that functions as the G2 recording electrode. The electric activity recorded by the G1 and G2 leads of the needle electrode passes through a differential amplifier and the voltage difference between them is displayed on an oscilloscope. The sound characteristics of the recorded responses are fed into an audio system. The standard needle examination includes a sampling of distal, middle, and proximal limb muscles of different root, plexus, and nerve origins, as well as paraspinal muscles. Three phases of the needle examination include needle insertion, rest, and activation, which together provide essential information about the state of maturation of a given peripheral nerve insult. The lesions that disrupt motor axons result in a dropout of individual *motor unit action potentials* (MUAPs) that contribute to the CMAP, whereas demyelinating lesions manifesting conduction block lead to abnormal CMAP responses observed only after stimulation at or above the lesion, with normal responses evoked distal to the lesion because of the lack of associated pathophysiologic effects.

Electrophysiologic patterns of peripheral neuropathy

Peripheral neuropathic disorders can be subdivided electrophysiologically into focal mononeuropathy, MNM, generalized polyneuropathy, sensory ganglioneuropathy, and cranial neuropathy. They are all associated with limited pathologic changes that include demyelination, axon loss, or a combination of the two depending on the rapidity of onset, underlying pathophysiologic condition, distribution, severity, acuteness of duration, and whether sensory or motor fibers are involved. Electrodiagnostic studies detect demyelinating conduction slowing, demyelinating conduction block, axon loss—induced conduction failure, or some combination thereof, and contribute to an understanding of the pathophysiologic nature and severity of an acquired mononeuropathy.

Chronic sensorimotor axonal loss polyneuropathy has a typical electrodiagnostic and temporal progression that parallels the clinical course. The pathologic process starts distally with a stocking distribution that evolves to a stocking-glove pattern. In its mildest form and excluding isolated sensory involvement, initial findings (i.e., fibrillation potentials) are noted distally in intrinsic foot muscles on needle EMG examination. The sural, superficial fibular sensory nerves, which are more sensitive to axon loss, are involved first, followed later by motor nerve involvement on needle EMG. Sustained denervation of intrinsic foot muscles leads to diminished motor NCV study response. The most prominent NCV study parameter of a demyelinating polyneuropathy is NCV slowing. This is characterized by prolonged sensory and motor peak latencies, with sensory NCV study results being more abnormal and often not elicited in the legs. Despite the predominant demyelinating pathophysiologic condition, a mild amount of fibrillation activity is often noted in needle EMG of the distal leg muscles, along with prominent chronic neurogenic MUAP changes. There are criteria for the separation of primary demyelinating processes from primarily axonal processes.[35] However, mixed demyelinating and axonal polyneuropathies show features of both axon loss and demyelination. Polyneuropathies variably involve sensory, motor, and autonomic axons; however, some affect only one type of fiber. Pure sensory polyneuropathy can be divided into acquired and hereditary forms, with less pronounced clinical severity in acquired forms and more pronounced distal and uniform involvement in the genetic types. The electrodiagnostic features of sensory ganglioneuropathy resembles pure sensory neuropathy with absent or reduced SNAP amplitudes.

Autonomic testing

Background

The ANS consists of a set of afferent pathways, a CNS integrating complex in the brain and spinal cord, and two distinct efferent limbs, sympathetic and parasympathetic, each with preganglionic and postganglionic neurons. The sympathetic nervous system fibers originating in the hypothalamus of the brain transit preganglionic sympathetic neural pathways located in the intermediolateral horn of the thoracic and lumbar spinal segments and elaborate short nerves that innervate postganglionic neurons in the prevertebral, paravertebral, and previsceral sympathetic ganglia. Postganglionic axons innervate effector organs. Postganglionic axons are generally thin and unmyelinated, measuring <5 micrometers (μm), and innervate smooth muscles of blood vessels, the heart, endocrine glands, and parenchymatous organs. Multiple neurotransmitters are involved in the integration of these responses, notably the monoamines epinephrine, norepinephrine, and serotonin. Postganglionic axons originating in thoracic and lumbosacral ganglia travel long distances to innervate the abdominal viscera and blood vessels of the legs, at times measuring >50 cm in length. Although parasympathetic and sympathetic effects have been traditionally regarded as antagonistic, it is now apparent that the interrelationship is more complex and context sensitive. For example, the specific effects of the autonomic innervation of a particular organ depend on not only the type of autonomic organ receptor present but also the level of preactivation at the time of neurotransmitter stimulation. The physiologic effects of a neurotransmitter can also be concentration dependent or vary with the number of receptors present in the end organ. Activation of the sympathetic nervous system evokes a diffuse response preparing the body for *"fight or flight"* situations requiring high metabolic demand and physical activity. Changes include increased myocardial contractility, HR, and BP; decreased GI motility; and shunting of blood flow away from nonessential organs. The parasympathetic nervous system regulates more restricted functions associated with resting activity, with the associated energy conservation expressed as decrease in HR and BP, pupillary constriction, and increased bronchial and GI activity, salivation, and lacrimation.

The *baroreceptor reflex* is the most important cardiovascular reflex for the control of rapid systolic BP oscillation.[36] It is triggered by the activation of both stretch receptors in the carotid sinus and aortic arch and afferent fibers that convey information along the glossopharyngeal and vagus nerves toward the solitary tract nucleus of the brainstem. The ANS acts upon three elements to maintain satisfactory control of BP: the heart, venous return, and systemic vascular resistance. Efferent arms of the ANS that communicate with these components are the sympathetic and parasympathetic innervation of the heart and the sympathetic innervation of the smooth muscles of peripheral blood vessels. A decrement in BP reduces the activity of vascular stretch receptors, thereby decreasing vagal excitation and inhibition of sympathetic activity. These changes result in reduced cardiovagal activity and increased sympathetic stimulation of blood vessels and the heart, leading to vasoconstriction, increased cardiac contractility, and tachycardia. This combination of cardiac and vascular adjustments ultimately restores BP to its original level, with a reverse process occurring in situations where BP is increased. These fine-tuning changes occur very quickly: cardiovagal activity changes HR in the first to second beat after changes in BP, whereas sympathetic influences on HR, myocardial contractility, and arterial vasomotor tone take several seconds to reach a clinical expression.

Autonomic diagnosis

Since the ANS regulates a wide range of biological functions, autonomic neuropathies in SS could potentially explain or contribute to a wide variety of symptoms (Table 9.3). As mentioned previously, autonomic symptoms may occur in up to 55% of SS patients.[7] However, the exact prevalence of autonomic neuropathies in SS has been difficult to determine because methods for screening and evaluation have differed among centers. Although generalized dysautonomia may rarely occur in SS,[37] the signs and symptoms usually vary according to the organs involved and whether there is greater impairment of sympathetic or parasympathetic control.

Orthostatic intolerance is one of the most disabling and frequently reported autonomic problems in SS and initial screening can easily be performed by office measurement of HR (reflects cardiovagal regulation) and BP (assesses sympathetic vasomotor tone) to look for variations with change in position. However, in situations when screening results are normal or near normal, a more sophisticated and sensitive assessment with electronic monitoring of HR and BP will usually be

Table 9.3 Signs and symptoms of autonomic nerve dysfunction reported in Sjögren's syndrome.

Cardiovascular
Arrhythmias
Dizziness
Heart palpitations
Lightheadedness
Orthostatic hypotension
Postural orthostatic tachycardia syndrome
Presyncope/syncope
Tachycardia

Gastrointestinal
Abdominal pain
Constipation
Diarrhea/frequent bowel movements
Dry mouth

Genitourinary
Urinary frequency or hesitancy

Ocular
Adie pupil
Dry eyes

Sudomotor
Heat intolerance
Hyperhidrosis
Hypohidrosis/anhidrosis

required. The 1996 Task Force report of the American Academy of Neurology evaluated the safety, reproducibility, ease of performance, and sensitivity of available ANS tests and issued various recommendations.[38] Tests most useful to evaluate parasympathetic function included HR variation during deep breathing with calculation of an expiratory and inspiratory ratio and HR variation during a Valsalva maneuver (VM) with calculation of the Valsalva ratio (VR). The recommendations for evaluation of sympathetic function included BP response to the VM, muscle contraction, and active standing. Sudomotor (relating to innervation of the sweat glands) testing of sympathetic skin response and quantitative sudomotor axon reflex test were also recommended.

The complex hemodynamic and autonomic changes induced by a VM depend on multiple interactions among BP, venous return, and the baroreflex, making the calculated VR sensitive to dysfunction of both the sympathetic and parasympathetic autonomic nervous system. Subjects are instructed to blow vigorously into a mouthpiece or mask applied over the mouth, sustaining a pressure of 40 mm Hg for 15 s while quantifying the expiratory force with a digital or aneroid manometer attached to the mask through a cannula. The VR is defined as the longest RR interval following completion of the maneuver divided by the shortest RR interval recorded during the strain phase (i.e., during the maneuver). In patients with autonomic neuropathies the VR will be increased and reflects parasympathetic dysfunction and impairment of vascular α-adrenergic innervation. Measurement of BP response to VM and other maneuvers are necessary for better assessment of the overall sympathetic function including cardiac β-adrenergic autonomic innervation.

Head-up tilt table test

Sympathetic control of vascular tone is essential for maintaining BP during standing or passive head-up tilting (HUT). The observed changes in turn provide valuable information on the integrity of the baroreflex and other autonomic reflexes. HUT is indicated in symptomatic patients in whom repeated office measurements fail to confirm the suspected diagnosis. HUT at 60 or 90 degrees and its gravitational stress evoke an immediate displacement of 500−1000 mL of blood to the lower part of the body, reducing BP and activating the baroreflex. This triggers adjustments in vascular tone and HR. After several seconds, a slight drop in BP generates a vagal inhibitory response and reflex tachycardia that reaches a peak at 15 seconds and is accompanied by progressive vasoconstriction. The recovery of BP subsequently induces reflex bradycardia that reaches a maximum at 30 seconds. Over the ensuing 1−2 minutes the BP remains steady in most subjects because of the combined sympathetic and cardiovagal adjustments. Most of the ANS changes related to standing occur within the first 5 minutes, while the long-term control of BP includes hormonal changes that influence vascular tone and fluid displacement. In normal subjects the initial active standing leads to a slight decrease in BP and increase in HR, whereas in those with orthostatic hypotension, BP is severely reduced in the first few seconds and minutes after active standing, accompanied by a reciprocal increase in HR. The criteria that define orthostatic postural hypotension vary slightly among different professional societies.[39] However, in general, the American Academy of Neurology, American Autonomic Society, and most other professional organizations define orthostatic hypotension as a decrease in systolic BP of at least 20 mm Hg (or >30 mmHg in the presence of hypertension) or a decrease in diastolic BP of at least 10 mm Hg within 3 min of standing.[39] A severe drop in BP should lead to consideration of poor vascular sympathetic tone and may be associated with either tachycardia or bradycardia, depending on the primary underlying cause of the hypotension. The sensitivity of the HUT table test for confirming neurally mediated syncope varies from 40% to 60%, with up to 50% of patients with a compatible clinical history demonstrating completely normal tilt-table test results.[34]

Postural orthostatic tachycardia syndrome

Patients with chronic orthostatic intolerance who experience symptoms associated with persistent and pronounced tachycardia (defined as an increase of >30 bpm or a total HR >120 bpm) within 10 min of standing or change in position are diagnosed with the *postural orthostatic tachycardia syndrome* (POTS). Normal subjects who undergo passive tilting from 0 to 60 degrees or 90 degrees will develop a slight transient drop in systolic, diastolic, and mean BPs that recovers in 1 minute with HR increases from 10 to 20 bpm, whereas those with severe adrenergic impairment have inadequate compensatory vasoconstriction leading to postural hypotension, persistent tachycardia, and a progressive fall in BP even during passive standing. In some cases of POTS, however, the BP response to this maneuver may be normal or slightly elevated while an uncomfortable rapid increase in heart rate persists.

Sweat testing

The regulation of body temperature is an important function of the ANS, and the control of sweating is essential for thermal homeostasis. Central and peripheral sudomotor sympathetic function is assessed by recording the responses of sweat glands to various types of stimuli. Such studies are especially useful in the early detection of small fiber neuropathies. Thermoregulatory sweat testing involves the application of a substance on the region of interest, which is capable of changing color when the body temperature is raised after placement in a room with elevated temperature or following exposure to a heating lamp to stimulate sweating in regions of the body under investigation. The most commonly employed substances are starch iodide and cornstarch with calcium carbonate, which change to a darker color on contact with sweat in contrast to areas with absent or decreased sweating, demonstrating topographic patterns of sudomotor disturbances. However, these studies are unable to differentiate central from peripheral autonomic disorders or those due to preganglionic or postganglionic sympathetic sudomotor disturbances.

Biopsies

Intraepidermal nerve fiber analysis

Over the past decade, specialized centers around the world have developed techniques to evaluate small sensory nerve fibers within the skin, which has facilitated the diagnosis of SFN, and has now become the procedure of choice for diagnosis of this condition in various populations. Fixed or unfixed skin punch biopsies are cut and processed for immunoperoxidase staining of IENFs with the antibody PGP9.5. An assessment is made to look for changes in normal IENF density and pattern of arborization of the nerve twigs within the epidermis and dermis and adjacent to the skin adnexal structures (Fig. 9.1). The cutaneous biopsy is safe and relatively painless and also the results derived from IENF analysis are diagnostically accurate, reproducible, and have a high correlation with clinical examination and electrodiagnostic and autonomic testing.

The procedure can be performed in an office setting where there is adequate lighting and privacy and a table that will accommodate the gowned patient who will be laying in a lateral decubitus position. There are two preferable sites, the distal leg and the proximal thigh, for the performance of epidermal nerve fiber analysis via a 3-mm punch biopsy, each with normative values for correlation to controls. It is important to avoid sites of prior trauma or earlier biopsy. A proximal thigh biopsy site is located 10 cm distal to the greater trochanter. The distal leg site for biopsy is located 10 cm proximal to the lateral malleolus. The number of IENFs are counted in five separate areas of the 3-mm tissue specimen and expressed as a mean value and range. Values that fall beneath the fifth percentile for age-matched controls are deemed significantly low; other findings including large swellings, horizontal branching, increased frequency of small swellings, and irregular distribution of IENFs along the dermal-epidermal junction also support the diagnosis of SFN (Fig. 9.1). Mention should be made of any cellular infiltrates in the dermis and epidermis, and the Congo red immunofluorescence test is routinely performed by most laboratories to search for amyloid deposits.

Cutaneous nerve biopsy

Presently, the major clinical indication to perform a cutaneous nerve biopsy is to confirm a suspected vasculitic neuropathy (Fig. 9.2). The reasons to perform a biopsy on patients with suspected nonvasculitic peripheral neuropathies have diminished because experience has shown that the structural abnormalities seen in other types of neuropathy are not specific for any disease process. Additionally, this is an invasive procedure usually associated with a permanent sensory deficit and, not uncommonly, neuralgia. In general, cutaneous nerve biopsies should be performed in centers that have designated laboratories and neuropathologists trained in the performance and interpretation of paraffin-embedded sections of muscle and nerve, frozen section histology, plastic embedding and preparation of semithin sections, and electron microscopy. The sural nerves and superficial fibular nerves are the most commonly biopsied via a full-thickness transection, and muscle tissue is simultaneously taken from the underlying soleus or peroneus brevis muscle to enhance the finding of inflammation and frank vasculitis.

The abnormalities found in peripheral nerves in various disease states can be categorized into disorders that primarily affect axons, myelin, and connective tissue elements, including blood vessels.[40] The most common forms of subacute or chronic

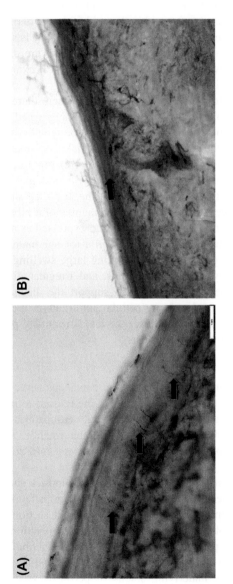

Both photomicrographs courtesy of Dr. Kurenai Tanji, Professor of Pathology in the Division of Neuropathology, Columbia University.

FIGURE 9.1

(A) Calf skin biopsy showing normal epidermal nerve fiber morphology and density (400x). Long epidermal branches (*arrows*) are relatively evenly distributed throughout the length of the specimen but not completely visualized by focusing on a single plain. (B) Abnormal 3-mm punch biopsy specimen (thigh) from a patient with Sjögren's syndrome showing significantly reduced nerve fiber density (arrow) in the epidermis (protein gene product 9.5, hematoxylin-eosin) (200x).

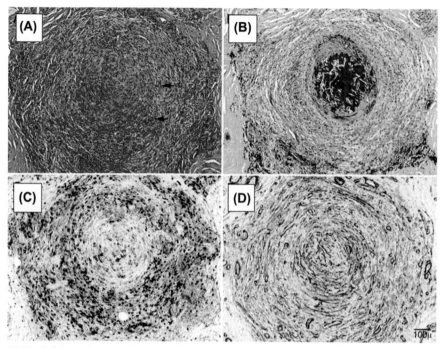

FIGURE 9.2

Serial transverse paraffin sections of a sural nerve biopsy showing necrotizing vasculitis in a larger arteriole. (A) Hematoxylin-eosin staining: shows inflammatory cell infiltration, fibrinoid necrosis (orange discoloration) (*arrows*), and luminal occlusion. (B) Masson trichrome staining: shows vessel wall destruction. (C) CD45 staining confirms the leukocyte infiltration. (D) Smooth muscle actin stain shows the fragmentation and destruction of muscle layers with loss of normal vessel wall architecture.

axonal degeneration (e.g., axonal sensorimotor polyneuropathy) are referred to as dying-back neuropathy or progressive distal axonopathy and are characterized by length-dependent degeneration beginning at the most distal portions of axons. The clinical correlate is involvement of the feet before the hands. In the chronic or late stages of axonal degeneration the principal morphologic features include a reduction in the number of myelinated axons and an increase in endoneurial connective tissue, without much evidence of the active axonal degeneration seen in the acute process. Occasional disintegrating fibers and macrophage activity may be seen. Degeneration and attempted regeneration may be seen in a given specimen. Axonal regeneration is characterized by the sprouting of thinly myelinated axonal extensions that form clusters of small, closely packed fibers and is best appreciated on semithin sections and electron microscopy. Teased nerve fiber preparations demonstrate the different stages of degeneration and regeneration where fragmentation and dissolution of the fiber may be seen at various stages of disintegration. Axonal atrophy is another pathologic finding observed in large fiber neuropathies and is characterized by a reduction in the cross-sectional diameter of the fiber with retention of its circular outline.

Axonal degeneration can also be seen in ganglionopathies (e.g., sensory ataxic neuronopathy, motor neuron disease) wherein the primary abnormality is thought to be in the cell body of the neuron. As this irreversible process occurs in the cell body, regeneration is impossible and the projecting axon degenerates, beginning at the most distal portions of the axon. In the case of destruction of an anterior horn cell neuron, the degeneration begins at the periphery or the most distal portions of the cell body, or toward the CNS, in a neuron located in the DRG in which the projections might be in the dorsal columns. The histologic appearance on light and electron microscopy is comparable to what was described earlier for dying-back axonal degeneration, except for the lack of regenerating axonal sprouts.

Primary demyelinating disorders of peripheral nerve (e.g., CIDP) are, by definition, those conditions in which the site of injury is directed to the myelin sheath or the sustaining Schwann cells. The principal morphologic manifestation of primary demyelination is segmental damage to myelin internodes in arbitrary sequence, while preserving others, with preservation of the axon at the site of myelin injury. Experimental animal studies have shown that demyelination begins at the node of Ranvier and proceeds with unwrapping and disintegration of the myelin. Subsequently, Schwann cells and macrophages phagocytize the broken down myelin. When demyelination involves only very short stretches of nerve fiber measuring <15 mm, the affected internode may be remyelinated by the surviving Schwann cell. Longer stretches of demyelination call upon proliferation of Schwann cells in order to remyelinate the segments. Segmental demyelination can be demonstrated well in tease fiber preparations. Semithin sections and electron microscopy of cross sections reveal naked axons. As the process of regeneration of the demyelinated segment proceeds, tease fiber preparations demonstrate shorter than normal distances between internodes, with relatively thin myelin sheaths that are disproportionately thinner than the axon diameter. Schwann cells proliferate along with their basement membranes and align concentrically around a thinly myelinated or demyelinated axon, which is otherwise intact. This process is referred to as *"onion bulb"* formation and is best appreciated on semithin sections and electron microscopy. Demyelinating pathology is also found in SS patients with polyradiculoneuropathy.

Evaluation of peripheral nerve also requires analysis of the connective tissue—supporting structures including blood vessels. Endoneurial connective tissue proliferation is seen in peripheral neuropathies of long-standing duration, irrespective of the cause or basic pathologic process. The epineurium is well assessed in plastic-embedded sections and may be the site of immune-mediated inflammation, with infiltration by inflammatory cells and vasculitis. Deposition of complement and membrane attack complex on vessel walls may be seen in certain forms of vasculitis using immunohistochemical stains. Patients undergoing cutaneous nerve biopsy should also be considered for a muscle biopsy at the same surgical site, such as the underlying soleus muscle when sampling the sural nerve or the peroneus brevis muscle if the superficial fibular sensory nerve is biopsied. This may increase the diagnostic yield for vasculitis.[41] The muscle will likewise be snap-frozen for histo-chemical analysis, stored in formalin for making paraffin sections, and placed in glutaraldehyde for electron microscopy. Careful analysis of the muscle biopsy tissue can provide valuable information on the involvement of skeletal muscles, to grade the severity of sensorimotor polyneuropathy, and to exclude inflammatory myopathy and vasculitis.

Lessons from clinicopathologic studies

Clinicopathologic studies dating back to the late 1960s have continuously expanded the spectrum of clinical manifestations from PNS and ANS involvement in SS and have described a wide variety of immunopathologic findings that suggest an immune-mediated process. Kaltreider and Talal[42] were among the first investigators to report the co-occurrence of more than one type of neuropathy within the same individual with SS and to document peripheral nerve vasculitis as a cause of SS sensorimotor polyneuropathy.

Kennett and Harding[43] characterized sensory ataxic neuronopathy as a slowly progressive ganglionopathy that can start assymetrically in both the upper and lower extremities. Simultaneously, Malinow and colleagues[24] published pathologic evi-dence that documented the presence of lymphocytic infiltration in the DRG of SS patients with sensory ataxic neuronopathies. These results were later confirmed by Griffin[25] who described lymphocytic infiltration of the dorsal roots and DRG, with degeneration of sensory neurons in mildly affected ganglia and neuronal loss in advanced cases.

Mellgren and colleagues[44] described the clinicopathologic features of 33 cases of SS and peripheral neuropathy evaluated by neurologic examinations, electrodiag-nostic studies, and sural nerve biopsies. Symmetric sensorimotor polyneuropathy occurred most frequently, followed by a symmetric sensory neuropathy. In 25% of cases a second neuropathy coexisted, including AN, mononeuropathy, or cranial neuropathy (especially trigeminal neuropathy); this was described in other reports as well.[43] The course of PNS involvement was slowly progressive,[44] except for a few patients who improved with prednisone therapy. Cutaneous nerve biopsies in 11 patients revealed perivascular inflammatory infiltrates, other vessel abnormalities, and necrotizing vasculitis (6 cases). Axonal degeneration predominated over demy-elination and was occasionally focal or multifocal.

More than a decade later, Mori and colleagues[11] described the clinicopathologic features of 92 SS patients with various peripheral neuropathies. The majority of pa-tients (92%) were diagnosed with SS after neurologic symptoms appeared. Fifty-five patients underwent sural nerve biopsies that revealed variable degrees of axonal loss. Predominantly large fiber loss was observed in sensory ataxic neuronopathy, whereas unmyelinated small fiber loss occurred in painful SFN. Angiitis and peri-vascular infiltrates were seen most frequently in MNM. The autopsy findings of one patient with sensory ataxic neuropathy showed not only severe large sensory neuron loss corresponding to dorsal root and posterior column involvement of the spinal cord but also severe sympathetic neuron loss. Degrees of neuron loss in DRG and sympathetic ganglia paralleled the segmental distribution of sensory and sweating impairment. Multifocal T-cell invasion was seen in DRG and sympathetic ganglia, perineurial space, and vessel walls in the nerve trunks. Based on these clinicopathologic observations and other findings, the authors suggested that sensory ataxic neuronopathy, painful SFN, and trigeminal neuropathy were due to a ganglionic neuronal disease process, whereas MNM and multiple cranial neuropathy were most likely caused by vasculitis.

Contemporaneously, Delalande and colleagues[4] described the clinicopathologic features of 82 patients with CNS and PNS SS. Interestingly, 25/82 (30%) had both CNS and PNS involvement. Based on the clinical and EMG features of the 51 PNS patients the most common patterns included distal axonal sensorimotor polyneuropathy ($n = 19$), cranial neuropathy ($n = 16$), pure sensory neuropathy ($n = 9$), multiple mononeuropathy ($n = 7$), and polyradiculoneuropathy ($n = 1$). Autonomic symptoms were observed in only three patients (bladder dysfunction) but screening for them was not systematically performed. Mononeuritis multiplex frequently occurred in patients with severe systemic complications of SS, including cutaneous vasculitis, Raynaud phenomenon and arthralgias. The course was characterized by acute or subacute onset with recurrent symptoms. Sural nerve biopsies performed in two such patients revealed lymphocytic infiltrates without necrotizing vasculitis. Serum cryoglobulins were detected in over 70% of patients with MNM and sensorimotor polyneuropathies.

Studies have also suggested a possible role for the humoral immune system in the pathogenesis of peripheral neuropathies in SS. In one small study, anti-ganglion neuron antibodies that recognized various proteins in DRG neurons were detected in SS patients with peripheral neuropathies but not in three other groups: healthy normal controls, SS patients who did not have neuropathies, and controls with vasculitic neuropathies who did not have SS.[45] Anti-acetylcholine receptor (AChR) antibodies that recognize the M3 muscarinic receptor (M3R) were later described in SS patients with PNS and ANS involvement.[46] In a mouse model, human antibodies to the M3R experimentally inhibited neuronally mediated contraction of smooth muscles throughout the GI tract and disrupted complex contractile motility patterns in the mouse colon. These autoantibodies were not active on tissue from knockout mice that lacked the M3R, providing compelling evidence of the direct interaction of patient autoantibodies with the M3R.[46] Such findings indicate that anti-M3R autoantibodies may be pathogenic and have the potential to cause panautonomic dysfunction of the GI tract in SS, ranging from reduced esophageal and gastric motor activity to altered colonic motility.

Microscopic vasculitis in peripheral nerve biopsies

Microscopic vasculitis or *microvasculitis* (Fig. 9.3) is defined as inflammation of the walls of the arteriae nervorum that typically affects vessels <40 μm in diameter,

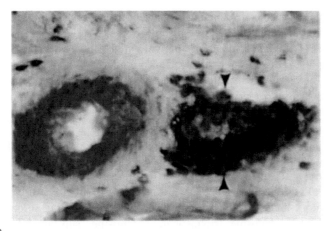

FIGURE 9.3

Microvasculitis. A focal intense collection of CD3[+] T cells (immunoperoxidase) efface the wall of a small epineurial blood vessel (*arrowheads*). In deeper sections (not shown) the same structure stains red in double-labeling with anti-actin smooth muscle antigen, a marker for the blood vessel wall (400X).

including the smallest arterioles, endoneurial capillaries, and venules.[47] It is frequently described in diabetics with various peripheral neuropathies[47–51] and rarely observed in patients with SS.[11,47] Although frequently implicated as a cause of diabetic neuropathies, its pathologic significance is not always clear. Cases that lack evidence of damage to the vessel wall or adjacent nerves would not meet the current Peripheral Nerve Society Guidelines for 'Definite" or "Probable" isolated peripheral nerve vasculitis.[52] The significance of this observation is exemplified by one report of a patient with diabetes, microvasculitis, and disabling symptoms who was treated with immunosuppressive therapy but suffered a progressively downhill course. At autopsy, no convincing pathologic evidence of isolated peripheral nerve vasculitis or systemic vasculitis was found, suggesting that microvasculitis was a nonspecific coincidental finding in the nerve biopsy from this case.[51] Thus further studies are needed before the finding of microvasculitis in a nerve biopsy from a patient with SS can be properly interpreted.

Pathophysiologic role of the sensory neuron

Extraordinary progress has been made in understanding the essential functions of sensory neurons that underlie the pathophysiologic changes in SS-associated PNS and ANS involvement. Peripheral neurons have historically been categorized into sensory and autonomic, with the former divided into large myelinated low-threshold receptors versus small-diameter high-threshold receptors for painful stimuli (nociception). However, the interpretation of molecular and morphologic studies has blurred the distinction between nociceptive and autonomic axons.[53] This has also led to an improved understanding of the neuropathic disturbances in SS and the related autoimmune connective tissue disorders.

The culprit is the small-diameter unmyelinated C-fiber, which does far more than sense pain. This evolutionarily primitive neuron functions bidirectionally with a distal axon terminal that not only transduces and transmits pain but also releases electric and paracrine chemical signals that maintain tissue homeostasis and the integrity of the skin.[54] Other C-fiber paracrine secretions modulate tissue responses to injury or threat. C-fibers release calcitonin gene—related peptide and substance P neuropeptides from their distal axon terminals. These trigger vasodilation, plasma protein extravasation, tissue edema, hemoconcentration, and leukocyte diapedesis.[55] C-fibers also modulate immune responses, with mast cells in close physical and chemical contact.[56] Signaling in C-fibers is in turn modified by inflammatory signals from different transmitters, including serotonin, histamine, glutamate, adenosine triphosphate, adenosine, substance P, calcitonin gene—related peptide, bradykinin, eicosanoids (such as prostaglandins, thromboxanes, leukotrienes, and endocannabinoids), nerve growth factor, and inflammatory cytokines. These transmitters bind to a variety of C-fiber surface receptors, including G protein—coupled receptors, transient receptor potential channels, acid-sensitive ion channels, two-pore potassium channels, and receptor tyrosine kinases,[57] that allow injury and inflammation to trigger and sensitize pain signaling. Cross talk between nociceptive and immune cells contributes to host defense and immune-mediated diseases.[58] Disturbed immunity underlies some cases of painful SFN.

In summary, transmitting pain signals is merely one part of the sensory neuron's role. To that end, the capillaries in sensory and somatic ganglia are fenestrated. This exposes the neuron cell bodies to blood-borne signals and also leaves them vulnerable to toxins, infections, and, most importantly, immune-mediated attack.[59,60]

Management and prognosis

A comprehensive neurologic assessment leads to an improved understanding of the underlying neuropathic disease process and helps the neurologist select an appropriate therapy. As discussed earlier, pathologic studies suggest that PNS involvement in SS is immune mediated and, therefore, potentially treatable with immunomodulating medications depending on the type of neuropathy and the stage of progression. A rheumatologic evaluation of the underlying systemic disease will sometimes also influence the choice of therapy. Clinical practice guidelines for the management of PNS and CNS SS are currently being developed by a national committee of experts under the auspices of the Sjögren's Syndrome Foundation, Inc. However, until these guidelines are completed, management decisions must be based on the results of uncontrolled studies, small case series/reports, and clinical experience from treating similar manifestations in related patient groups. Treatment algorithms have been reviewed.[28]

Treatment of peripheral neuropathies

Conservative measures

Some patients with mild sensory neuropathies due to SFN or axonal sensory neuropathy do well with symptomatic treatment using therapeutic doses of gabapentin or pregabalin; serotonin reuptake inhibitors (e.g., duloxetine, venlafaxine) can be substituted or added as needed.[61,62] Tricyclic antidepressants (e.g., amitriptyline), unless used in very low doses, are best avoided in this population because anticholinergic side effects can exacerbate sicca symptoms. Secondary amine tricyclics (e.g., nortriptyline, desipramine) are sometimes better tolerated. For all neuropathies, once improvement is seen, physical and occupational therapy, including gait and balance training, should be initiated if the patient has functional deficits.

Corticosteroids

Corticosteroids are widely prescribed because of their rapid onset of action and wide array of inhibitory effects on various inflammatory and immune responses. These effects include the ability to decrease vascular permeability, to inhibit migration/activation of inflammatory cells to sites of tissue injury, to inhibit polymorphonuclear and mononuclear cell function, and to inhibit various inflammatory mediators such as kinins, histamine, and prostaglandins. Steroids also have broad effects on antigen processing. This treatment is considered the first-line therapy for vasculitic peripheral neuropathies and multiple cranial neuropathies caused by vasculitis.[4,63] Some authors also recommend corticosteroids, with or without intravenous immunoglobulin (IVIg), as the first-line therapy for sensory ataxic neuronopathies[28,64]; however, this strategy has yielded variable results.[65,66] Most patients with axonal sensory or sensorimotor neuropathies do not respond well to this treatment.[34] Likewise, response to corticosteroids for most patients with SFNs is generally poor.[67] Under ideal circumstances, steroid treatment (e.g., prednisone, 1 mg/kg/day followed by a taper) should be limited to 3–6 months while attempts are made to find steroid-sparing agents (vide infra) with less toxicity. Divided doses of prednisone probably have a more potent immunosuppressive and antiinflammatory effect than a single high daily morning dose and should be administered during the first 2 weeks of therapy. Alternatively, pulse therapy using 1000 mg of intravenous (IV) methylprednisolone daily for 3–4 days on a monthly basis for the first 2–3 months is generally well tolerated, efficacious, and associated with fewer side effects than high-dose long-term oral therapy. For patients whose disease activity is under good control, efforts should be made as soon as possible to taper oral steroid therapy to an alternate day regimen in order to reduce long-term toxicity, in particular, hypothalamic pituitary axis suppression, steroid myopathy, and osteoporosis.

Cyclophosphamide

Cyclophosphamide is typically used in conjunction with corticosteroids to induce remission in patients with vasculitic neuropathies (e.g., mononeuropathy multiplex) and more severe systemic disease (e.g., CNS involvement), and 1–2 months of therapy may be required before any benefit is observed. One case report also suggested benefit when IV pulse cyclophosphamide was used as monotherapy for the treatment of SS-associated dorsal root ganglionitis.[68] Cyclophosphamide is a cytotoxic alkylating agent that induces the formation of cross-links between and within DNA strands and interferes with mitosis and cell replication. The immunosuppressive effects of cyclophosphamide stem from the absolute suppression of B and T cells, with consequent effects on both cell-mediated and humoral immunity, respectively. The recommended initial dose of IV pulse cyclophosphamide varies from 0.5 to 0.7 g/m^2 at 2-week intervals and is given initially on days 1, 15, and 30, then continued every 3 weeks until remission is obtained. A change to the use of other immunosuppressants for long-term maintenance therapy is important because cyclophosphamide is associated with numerous toxicities including infections, hemorrhagic cystitis, bladder fibrosis, bone marrow suppression, ovarian failure, bladder cancer, and hematologic malignancies.

Other immunosuppressants

Azathioprine and methotrexate may be utilized as corticosteroid-sparing agents for any steroid-responsive neuropathy or as maintenance therapy following treatment with cyclophosphamide. They may be used as single agents or in combination with other immunosuppressants. Azathioprine is an antimetabolite and purine analogue that interferes with DNA synthesis. It is associated with decreased numbers of B and T cells, as well as decreased B-cell proliferative responses and antibody synthesis. It also inhibits natural killer cell activity. It can be used for the treatment of internal organ problems in SS as well as PNS and CNS manifestations and is dosed at 2–3 mg/kg body weight administered once daily. Many experts agree that efficacious dosing is reflected by elevation of the mean corpuscular volume or can be assessed by measurement of 6-thioguanine levels, when available.[69,70] Methotrexate is an antimetabolite that inhibits folic acid metabolism and may be considered in selected patients who are intolerant to corticosteroids and azathioprine. It is also used to treat the rheumatic manifestations of SS (Chapter 11) and dosed 7.5–25 mg weekly following a regimen similar to that used for rheumatoid arthritis. Although neither azathioprine nor methotrexate is cited in the literature as primary therapy for SS-associated polyneuropathy, either may play a role in adjunctive or maintenance therapy, particularly in vasculitic neuropathies.

Mycophenolate mofetil is recommended as an alternative to azathioprine and methotrexate and has been utilized as the second-line therapy for patients with sensory ataxic neuronopathy/ganglionopathy who have failed other treatments.[71,72] It is the prodrug of mycophenolic acid and inhibits inosine monophosphate dehydrogenase required for the synthesis of DNA, thereby affecting proliferating T- and B-cells. It is administered in doses starting at 500 mg twice daily and slowly increased to 3000 mg/day in two divided doses. A pilot study[73] evaluated the efficacy and safety of mycophenolate mofetil in SS refractory to other immunosuppressive agents, noting that it was well tolerated in 8 of 11 patients; it may also be used to treat renal or interstitial lung disease in SS.[74]

Plasma exchange

Plasma exchange is a second-line treatment for all types of peripheral neuropathy refractory to conventional regimens, especially when there is a need for prompt control of disease activity. In 2010 the American Society for Apheresis updated its evidence-based review on indications for therapeutic apheresis.[75] The American Academy of Neurology completed its review of plasmapheresis in neurologic disorders the same year and published its findings in 2011.[76] Over the last 10 years, the Cochrane collaboration has been performing reviews of plasma exchange in neurologic disorders but it has been doing this for individual diseases rather than for the treatment as a whole.[77] In general, the different groups came to very similar conclusions using slightly different methods of assessment.[78] The diseases with the best data on efficacy include acute inflammatory demyelinating polyneuropathy or CIDP and paraproteinemic polyneuropathies, both of which may occur in SS albeit rarely. Additionally, five to nine sessions of plasmapheresis was reported to be effective in the treatment of two of four women with acute and subacute SS-associated sensory ataxic neuronopathy, demonstrating a favorable response within 2 weeks of therapy in those so treated.[79]

Immunoglobulin therapy

High-dose IVIg is a safe and well-tolerated treatment compared with standard corticosteroid and immunosuppressive therapy. It is recommended as the treatment for painful SFNs in SS patients in whom more conservative therapies fail or who exhibit progressive symptoms.[11,28,80–82] In some cases the response to treatment may be dramatic.[80] This therapy has also been used to successfully manage patients with axonal sensory or sensorimotor polyneuropathies who experience severe sensory symptoms or motor deficits.[11,83] As mentioned earlier, IVIg with or without corticosteroids is frequently prescribed as the first-line therapy for sensory ataxic neuronopathies, although the response may be variable.[66,71,83] One series reported benefit from using IVIg in 4 of 4 patients with radiculoneuropathy.[11] IVIg has also been recommended in cases of treatment-resistant vasculitic neuropathies related to SS and other causes.[84]

The immune-modulating and antiinflammatory actions of IVIg may be seen as early as 1 month after initiation of therapy and are cumulative; the duration of therapy is guided by clinical response and various dosing regimens have been published. Typically doses of 2 g/kg body weight per month are administered in weekly divided doses via slow drip or, alternatively, given as 0.4 g/kg/day for five consecutive days once monthly. Side effects are common and include transient headaches, fever, chills, rash, erythema, flushing, nausea, myalgias, arthralgias, abdominal cramps, chest or back pain, and, rarely, aseptic meningitis or anaphylaxis (especially in patients who are deficit in IgA). The two most important cautionary steps to assure uneventful and safe administration are adequate oral and IV prehydration and an infusion rate that does not exceed 10 g per hour. Additional strategies to manage side effects include the use of premedications and PRN medications for certain symptoms or a change to a different IVIg product. Subcutaneous immunoglobulin

(SCIg) administered at home with an infusion pump is sometimes preferred in patients with intolerable side effects from IVIg. However, the feasibility of using this therapeutic option in a given individual varies according to the total monthly dose of immunoglobulin that is required.

Biological therapy

Rituximab is a genetically engineered chimeric murine-human monoclonal IgG1 that recognizes the CD20 antigen on the surface of B-cells and is FDA-approved for the treatment of rheumatoid arthritis and antineutrophil cytoplasmic antibody—associated vasculitis. It depletes B cells through three main mechanisms: antibody-dependent cell-mediated cytotoxicity, complement-mediated cytotoxicity, and induction of apoptosis. IV rituximab is most useful in SS for the treatment of peripheral neuropathies caused by cryoglobulinemia and/or vasculitis[85,86] and is recommended for other SS-related problems as well.[87] It is usually given as two 1000-mg doses spaced 2 weeks apart. In the French Autoimmunity and Rituximab (AIR) registry, 9/10 (90%) SS patients with PNS involvement associated with cryoglobulinemia and/or vasculitis showed improvement in as early as 3 months compared ($P = .03$) with 2/7 (29%) patients who lacked these features. Rankin scores and ESSDAI scores also significantly improved in the first group when compared with the second group. Of the two responders in the second group, one had an axonal sensorimotor neuropathy, whereas the other had a painful SFN. Another case report also documented sustained remission of an axonal sensorimotor polyneuropathy associated with an IgM-κ monoclonal gammopathy in SS following treatment with rituximab.[88]

Tumor necrosis factor (TNF)-α inhibitors can be used to treat the rheumatic manifestations of SS, particularly in patients with overlapping features of rheumatoid arthritis.[87] As TNF-α regulates nicotinic responses in mixed cultures of sympathetic neurons and nonneuronal cells, there is a rationale for using these therapies in neuropathies as well.[89] In one study, anti-TNF-neutralizing antibodies reduced pain-related behavior in two different mouse models of painful mononeuropathy.[90] Infliximab was reportedly effective for the treatment of an SS-associated sensory neuropathy in a single case report[91] of a patient who received infusions of 3 mg/kg at weeks 0, 2, 6 and for every 12 weeks thereafter, without adverse side effects. Paradoxically, however, it has also been reported that SFNs can develop as a complication of TNF-α inhibitor therapy for rheumatoid arthritis.[92]

Autonomic involvement

As ANS dysfunction is most often described in SS patients with sensory neuropathies, the treatment is mostly symptomatic, and systemic therapy, when utilized, is directed at the underlying sensory neuropathy. Treatment algorithms have been most widely described for orthostatic hypotension and POTS.

The nonpharmacologic treatment of orthostatic intolerance, a frequent and often devastating feature of dysautonomia in SS, includes increased hydration and liberalization of dietary salt intake to increase blood volume in order to decrease baroreceptor sensitivity. Typical regimens include 2 L of water and 175–250 mEq of salt tablets daily. Reconditioning exercises increase plasma volume, muscle mass, and vascular tone, thereby decreasing blood pooling in the legs while standing. Avoidance of hot ambient temperatures and alcohol, which result in vasodilatation, and the use of compressive hosiery can offset the symptoms of severe hypotension. Use of medications that may aggravate orthostatic intolerance should be discontinued.

The mainstay of pharmacologic therapy for hypotension is fludrocortisone, a synthetic adrenocortical steroid that increases salt absorption from the kidney tubules and leads to an increase in BP through an increase in the total fluid volume; alternatively, midodrine, an adrenaline agonist that increases peripheral vascular resistance, may also be used to manage low BP. The starting dose of fludrocortisone is 0.1 mg once or twice daily (at 7 a.m. and/or 2 p.m.), with increases as needed, to 0.3 mg once or twice daily. Full benefit requires a high dietary salt and fluid intake. Dosing of midodrine is begun at 2.5–5 mg, one to two tablets every 3 hours. Droxidopa, a synthetic amino acid precursor that is a prodrug to the neurotransmitter norepinephrine may also be considered. Unlike midodrine, it is capable of crossing the blood-brain barrier, making it more desirable in refractory patients. The efficacy of droxidopa in improving BP occurs with a starting dose of 60 mg and it may be combined with low-dose midodrine (5 mg) for a more potent and sustained response.

Pyridostigmine is an acetylcholinesterase inhibitor that promotes ganglionic and neural transmission in both sympathetic and parasympathetic nerves[93] and may improve standing HR, diastolic BP, and symptoms of orthostatic intolerance in some patients with POTS.[94] Its use is limited by significant GI side effects. Low to moderate doses of β-blockers (e.g., propranolol) can also be used to manage symptomatic tachycardia in POTS.

The short-term benefit of IVIG for orthostatic intolerance is most likely due to concomitant prehydration with saline that is prescribed to expand the intravascular fluid volume and offset drug-induced side effects. The long-term benefit of IVIG for autonomic neuropathies remains unclear, as anecdotal reports and small case series have reported conflicting results.[11,95–97]

GI motility problems related to AN are treated as outlined in Chapter 11.

Conclusions

Peripheral and autonomic nerve manifestations frequently occur in SS and adversely affect patients' quality of life. Painful SFN and axonal sensory or sensorimotor neuropathies are most common. ANs frequently coexist with sensory neuropathies. Mononeuritis multiplex, multiple cranial neuropathies, and asymmetric axonal sensory or sensorimotor neuropathies are most frequently associated with peripheral nerve vasculitis. Disability from neuropathies in SS is due to motor deficits, ataxia, and chronic pain. A better understanding of the underlying pathophysiologic condition, including the mechanisms that cause chronic pain, and the interrelationship of various neuropathic clinical syndromes in SS will undoubtedly lead to more targeted and effective therapy in the future.

References

1. Alexander E, Provost T, Stevens M, Alexande G. Neurologic complications of primary Sjögren's syndrome. *Medicine.* 1982;61:247–257.
2. Carvajal Alegria G, Guellec D, Devauchelle-Pensec V, Saraux A. Is there specific neurological disorders of primary Sjögren's syndrome? *Jt Bone Spine.* 2015;82(2): 86–89.
3. Jamilloux Y, Magy L, Hurtevent JF, Gondran G, de Seze J, Launay D, Ly K, Lambert M, Hachulla E, Hatron P-Y, Vidal E, Fauchais A-L. Immunological profiles determine neurological involvement in Sjögren's syndrome. *Eur J Intern Med.* 2014;25:177–181.
4. Delalande S, De Seze J, Fauchais AL, Hachulla E, Stojkovic T, Ferriby D, Dubucquoi S, Pruvo JP, Vermersch P, Hatron PY. Neurologic manifestations in primary Sjögren syndrome: a study of 82 patients. *Medicine.* 2004;83(5):280–291.
5. Lafitte C, Amoura Z, Cacoub P, Pradat-Diehl P, Picq C, Salachas F, Léger JM, Piette JC, Delattre JY. Neurological complications of primary Sjögren's syndrome. *J Neurol.* 2001; 284(7):577–584.
6. Tobón GJ, Pers JO, Devauchelle-Pensec V, Youinou P. Neurological disorders in primary Sjögren's syndrome. *Autoimmune Dis.* 2012;2012:645967.
7. Newton JL, Frith J, Powell D, Hackett K, Wilton K, Bowman S, Price E, Pease C, Andrews J, Emery P, Hunter J, Gupta M, Vadivelu S, Giles I, Isenberg D, Lanyon P, Jones A, Regan M, Cooper A, Moots R, Sutcliffe N, Bombardieri M, Pitzalis C, McLaren J, Young-Min S, Dasgupta B, Griffiths B, Lendrem D, Mitchell S, Ng WF. UK primary Sjögren's syndrome registry. Autonomic symptoms are common and are associated with overall symptom burden and disease activity in primary Sjögren's syndrome. *Ann Rheum Dis.* 2011;71(12):1973–1979.
8. Suarez GA, Opfer-Gehrking TL, Offord KP, Atkinson EJ, O'Brien PC, Low PA. The Autonomic Symptom Profile: a new instrument to assess autonomic symptoms. *Neurology.* 1999;52(3):523–528.
9. Andonopoulos AP, Christodoulou J, Ballas C, Bounas A, Alexopoulos D. Autonomic cardiovascular neuropathy in Sjögren's syndrome. A controlled study. *J Rheumatol.* 1998; 25(12):2385–2388.
10. Koh J, Kwok S-K, Lee J, Park S-H. Autonomic dysfunction in primary Sjögren's syndrome: a prospective cohort analysis of 154 Korean patients. *Korean J Intern Med.* 2017;32(1):165–173.
11. Mori K, Iijima M, Koike H, Hattori N, Tanaka F, Watanabe H, Katsuno M, Fujita A, Aiba I, Ogata A, Saito T, Asakura K, Yoshida M, Hirayama M, Sobue G. The wide spectrum of clinical manifestations in Sjögren's syndrome-associated neuropathy. *Brain.* 2005;128:2518–2534.
12. Sobue G, Yasuda T, Kachi T, Sakakibara T, Mitsuma T. Chronic progressive sensory ataxic neuropathy: clinicopathological features of idiopathic and Sjögren's syndrome-associated cases. *J Neurol.* 1993;240(1):1–7.

13. Mori K, Iijima M, Sugiura M, Koike H, Hattori N, Ito H, Hirayama M, Sobue G. Sjögren's syndrome associated painful sensory neuropathy without sensory ataxia. *J Neurol Neurosurg Psychiatry*. 2003;7499:1320−1322.

14. Rafai MA, Boulaajaj FZ, Moutawakil F, Addali N, El Moutawakkil B, Fadel H, Hakim K, Bourezgui M, Sibai M, El Otmani H, Slassi I. Neurological manifestations revealing primitive Gougerot-Sjögren syndrome: 9 cases. *Jt Bone Spine*. 2009;76(2): 139−145.

15. Gøransson LG, Herigstad A, Tjensvoll AB, Harboe E, Mellgren SI, Omdal R. Peripheral neuropathy in primary sjogren syndrome: a population-based study. *Arch Neurol*. 2006; 63(11):1612−1615.

16. Andonopoulos AP, Lagos G, Drosos AA, Moutsopoulos HM. The spectrum of neurological involvement in Sjögren syndrome. *Br J Rheumatol*. 1990;29:21−23.

17. Perzyńska-Mazan J, Maślińska M, Gasik R. Neurological manifestations of primary Sjögren's syndrome. *Reumatologia*. 2018;56(2):99−105.

18. Colaci M, Cassone G, Manfredi A, Sebastiani M, Giuggioli D, Ferri C. Neurologic complications associated with Sjogren's disease: case reports and modern pathogenic dilemma. *Case Rep Neurol Med*. 2014;2014:590292.

19. Chan AC, Wilder-Smith EP. Small fiber neuropathy: getting bigger!. *Muscle Nerve*. 2016;53:671−682.

20. Haensch CA, Tosch M, Katona I, Weis J, Isenmann S. Small-fiber neuropathy with cardiac denervation in postural tachycardia syndrome. *Muscle Nerve*. 2014;50(6), 956−561.

21. Font J, Ramos-Casals M, de la Red G, Pou A, Casanova A, Garcia-Carrasco M, Cervera R, Molina JA, Valls J, Bové A, Ingelmo M, Graus F. Pure sensory neuropathy in primary Sjogren's syndrome. Longterm prospective followup and review of the literature. *J Rheumatol*. 2003;30(7):1552−1557.

22. Gregg EW, Sorlie P, Paulose-Ram R, Gu Q, Eberhardt MS, Wolz M, Burt V, Curtin L, Engelgau M, Geiss L, 1999−2000 National Health And Nutrition Examination Survey. Prevalence of lower-extremity disease in the US adult population >=40 years of age with and without diabetes: 1999−2000 national health and nutrition examination survey. *Diabetes Care*. 2004;27(7):1591−1597.

23. Bakkers M, Faber CG, Hoeijmakers JGJ, Lauria G, Merkies IS. Small-fiber, large impact: quality of life in small-fiber neuropathy. *Muscle Nerve*. 2014;49(3):329−336.

24. Malinow K, Yannakakis GD, Glusman SM, Edlow DW Griffin J, Powell DL, Ramsey-Goldman DR, Eidelman BH, Medsger Jr TA, Alexander E. Subacute sensory neuronopathy secondary to dorsal root ganglionitis in primary Sjögren's syndrome. *Ann Neurol*. 1986;20(4):535−537.

25. Griffin JW, Cornblath DR, Alexander E, Campbell J, Low PA, Bird S, Feldman EL. Ataxic sensory neuropathy and dorsal root ganglionitis associated with Sjögren's syndrome. *Ann Neurol*. 1990;27(3):304−315.

26. Mori K, Koike H, Misu K, Hattori N, Ichimura M, Sobue G. Spinal cord magnetic resonance imaging demonstrates sensory neuronal involvement and clinical severity in neuronopathy associated with Sjögren's syndrome. *J Neurol Neurosurg Psychiatry*. 2001;71(4):488−492.

27. Birnbaum J, Duncan T, Owoyemi K, Wang KC, Carrino J, Chhabra A. Use of a novel high-resolution magnetic resonance neurography protocol to detect abnormal dorsal root Ganglia in Sjogren patients with neuropathic pain: case series of 10 patients and review of the literature. *Medicine*. 2014;93(3):121−134.

28. McCoy S, Baer A. Neurological complications of Sjögren's syndrome: diagnosis and management. *Curr Treatm Opt Rheumatol*. 2017;3(4):275–288.
29. Grant I, Hunder G, Hamburger H, Dyck P. Peripheral neuropathy associated with sicca complex. *Neurology*. 1997;48:855–862.
30. Awad A, Mathew S, Katirji B. Acute motor axonal neuropathy in association with Sjögren syndrome. *Muscle Nerve*. 2010;42(5):828–830.
31. Mochizuki H, Kamakura K, Masaki T, Hirata A, Nakamura R, Motoyoshi K. Motor dominant neuropathy in Sjögren's syndrome: report of two cases. *Intern Med*. 2002; 41:142–146.
32. Zahlane S, Louhab N, El Mellakh M, Kissani N. Anterior horn syndrome: a rare manifestation of primary Sjögren's syndrome. *Jt Bone Spine*. 2016;83(4):448–450.
33. Ferrante M. Electrodiagnostic studies in motor disorders [Chapter 5]. In: Younger DS, ed. *Motor disorders*. 3rd ed. Connecticut: (E-Book). Rothstein Publishers; 2015:83–106.
34. Gutierrez J, Younger DS. *Autonomic electrophysiologic assessment* [Chapter 7]. *Motor disorders*. 3rd ed. Connecticut: (E-Book). Rothstein Publishers; 2015:117–128.
35. Bromberg MB. Review of the evolution of electrodiagnostic criteria for chronic inflammatory demyelinating polyradiculo-neuropathy. *Muscle Nerve*. 2011;43:780–794.
36. Wieling W, Shepherd JT. Initial and delayed circulatory responses to orthostatic stress in normal humans and in subjects with orthostatic intolerance. *Int Angiol*. 1992;11:69–82.
37. Sakakibara R, Hirano S, Asahina M, Sawai S, Nemoto Y, Hiraga A, Uchiyama T, Hattori T. Primary Sjogren's syndrome presenting with generalized autonomic failure. *Eur J Neurol*. 2004;11:635–638.
38. Assessment: clinical autonomic testing report of the therapeutics and technology assessment subcommittee of the American Academy of neurology. *Neurology*. 1996;46: 873–888.
39. Frith J. Diagnosing orthostatic hypotension: a narrative review of the evidence. *Br Med Bull*. 2015;115(1):123–134.
40. De Girolami U, Carlini P, Amato AA, Younger DS. Muscle and nerve biopsy pathology [Chapter 8]. In: Younger DS, ed. *Motor disorders*. 3rd ed. Connecticut: (E-Book). Rothstein Publishers; 2015:129–145.
41. Agadi JB, Raghav G, Mahadevan A, Shankar SK. Usefulness of superficial peroneal nerve/peroneus brevis muscle biopsy in the diagnosis of vasculitic neuropathy. *J Clin Neurosci*. 2012;19(10):1392–1396.
42. Kaltreider HL, Talal N. The neuropathy of Sjögren's syndrome: trigeminal nerve involvement. *Ann Intern Med*. 1969;70:751–762.
43. Kennett RP, Harding AE. Peripheral neuropathy associated with the sicca syndrome. *J Neurol Neurosurg Psychiatry*. 1986;49:90–92.
44. Mellgren SI, Conn DL, Stevens JC, Dyck PJ. Peripheral neuropathy in primary Sjögren's syndrome. *Neurology*. 1989;39(3):390–394.
45. Murata Y, Maeda K, Kawai H, Terashima T, Okabe H, Kashiwagi A, Yasuda H. Antiganglion neuron antibodies correlate with neuropathy in Sjögren's syndrome. *Neuroreport*. 2005;16(7):677–681.
46. Park K, Haberberger RV, Gordon TP, Jackson MW. Antibodies interfering with the type 3 muscarinic receptor pathway inhibit gastrointestinal motility and cholinergic neurotransmission in Sjögren's syndrome. *Arthritis Rheum*. 2011;63(5):1426–1434.
47. Gwathmey KG., Tracy JA., Dyck PJB.. Peripheral nerve vasculitis: classification and disease associations. In. Younger DS. The vasculitides; 2nd ed.. vol. 2. Nova Science: New York, 241-267. [Chapter 12].

48. Younger DS, Rosoklija G, Hays AP, Trojaborg W, Latov N. Diabetic peripheral neuropathy: a clinicopathologic and immunohistochemical analysis of sural nerve biopsies. *Muscle Nerve.* 1996;19(6):722−727.

49. Dyck PJB, Windebank AJ. Diabetic and nondiabetic lumbosacral radiculoplexus neuropathies: new insights into pathophysiology and treatment. *Muscle Nerve.* 2002;25: 477−491.

50. Younger DS. Diabetic neuropathy: a clinical and neuropathological study of 107 patients. *Neurol Res Int.* 2010;2010, 140379.

51. Younger DS. Diabetic lumbosacral radiculoplexus neuropathy: a postmortem studied patient and review of the literature. *J Neurol.* 2011;258:1364−1367.

52. Collins MP, Dyck PJ, Gronseth GS, Guillevin L, Hadden RD, Heuss D, Léger JM, Notermans NC, Pollard JD, Said G, Sobue G, Vrancken AF, Kissel JT. Peripheral Nerve Society. Peripheral Nerve Society Guideline on the classification, diagnosis, investigation, and immunosuppressive therapy of non-systemic vasculitic neuropathy: executive summary. *J Peripher Nerv Syst.* 2010;15:176−184.

53. Oaklander AL. Immunotherapy prospects for painful small-fiber sensory neuropathies and ganglionopathies. *Neurotherapeutics.* 2015;13(1):108−117.

54. Fink E, Oaklander AL. Small-fiber neuropathy: answering the burning questions. *Sci Aging Knowl Environ.* 2006;2006(6):pe7.

55. Hsieh ST, Lin WM. Modulation of keratinocyte proliferation by skin innervation. *J Investig Dermatol.* 1999;113:579−586.

56. Levine J, Dardick SJ, Basbaum AI, Scipio E. Reflex neurogenic inflammation 1. Contribution of the peripheral nervous system to spatially remote inflammatory responses that follow injury. *J Neurosci.* 1985;5:1380−1386.

57. Egan CL, Viglione-Schneck MJ, Walsh LJ, Green B, Trojanowski J, Whitaker-Menezes D, Murphy G. Characterization of unmyelinated axons uniting epidermal and dermal immune cells in primate and murine skin. *J Cutan Pathol.* 1998;25:20−29.

58. Basbaum AI, Bautista DM, Scherrer G, Julius D. Cellular and molecular mechanisms of pain. *Cell.* 2009;139(2):267−284.

59. McMahon SB, Russa FL, Bennett DL. Crosstalk between the nociceptive and immune systems in host defence and disease. *Nat Rev Neurosci.* 2015;19:389−402.

60. Kuntzer T, Antoine JC, Steck AJ. Clinical features and pathophysiological basis of sensory neuronopathies (ganglionopathies). *Muscle Nerve.* 2004;30:255−268.

61. Moulin DE, Clark AJ, Gilron I, Ware MA, Watson CP, Sessle BJ, Coderre T, Morley-Forster PK, Stinson J, Boulanger A, Peng P, Finley GA, Taenzer P, Squire P, Dion D, Cholkan A, Gilani A, Gordon A, Henry J, Jovey R, Lynch M, Mailis-Gagnon A, Panju A, Rollman GB, Velly A, Pain Society C. Pharmacological management of chronic neuropathic pain − consensus statement and guidelines from the Canadian Pain Society. *Pain Res Manag.* 2007;12(1):13−21.

62. Dworkin RH, O'Connor AB, Backonja M, Farrar JT, Finnerup NB, Jensen TS, Kalso EA, Loeser JD, Miaskowski C, Nurmikko TJ, Portenoy RK, Rice AS, Stacey BR, Treede RD, Turk DC, Wallace MS. Pharmacologic management of neuropathic pain: evidence-based recommendations. *Pain.* 2007;132(3):237−251.

63. Schaublin GA, Michet Jr CJ, Dyck PJ, Burns TM. An update on the classification and treatment of vasculitic neuropathy. *Lancet Neurol.* 2017;4(12):853−865.

64. Sheikh SI, Amato AA. The dorsal root ganglion under attack: the acquired sensory ganglionopathies. *Pract Neurol.* 2010;10:326−334.

65. Berkowitz AL, Samuels MA. The neurology of Sjögren's syndrome and the rheumatology of peripheral neuropathy and myelitis. *Pract Neurol.* 2014;14(1):14−22.

66. Takahashi Y, Takata T, Hoshino M, Sakurai M, Kanazawa I. Benefit of IVIG for long-standing ataxic sensory neuronopathy with Sjögren's syndrome. IV immunoglobulin. *Neurology.* 2003;60(3):503−505.

67. Birnbaum J. Peripheral nervous system manifestations of Sjögren syndrome: clinical patterns, diagnostic paradigms, etiopathogenesis, and therapeutic strategies. *Neurologist.* 2010;16(5):287−297.

68. Kastrup O, Maschke M, Diener HC. Pulse-cyclophosphamide in the treatment of ataxic sensory and cranial neuropathy associated with Sjögren syndrome [Letter]. *Clin Neurol Neurosurg.* 2005;107:440−441.

69. Decaux G, Prospert F, Horsmans Y, Desager JP. Relationship between red cell mean corpuscular volume and 6-thioguanine nucleotides in patients treated with azathioprine. *J Lab Clin Med.* 2000;135(3):256−262.

70. Yang N, Jiang Q. Measuring clinical efficacy of azathioprine in myasthenia gravis with mean corpuscular volume. *Neurology.* 2016;86(16 Supplement). P5.036.

71. Pereira PR, Viala K, Maisonobe T, Haroche J, Mathian A, Hié M, Amoura Z, Cohen Aubart F, et al. Sjögren sensory neuronopathy (Sjögren Ganglionopathy): long-term outcome and treatment response in a series of 13 cases. *Medicine.* 2016;95(19):e3632.

72. Danieli M, Pettinari L, Morariu R, Monteforte F, ogullo F. Intravenous immunoglobulin and mycophenolate mofetil for long-standing sensory neuronopathy in Sjögren's syndrome. *Case Reports Immunol.* 2012;2012:186320.

73. Willeke P, Schluter B, Becker H, Schotte H, Domschke W, Gaubitz M. Mycophenolate treatment in patients with primary Sjögren's syndrome: a pilot trial. *Arthritis Res Ther.* 2007;9:R115.

74. Vivino FB, Bunya VY, Massaro-Giordano G, Johr CR, Giattino SL, Schorpion A, Shafer B, Peck A, Sivils K, Rasmussen A, JA C, He J, Ambrus Jr JL. Sjögren's syndrome: an update on disease pathogenesis, clinical manifestations and treatment. *Clin Immunol.* 2019;203:81−121.

75. Szczepiorkowski ZM, Winters JL, Bandarenko N, Kim HC, Linenberger ML, Marques MB, Sarode R, Schwartz J, Weinstein R, Shaz BH. Guidelines on the use of therapeutic apheresis in clinical practice—evidence-based approach from the apheresis applications committee of the American society for apheresis. *J Clin Apher.* 2010;25: 83−177.

76. Cortese I, Chaudhry V, So YT, Cantor F, Cornblath DR, Rae-Grant A. Assessment subcommittee of the American Academy of neurology: report of the therapeutics and technology evidence-based guideline update: plasmapheresis in neurologic disorders. *Neurology.* 2011;76:294−300.

77. Mehndiratta MM, Hughes RAC, Agarwal P. Plasma exchange for chronic inflammatory demyelinating polyradiculoneuropathy. *Cochrane Database Syst Rev.* 2004, CD003906.

78. Cortese I, Cornblath DR. Therapeutic plasma exchange in neurology: 2012. *J Clin Apher.* 2013;28:16−19.

79. Chen WH, Yeh JH, Chiu HC. Plasmapheresis in the treatment of ataxic sensory neuropathy associated with Sjögren's syndrome. *Eur Neurol.* 2001;45(4):270−274.

80. Kizawa M, Mori K, Iijima M, Koike H, Hattori N, Sobue G. Intravenous immunoglobulin treatment in painful sensory neuropathy without sensory ataxia associated with Sjögren's syndrome. *J Neurol Neurosurg Psychiatry.* 2006;77:967−969.

81. Wakasugi D, Kato T, Gono T, Ito E, Nodera H, Kawaguchi Y, Yamanaka H, Hara M. Extreme efficacy of intravenous immunoglobulin therapy for severe burning pain in a patient with small fiber neuropathy associated with primary Sjögren's syndrome. *Mod Rheumatol.* 2009;19(4):437−440.

82. Morozumi S, Kawagashira Y, Iijima M, Koike H, Hattori N, Katsuno M, Tanaka F, Sobue G. Intravenous immunoglobulin treatment for painful sensory neuropathy associated with Sjogren's syndrome. *J Neurol Sci.* 2009;279(1−2):57−61.

83. Rist S, Sellam J, Hachulla E, Sordet C, Puechal X, Hatron PY, Benhamou CL, Sibilia J, Mariette X, Club Rhumatismes et Inflammation. Experience of intravenous immunoglobulin therapy in neuropathy associated with primary Sjögren's syndrome: a national multicentric retrospective study. *Arthritis Care Res.* 2011;63(9):1339−1344.

84. Levy Y, Uziel Y, Zandman G, Amital H, Sherer Y, Langevitz P, Goldman B, Shoenfeld Y. Intravenous immunoglobulins in peripheral neuropathy associated with vasculitis. *Ann Rheum Dis.* 2003;62:1221−1223.

85. Seror R, Sordet C, Guillevin L, Hachulla E, Masson C, Ittah M, Candon S, Le Guern V, Aouba A, Sibilia J, Gottenberg JE, Mariette X. Tolerance and efficacy of rituximab and changes in serum B cell biomarkers in patients with systemic complications of primary Sjögren's syndrome. *Ann Rheum Dis.* 2006;66:351−357.

86. Mekinian A, Ravaud P, Hatron PY, Larroche C, Leone J, Gombert B, Hamidou M, Cantagrel A, Marcelli C, Rist S, Breban M, Launay D, Fain O, Gottenberg JE, Mariette X. Efficacy of rituximab in primary Sjögren's syndrome with peripheral nervous system involvement: results from the AIR registry. *Ann Rheum Dis.* 2012;71(1): 84−87.

87. Carsons SE, Vivino FB, Parke A, Carteron N, Sankar V, Brasington R, Brennan MT, Ehlers W, Fox R, Scofield H, Hammitt KM, Birnbaum J, Kassan S, Mandel S. Treatment guidelines for rheumatologic manifestations of Sjögren's syndrome: use of biologic agents, management of fatigue, and inflammatory musculoskeletal pain. *Arthritis Care Res.* 2017;69(4):517−527.

88. Pertovaara M, Korpela M. Sustained response to rituximab in a patient with Sjögren's syndrome and severe refractory polyneuropathy. *Clin Exp Rheumatol.* 2012;30:808.

89. Soliven B, Wang N. Tumor necrosis factor-α regulates nicotinic responses in mixed cultures of sympathetic neurons and nonneuronal cells. *J Neurochem.* 1995;64:883−894.

90. Sommer C, Lindenlaub T, Teuteberg P, et al. Anti-TNF-neutralizing antibodies reduce pain-related behavior in two different mouse models of painful mononeuropathy. *Brain Res.* 2001;913:86−89.

91. Caroyer J-M, Manto MU, Steinfeld SD. Severe sensory neuronopathy responsive to infliximab in primary Sjogren syndrome. *Neurology.* 2002;59:1113−1114.

92. Birnbaum J, Clifton O, Bingham C. Non-length-dependent and length-dependent small-fiber neuropathies associated with tumor necrosis factor (TNF)-inhibitor therapy in patients with rheumatoid arthritis: expanding the spectrum of neurological disease associated with TNF-inhibitors. *Semin Arthritis Rheum.* 2014;43(5):638−647.

93. Gales B, Gales M. Pyridostigmine in the treatment of orthostatic intolerance. *Ann Pharmacother.* 2007;41:314−318.

94. Kanjwal K, Karabin K, Sheikh M, Elmer L, Kanjwal Y, Saeed B, Grubb B. Pyridostigmine in the treatment of postural orthostatic tachycardia: a single-center experience. *Pacing Clin Electrophysiol.* 2011;34(6):750−755.

95. Dupond J-L, Helder g, Wazieres B. Five year efficacy of intravenous gammaglobulin to treat dysautonomia in Sjögren's syndrome. *Am J Med.* 1999;106:125.

96. Cook G, Landau M. Empiric treatment of suspected autoimmune autonomic neuropathies. *Neurology*. 2016;86(16 Supplement) (P5.110).

97. Gibbons C, Vernino S, Freeman F. Combined immunomodulatory therapy in autoimmune autonomic ganglionopathy. *Arch Neurol*. 2008;65(2):213−217.

Diagnosis and management of central nervous system Sjögren's syndrome

10

**Pantelis P. Pavlakis, MD, PhD[1], Theresa Lawrence—Ford, MD[2],
Shalini Mahajan, MD[3], Janet Lewis, MD[4], Arun Varadhachary, MD[5], Ianna Briggs[6],
Elisabeth Goldberg, LMFT[6], Daniel J. Wallace, MD, FACP, MACR[7],
Steven Mandel, MD[8]**

[1]Assistant Attending, Department of Neurology, Hospital for Special Surgery, New York, NY, United States; [2]Medical Director, CEO, Rheumatology, North Georgia Rheumatology Group, Gwinnett County, GA, United States; [3]Assistant Professor, Department of Neurology, Cedars Sinai Medical Center Los Angeles, CA, United States; [4]Associate Professor, Chief, Division of Rheumatology, University of Virginia, Charlottesville, VA, United States; [5]Associate Professor of Neurology, Washington University School of Medicine in St. Louis, Saint Louis, MO, United States; [6]PLLC, Research Assistant, Neurology, Zuckerberg School of Medicine, New York City, NY, United States; [7]Associate Director, Rheumatology Fellowship Program, Board of Governors, Cedars-Sinai Medical Center, Professor of Medicine, David Geffen School of Medicine at UCLA, Los Angeles, CA, Unites States; [8]Clinical Professor of Neurology, Donald and Barbara Zucker School of Medicine at Hofstra/Northwell, Lenox Hill Hospital, New York City, NY, United States

Prevalence

Large-scale population studies have estimated the frequency of central nervous system (CNS) disease among Sjögren's syndrome (SS) patients at 2%−5%.[1,2] However, the prevalence of CNS involvement in SS remains controversial, with other studies showing wide variation. This variation can be accounted for by the differences in both the diagnostic criteria for SS and what constitutes a neurologic manifestation of SS. Additional selection bias of patients referred for studies may also impact cohort results. CNS manifestations may often precede the diagnosis of SS, which further contributes to the challenges in determining its frequency.[1]

Pathophysiology

Although there has been a concerted effort in describing the pathogenesis of CNS manifestations in SS, the mechanisms responsible for most syndromes are generally unknown. Several hypotheses have been proposed to address the underlying pathogenetic mechanisms. As there is significant diversity among the clinical phenotypes observed, it is reasonable to assume that discrete pathogenetic mechanisms may lead to different clinical syndromes. Elaine Alexander, MD, and her group at the Johns Hopkins University were the first to describe the association of CNS disease with SS.[3] Since then, extensive evidence has been compiled to suggest that the mechanisms that cause these manifestations are immune-mediated.

The underlying cause of the dysregulated immune response against self is unknown. However, Alexander et al.[4] felt that it was inherent that the brain, as a part of the nervous system, would not be spared from potential extraglandular complications and the resultant inciting events.

The presence of serum autoantibodies in CNS disease associated with SS has been documented, and they include antinuclear antibodies (ANAs), rheumatoid factor, anti-SSA/-Ro antibodies, and anti-SSB/La antibodies.[4] However, lack of positivity for antibodies does not exclude a diagnosis. It has been shown that CNS complications occur with approximately equal frequency in patients who are SSA positive or negative,[5] although antibody-positive patients were initially reported to have a more aggressive form of the disease.[4] It has also been observed, however, that patients with CNS involvement have the same immunogenetic HLA class II DRB1 genetic profile as patients without CNS disease, regardless of the SSA antibody status. Alexander et al. evaluated the cerebrospinal fluid (CSF) of patients with active CNS-SS disease and found mononuclear pleocytosis, elevated protein levels, and an elevated IgG index with one or more oligoclonal bands, suggesting a breach of the blood-brain barrier by inflammatory lymphocyte infiltration and resultant synthesis of intrathecal IgG antibodies.[4]

In preclinical studies, Bacman et al.[6] identified the presence of IgG autoantibodies against M3 muscarinic acetylcholine receptors (mAChR). These autoantibodies have been linked to secretory dysfunction of exocrine glands[7–9] and also interact with cerebral mAChRs expressed on the surface of cells in the frontal cortex.[10] The presence of these antibodies reveals agonist activity associated with M1 and M3 mAChR activation, thus promoting nitrous oxide (NO) and prostaglandin biosynthesis.[11] Cumulatively, these findings suggest that anti-mAChR antibodies could promote pathologic neuroinflammation in the cerebral cortex. However, the presence and pathogenetic role of these antibodies is yet to be confirmed in patients with SS and CNS involvement.

Autoantibodies against ion channels or neuronal surface neurotransmitter receptors are known to cause autoimmune encephalitis syndromes in patients without systemic autoimmune disease.[12] Antibodies against N-acetyl-D-glutamate receptor 2 (NR2) glutamate receptors have been identified in patients with systemic lupus erythematosus (SLE) and less frequently in those with SS. However, studies have failed to associate the presence of these autoantibodies with specific neurologic syndromes in SS.[13]

Autoinvasive lymphocytes will likely enter the exocrine glands and other tissues such as the brain, induce cell destruction, and activate proinflammatory cytokines, autoantibodies, and matrix metalloproteinases.[14,15] Intrathecal activation of the terminal pathway of complement has also been documented.[16,17] One such hypothesis is that direct infiltration of the CNS by mononuclear cells is responsible for the neurologic disease.[18] Support to this hypothesis comes from CSF abnormalities of patients with CNS disease, showing evidence of blood-brain barrier breach and intrathecal inflammation, as described earlier.

Additionally, the vascular injury seen in CNS disease in SS may be related to microvasculopathy from endothelial damage mediated by antineuronal antibodies and anti-Ro antibodies, leading to small infarcts.[4,15] In these patients, positive serum anti-SSA autoantibodies were associated with more severe neurologic disease and signs of small vessel vasculitis on cerebral angiography. However, both anti-SSA-positive and anti-SSA-negative SS patients can develop CNS involvement. No biomarker has yet been unequivocally associated with CNS involvement.[19] Antineutrophil cytoplasmic antibodies and anticardiolipin antibodies have not been found to be associated with CNS involvement in SS.[17] It has been proposed that ischemia secondary to small vessel vasculitis may be responsible for some of the signs and symptoms in CNS involvement in SS. According to angiographic studies, ischemia may play a role secondary to diffuse small vessel vasculitis.[16,20–22] Morreale et al.[23] reported ultrasonographic abnormalities suggestive of microvasculopathy in a case series of primary SS patients undergoing transcranial Doppler ultrasound. These were associated with cognitive dysfunction and psychiatric symptoms as well as the presence of anti-Ro antibodies, but not with the presence of vasculitic brain lesions. These abnormalities suggest possible endothelial dysfunction of the cerebral microcirculation and not a hypercoagulable state as seen in the antiphospholipid syndrome.

Major clinical syndromes
Focal/multifocal disease

Focal or multifocal neurologic deficits, localized to the CNS, have been described in patients with primary SS.[3,17,24] Presenting manifestations vary depending on the area of the nervous system affected and can include aphasia, dysarthria, focal/multifocal weakness or sensory loss, ataxia, myelopathy, or optic neuritis (see Table 10.1). As focal or multifocal neurologic deficits are thought to represent either vasculitis or demyelination, their onset is typically subacute, but individual presentations may vary. They may be the presenting manifestation of SS or may be associated with systemic disease; in the latter case, these are often associated with symptoms, or serologic markers of active systemic disease, which can be helpful in differentiating them from other mimic syndromes (see Tables 10.2 and 10.3).

Demyelinating syndromes secondary to SS include optic neuritis, transverse myelitis, and multiple sclerosis (MS)-like disease. Additionally, coexisting bona fide neuromyelitis optica (NMO) and MS can be seen in patients with primary SS. Optic neuritis typically presents with acute, or subacute, onset of vision loss and blurry vision with or without eye pain. Corresponding pupillary abnormalities (poorly reactive or nonreactive pupil, afferent pupillary defect) and papilledema are present on examination. Myelopathy typically presents with motor deficits spanning from the affected segments to the segments below, and a sensory level. Gait instability and/or paresis are present in more severe cases, depending on the extent of cord involvement. Sphincter abnormalities, initially in the form of urinary

Table 10.1 Central neurologic syndromes associated with Sjögren's syndrome.

Focal disease	Diffuse disease
Focal/multifocal deficits	Aseptic meningitis
MS-like disease/NMO	Cognitive dysfunction
Optic neuropathy	Psychiatric manifestations
Myelopathy	Seizures
Motor neuronopathy	
Cerebellar ataxia	
Asymptomatic white matter disease	

MS, *multiple sclerosis;* NMO, *neuromyelitis optica.*

Table 10.2 Differentiation of SS-associated demyelinating disease from MS and NMO.

	SS with CNS involvement	MS	NMO
Clinical or serologic features of active systemic disease Imaging findings	May be present or absent	Absent	Absent
Brain white matter lesions	Location, orientation, and morphology may vary	Typically ovoid Oriented perpendicular to ventricles	Location, orientation, and morphology may vary
Cord lesions	Cord lesions spanning less than three spinal segments	Cord lesions spanning less than three spinal segments	Cord lesions spanning more than three spinal segments
Other characteristic findings	Basal ganglia lesions	Corpus callosum lesions Posterior fossa lesions more common Central vein sign	Hypothalamic lesions
Oligoclonal bands	Usually absent or <3 Unlikely if >10	Usually >3 Highly predictive if >10	Usually absent or <3
NMO-IgG (aquaporin-4 antibodies)	Negative	Negative	Positive in 80% of cases

CNS, *central nervous system;* MS, *multiple sclerosis;* NMO, *neuromyelitis optica;* SS, *Sjögren's syndrome.*

Table 10.3 Differential diagnosis of central nervous system Sjögren's syndrome.

Focal disease	
Focal/multifocal deficits	Other systemic autoimmune diseases (i.e., systemic lupus erythematosus, antiphospholipid syndrome, sarcoidosis, Behcet disease) Stroke (in cases with acute onset of symptoms) Primary CNS vasculitis Infectious (HSV, VZV, CMV, HIV, progressive multifocal leukoencephalopathy) Septic embolism/endocarditis ADEM Multiple sclerosis Prion disease (Creutzfeldt-Jakob disease) Paraneoplastic Metabolic disorders
Optic neuropathy	Other systemic autoimmune diseases Temporal arteritis MS NMO Anterior ischemic optic neuropathy Toxic (ethambutol, methanol toxicity) Hereditary (Leber hereditary optic neuropathy)
Myelopathy	Idiopathic transverse myelitis MS NMO Paraneoplastic Infectious/postinfectious (enterovirus, EBV, CMV, HTLV, HIV, *Brucella*) Metabolic (vitamin B_{12} and copper deficiency, adrenomyeloneuropathy) Spinal stenosis
Motor neuronopathy (ALS-like syndrome)	ALS Multifocal motor neuropathy Demyelinating disease (MS, NMO) Other systemic autoimmune diseases Myasthenia gravis (in cases with prominent bulbar involvement) Metabolic (copper deficiency, adrenomyeloneuropathy, primary hyperparathyroidism) Infectious/postinfectious (HTLV, WNV)
Cerebellar ataxia	Stroke Infectious/postinfectious Multiple sclerosis ADEM Paraneoplastic Prion disease (Creutzfeldt-Jakob disease) Toxic (alcohol, phenytoin, lithium, barbiturates) Cerebellar tumors

Continued

Table 10.3 Differential diagnosis of central nervous system Sjögren's syndrome.—*cont'd*

Focal disease		
Asymptomatic white matter disease	Neurodegenerative diseases (olivopontocerebellar degeneration) Hereditary (spinocerebellar ataxias, Friedreich ataxia)
	Vascular risk factors (diabetes mellitus, hypertension, hyperlipidemia) Migraines Traumatic brain injury

Diffuse disease	
Aseptic meningitis	Other systemic autoimmune diseases (sarcoidosis, rheumatoid pachymeningitis) Infectious meningitis (HSV, Coxsackie virus, LCMV, mumps, CMV, HIV, Lyme disease, *Coxiella*, leptospirosis, *Cryptococcus*, syphilis, tuberculosis) Meningeal carcinomatosis Medications (intravenous immunoglobulin, NSAIDs) Primary CNS vasculitis
Cognitive dysfunction/ psychiatric manifestations/ seizures	Primary neurodegenerative diseases (Alzheimer disease, frontotemporal dementia, vascular dementia) Other autoimmune diseases Toxic-metabolic encephalopathy (medications, liver disease, kidney disease, electrolyte disturbances, non-CNS infections, vitamin B_{12} deficiency, thiamine deficiency, uncontrolled hypothyroidism) Infectious meningoencephalitis (acute/subacute onset) Autoimmune encephalitis (acute/subacute onset or rapidly progressive cognitive dysfunction)

ADEM, *acute disseminated encephalomyelitis*; ALS, *amyotrophic lateral sclerosis*; CMV, *cytomega-lovirus*; CNS, *central nervous system*; EBV, *Epstein-Barr virus*; HIV, *human immunodeficiency virus*; HSV, *herpes simplex virus*; HTLV, *human T-lymphotropic virus*; LCMV, *lymphocytic choriomeningitis virus*; MS, *multiple sclerosis*; NMO, *neuromyelitis optica*; NSAIDs, *nonsteroidal antiinflammatory drugs*; SS, *Sjögren's syndrome*; VZV, *varicella zoster virus*; WNV, *West Nile virus*.

retention and later in the form of hyperactive bladder and urge incontinence, are also typically present. Hyperreflexia and spasticity can be seen below the affected segments, although these are usually not evident in the acute phase.

NMO and MS may also overlap with SS and are further discussed later. There is significant overlap in the clinical and imaging features of these syndromes, which makes their distinction challenging in clinical practice (also see Table 10.2). Presence of active systemic disease usually favors a cause secondary to SS, whereas findings of longitudinally extensive transverse myelitis (LETM), myelitis spanning more than three spinal segments) or aquaporin-4 antibodies are strongly predictive of NMO. Increased white matter lesion burden can also be seen on brain MRI of patient's with SS, without correlating neurologic deficits.

Cerebellar ataxia and degeneration have also been described in patients with SS.[25,26] Onset may be acute, subacute, or more insidious. Patients may complain of clumsiness or incoordination, imbalance, speech or swallowing problems, vertigo, or nausea. Intention tremor, dysdiadochokinesia, gait instability, extraocular movement abnormalities, or dysarthria may be present on examination. Cerebellar atrophy, or signal abnormalities, can be present on MRI.

A motor neuronopathy has been described to occur rarely in patients with SS.[24,27,28] Patients present with progressive weakness, atrophy, muscle twitching due to fasciculations and upper motor neuron signs, and otherwise identical clinical and electrodiagnostic features of amyotrophic lateral sclerosis. However, there have been isolated cases reported with unusually protracted, slowly progressive disease.[27]

Demyelinating syndromes
Neuromyelitis optica

NMO is a demyelinating disease of the central nervous system, typically presenting as optic neuritis and/or longitudinally extensive transverse myelitis (LETM).[29] Brain involvement ranges from minimal to typically silent white matter lesions, which do not fulfill criteria for multiple sclerosis (MS).[29] NMO was initially regarded as a variant of MS (opticospinal MS). However, after the discovery that a specific immunofluorescence pattern of serum reactivity against Virchow's spaces, brain vessels and pia matter (i.e. NMO-IgG) [30] was caused by antibodies against the water channel aquaporin-4,[31] NMO is now considered a separate entity with distinct clinicopathological features and response to immunomodulatory treatments.[32] Apart from the typical presentation described earlier, the spectrum of NMO can include other manifestations such as intractable vomiting, hiccups, and acute brainstem syndromes; narcolepsy or endocrinopathies can also be seen due to hypothalamic involvement.[33] Cases of NMO with SS have also been reported to present with tumefactive cerebral involvement.[34,35] NMO typically follows a relapsing course and is considered to have a worse prognosis than MS.[32]

According to the 2015 International Consensus Diagnostic Criteria for NMO,[36] diagnosis can be made in patients with positive NMO-IgG/anti-aquaporin-4 antibodies and typical clinical syndromes including optic neuritis, LETM, brainstem syndromes, and symptomatic narcolepsy. The diagnosis can also be made in seronegative patients who manifest two of the typical clinical syndromes, if other causes are excluded and specific imaging criteria are met.[36] It is important to differentiate NMO from MS, as their response to immunomodulatory treatments differs; relapsing-remitting MS responds to interferon beta-1b treatment and other disease-specific immunomodulatory agents, whereas NMO responds better to immunosuppressive agents such as rituximab and azathioprine than to interferon beta-1b.[32]

The overlap between systemic autoimmune diseases, including SS, and NMO has been long known. Organ-specific and systemic autoimmune diseases are present in up to one-third of patients with NMO with a relapsing course.[36] SS and SLE, in particular, seem to be common autoimmune comorbidities.[37,38] Conversely, antibodies against aquaporin-4 have been detected in patients with SS and optic neuritis, and/or LETM , who fulfill the diagnostic criteria for NMO.[39,40] SS and NMO have also been reported to coexist in the pediatric population.[41]

There is also significant overlap in serologic findings among transverse myelitis, NMO, and systemic autoimmune diseases. Anti-Ro antibodies have been found in idiopathic transverse myelitis cases in the absence of other features suggestive of NMO or SS.[42] Various autoantibodies, such as ANAs and anti-Ro antibodies, have been found in patients with NMO even in the absence of systemic autoimmune diseases.[38,43] In a study of 153 patients with NMO spectrum disorder (NMOSD), ANAs were found in 43.8% and anti-Ro antibodies in 15.7% of patients, whereas only 5 patients fulfilled the diagnostic criteria for SS or SLE.[38]

Aquaporin-4 antibodies have a high specificity for NMOSDs, as they are rarely found in patients without neurologic involvement.[38,44] Therefore testing for the presence of aquaporin-4 antibodies in the absence of suggestive clinical manifestations or imaging findings is of low diagnostic yield. The presence of systemic autoantibodies in patients with NMO has been established and reproduced by many studies. However, occasionally, the presence of systemic antibodies does not signify systemic autoimmune disease, as the antibodies have also been reported to be present in healthy individuals over the age of 60 years [45]; this observation should be taken into account in the approach to a patient with NMOSD.

It is unclear whether patients with overlapping NMO and SS have distinct clinical features, compared to their counterparts without neurologic or systemic autoimmune diseases. Although earlier studies suggested that a concurrent history of autoimmune diseases is associated with decreased survival among patients with NMO,[46] other studies have yielded conflicting results. Another study showed no difference in clinical characteristics between patients with NMO with and without autoimmune diseases; however, when comparing patients with idiopathic NMO and those with NMO and systemic autoimmune diseases, motor deficits were encountered more frequently in the former group.[47]

In one study, patients with NMO and systemic autoimmune diseases were reported to have brain imaging lesions more frequently than those with idiopathic NMO.[47] However, another study reported different results.[48]

In a cohort of patients with NMO, 10% of whom also had SS, ANA positivity was associated with slower progression of neurologic disease.[49] Two more studies compared patients with NMO and SS overlap with those with NMO alone and also yielded conflicting results; in the first study, patients with SS and NMO had higher relapse rate and more severe visual impairment, measured by visual acuity and visual evoked potentials, than patients with NMO alone.[50] However, the second study showed no difference in clinical features and rate of progression of NMO among the two groups.[51] In a large series of SS patients, NMO was associated with younger age at the time of SS diagnosis, significantly less frequent sicca symptoms, and less frequent extraglandular manifestations including arthritis, Raynaud phenomenon, interstitial lung disease, and renal tubular acidosis.[52]

Whether the two nosologic entities are causally linked remains unclear. However, the fact that the majority of NMO cases occur in the absence of systemic autoimmune diseases and the high specificity of aquaporin-4 antibodies for the NMOSD clinical phenotype suggest that overlap cases probably represent a mere coexistence of two distinct autoimmune diseases rather than a causal link. Nevertheless, there are studies demonstrating common immunologic pathways involved in the two conditions; a study reported histopathologic evidence of salivary gland inflammation in 20 of 25 patients presenting with LETM or NMO, while only 4 fulfilled the diagnostic criteria for SS.[53] Another histopathologic study involving patients with NMO and SS-NMO overlap found no expression of aquaporin-4 in patients' salivary glands. However, there was disruption in the distribution of expressed aquaporin-5 in patients with poor salivation.[54] Although aquaporin-4 antibodies are not found in SS patients without neurologic involvement, antibodies against other aquaporins (aquaporin-8 and aquaporin-9) have been detected in sera of patients with SS without neurologic involvement,[55] suggesting that epitope spreading could be one potential mechanism in patients with SS and NMO overlap. Common cytokine expression profiles, including B cell—activating factor and Th17, have been reported in SS and NMO,[56–59] as have polymorphisms of *TNFSF4*.[60]

Multiple sclerosis

MS is an autoimmune, demyelinating disease of the CNS. It usually follows a relapsing course with incomplete resolution in-between flares in the earlier stages.[61] Dispersion in both space (anatomically) and time, of two otherwise unexplained events consistent with demyelination, is usually required for diagnosis, along with specific imaging criteria that should be met.[62] A number of patients eventually follow a progressive course later in the disease, with or without relapses, whereas 15% of patients follow a primary progressive course from disease onset.[61]

It is important to differentiate MS from neurologic manifestations of systemic autoimmune diseases, as there are a number of approved treatments for MS,[61] the efficacy of which has not been proven in other disease mimics. The differentiation between MS and other systemic diseases is usually made by means of existing diagnostic criteria [62] and is often a diagnosis of exclusion in clinical practice. However, this distinction has proven to be too simplistic at times.

The clinical overlap between MS and SS was first reported in 1986 when 20 patients, already having MS, with typical clinical, imaging, and CSF findings, including oligoclonal bands, were also found to fulfill the diagnostic criteria for SS.[63] The prevalence of SS among patients with MS has been reported to range between 0.9% and 3.3%,[64–66] including a large cohort of 440 patients with MS,[66] which is approximately the prevalence of SS in the general population. Another larger scale study involving 192 patients with MS did not find any patients with clinical features of SS.[67] On the other hand, a study including only patients with primary progressive MS reported a relatively high prevalence of SS, with 10/60 patients with primary progressive MS fulfilling the criteria for SS.[68]

The presence of SS has been associated with significantly greater disability and visual symptoms among patients with MS.[66] White matter lesions, a hallmark imaging finding of MS, can also be seen on MRI in patients with SS, both asymptomatic and with neurologic disease. Although there are imaging criteria for the diagnosis of MS, at times, these conditions can be difficult to differentiate. The imaging findings of SS, their relation to MS, and the differentiation between the two diseases by means of imaging are further discussed in the Laboratory and Imaging sections of this chapter and summarized in Table 10.2.

There are several confounding factors hindering our ability to better understand the links between MS and SS with CNS involvement and to interpret the findings of the abovementioned studies. One factor is that the majority of these studies are retrospective including patients who were evaluated before the description of NMO. Therefore it is not unreasonable to assume that a number of patients initially diagnosed with MS could now be classified as having NMO, which also often tends to frequently coexist with SS.

One study reported ANAs and anti-Ro antibodies in 23.8% and 7% of MS patients, respectively, while none of the anti-Ro-positive patients had any clinical features of SS.[69] However, long-term interferon beta-1b treatment is known to induce autoantibodies and autoimmune disease and there have been cases of SS becoming clinically apparent both shortly after [70] interferon beta-1b treatment and after long-term treatment.[71] Autonomic dysfunction, which can cause sicca symptoms, has also been reported in patients with MS [72] and has been found to correlate with more rapid disease progression, which can further complicate the distinction between the two.

Diffuse disease

Aseptic meningitis can present in SS patients with headache, photophobia, nausea, vomiting, and nuchal rigidity.[73] Multiple cranial neuropathies can also be an accompanying feature, the presence of which should raise the suspicion of meningeal involvement.[73] Cognitive symptoms are common complaints of patients with systemic autoimmune disease, including SS. These can be confounded by other symptoms and processes such as coexisting pain, fatigue, and depression.[74] However, cognitive dysfunction has been demonstrated in studies involving cognitive testing of patients with such complaints, ranging from mild cognitive dysfunction to dementia, or severe encephalopathy.[75,76] Interestingly, one study showed a slightly increased, 1.2-fold, risk of dementia among patients with primary SS even after adjusting for other risk factors and neurodegenerative diseases.[77] In the nonacute setting, neuropsychologic testing can be helpful in assessing a patient with symptoms or signs of cognitive dysfunction; it provides an objective means of evaluating different cognitive functions, including memory, in a quantifiable manner that can be tracked after treatment. In addition, it can discern and differentiate between different underlying causes including neurodegenerative diseases and mood disorders, if present.[78] Apart from cognitive symptoms and dysfunction, other neuropsychiatric symptoms have been described, including depression, anxiety, and personality disorders, whereas manic features and psychosis were not observed in patients with SS.[79,80]

Seizures are rarely seen in patients with primary SS. However, they have been reported in various case series describing patients with SS and CNS involvement.[17,24] These may present as complex partial, including temporal lobe, or generalized seizures.[24] It is unclear whether seizures represent the mere coexistence of epilepsy and SS, as epilepsy may affect up to 1% of the general population, or they represent a sequela of structural brain damage such as microinfarctions from vasculitis. Nevertheless, in the acute setting, they represent a medical emergency requiring prompt evaluation, especially in patients with active systemic disease.

Neurodiagnostic studies

Serologic findings such as elevated erythrocyte sedimentation rate and C-reactive protein levels and low C4 complement levels may reflect the underlying systemic disease state.[81] Active neurologic disease or new neurologic deficits in a patient with established SS and active systemic disease usually suggests an extraglandular manifestation of SS rather than a distinct primary neurologic disease. However, serologic findings should be considered with caution and in the context of each clinical presentation because, apart from SS, it is not uncommon to encounter autoantibodies, such as ANA, anti-Ro, and anti-La, in other neurologic conditions that may mimic SS, such as MS, NMO, and idiopathic myelitis.[42]

Increased CSF white blood cell count and elevated CSF protein levels may occur in SS patients with neurologic disease.[24] Elevation of the IgG index and the presence of oligoclonal bands have been reported in both SS-related CNS disease [24] and MS. However, the presence of three or more oligoclonal bands is more suggestive of a diagnosis of MS than SS; additionally, the presence of more than 10 bands in the CSF is almost pathognomonic of MS.[82]

Periventricular or subcortical brain white matter lesions have been reported in patients with SS [17,83] (Fig. 10.1). A number of studies have reported increased white matter disease burden, compared with healthy controls, in SS patients both with CNS involvement [84] and without neurologic symptoms.[83] Therefore we recommend the use of gadolinium-enhanced MRI in cases of suspected active neurologic disease. Among patients with headaches, patients with a diagnosis of SS were found to have more lesions in subcortical regions, basal ganglia, and infratentorial regions when compared with patients without a diagnosis of SS.[85] However, the aggregate of white matter lesions was not significantly different between the two groups. Other studies have also reported no significant difference in white matter disease burden between SS patients and controls.[86] Given the discrepancies between published studies, white matter abnormalities, as an isolated finding, are not considered pathognomonic of CNS disease; however, in the presence of new, or progressive, neurologic deficits, the presence of such abnormalities can suggest active neurologic

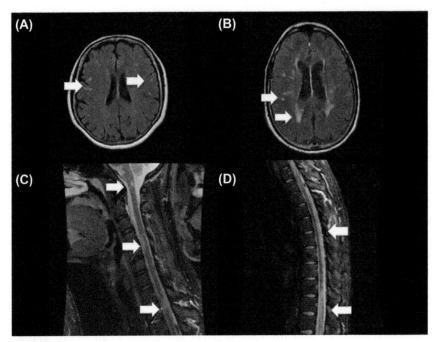

FIGURE 10.1

(A) T2-weighted fluid-attenuated inversion recovery (FLAIR) brain MRI showing nonspecific white matter lesions (*arrows*) commonly seen in Sjögren's syndrome. (B) T2-weighted FLAIR brain MRI of a patient with multiple sclerosis, showing periventricular, perpendicularly oriented white matter lesions. (C) T2-weighted FLAIR cervical spine MRI of a patient with multiple sclerosis and cervical myelitis, as well as a medullary lesion (*arrows*). (D) T2-weighted FLAIR thoracic spine MRI of a patient with multiple sclerosis and myelitis.

disease and should prompt further workup. Overall, the clinical evaluation of patients with white matter lesions is multifaceted and should be correlated with other factors such as the patient's age, vascular risk factors, history of migraines, and history of head trauma, all of which may significantly influence white matter disease prognosis. White matter lesions in SS may mimic MS or other inflammatory vasculopathies. White matter lesions associated with MS tend to have a periventricular location and perpendicular orientation (Fig. 10.1). Corpus callosum involvement, a hallmark of MS, is rare in SS.[24] In addition, studies report that perivenular localization of white matter lesions ("central vein sign") is typical of MS and can accurately differentiate this from other inflammatory neurologic conditions, including SS,[87] perhaps reflecting the underlying pathology of MS, which also includes perivenular lymphocytic infiltrates. On the other hand, basal ganglia involvement is more often seen in SS with CNS involvement than in other disease mimics (see Table 10.2).[24]

CNS vasculitis, regardless of the cause, may also be associated with subcortical white matter lesions. Serologic and CSF studies are useful in evaluating systemic and CNS disease, respectively.[88] Cerebral vessel imaging can be a useful confirmation of the pathologic condition, with cerebral angiography being the most sensitive imaging modality.[88] As vasculitis is pathologically defined, meningeal and brain biopsy can provide definitive diagnosis in ambiguous cases.[88] However, this is an invasive diagnostic modality typically reserved for only the most diagnostically challenging cases.

Electroencephalography and brain MRI should be performed in cases of suspected seizures and in prolonged or atypical cases of encephalopathy. CSF analysis can be considered in cases with focal neurologic deficits, or concurrent active disease, after mass lesions are ruled out by brain imaging, as it may be a presenting symptom of CNS vasculitis.[88] CSF analysis is also helpful in excluding other conditions with similar presentation, such as viral or autoimmune encephalitis.

In cases of myelitis, spinal cord imaging with gadolinium is recommended to confirm the diagnosis and to differentiate between different causes; longitudinally extensive lesions spanning three or more spinal segments are typical of NMO.[33] Brain MRI can be useful to evaluate the associated white matter lesions, which can be helpful in diagnosing MS or NMO based on their distribution pattern. Serologic and CSF studies can be helpful to discriminate from other causes (i.e., infectious, paraneoplastic).

In cases of cognitive impairment, screening for the underlying related medical conditions should include renal and liver function tests, thyroid function tests, assessing vitamin B_{12} levels, and screening for depression.[89] In cases of rapidly progressive cognitive dysfunction, brain MRI and further serologic and CSF studies are useful to differentiate among infectious, autoimmune, and prion-related diseases.[90] In patients with SS, brain imaging can be helpful to assess for further CNS involvement. Hippocampal atrophy has been reported in patients with SS and cognitive impairment, which was associated with the presence of NR2-glutamate receptor antibodies.[91] However, the clinical significance of these antibodies remains unclear. Abnormalities on single-photon emission computed tomography [92] and white matter microstructure alterations, evaluated by diffusion tensor imaging,[93] have also been reported in SS patients and have been correlated with cognitive dysfunction.

Treatment

Unfortunately, there are no randomized, double-blind, placebo-controlled trial results upon which to base the treatment decisions for CNS SS. Clinical practice guidelines for management of neurologic SS are currently being developed under the auspices of the Sjögren's Syndrome Foundation, Inc. but will largely be derived from uncontrolled studies, case series, and consensus expert opinion. At present, treatment algorithms are based on the acuity, severity, and progression of neurologic symptoms, patient comorbidities, and SS disease activity in other organs. The overall approach roughly parallels the same algorithms used to treat CNS SLE.

Symptoms and deficits may present acutely and progress rapidly with a grave impact on patients' morbidity and level of function. Apart from the direct effects on patients' health and well-being from CNS disease, there may be additional complications related to the neurologic deficit that further increase morbidity and mortality. For example, dysphagia can increase the risk of aspiration pneumonia and urinary retention following transverse myelitis can increase the risk of urinary tract infections and sepsis. Therefore timely diagnosis and initiation of appropriate therapy are essential to prevent or reduce permanent neurologic deficits. A multidisciplinary approach can also be helpful to rule out SS mimics and improve therapeutic outcomes.

In addition to SS patients with acute neurologic syndromes, patients with progressive deficits involving the CNS are likely to have inflammatory neurologic disease and would benefit from immunomodulatory treatment once infectious causes have been excluded. A practical rule of thumb is to consider immunotherapies in patients with acute or subacute onset, or progressive deficits, especially if there is clinical or serologic evidence of active systemic disease. However, as neurologic manifestations may be the presenting feature of, or even precede, systemic disease, the latter may not always be present.

In cases of active focal, or multifocal disease, including transverse myelitis, high-dose intravenous pulse corticosteroids for 3—5 days followed by high-dose oral steroids (e.g., prednisone, 1 mg/kg/day) for a month with eventual taper is usually considered as the first-line therapy. As it is uncommon to achieve remission with steroids alone, this treatment is usually supplemented with immunosuppressive therapy such as azathioprine (1—2.5 mg/kg/day) or intravenous pulse cyclophosphamide, depending on the disease severity.[91] In one small case series, treatment with intravenous rituximab was also used with varying degrees of success[94] and a more favorable adverse effect profile. Plasma exchange, or other agents, including mycophenolate mofetil and methotrexate has also been tried with variable results. Cases of suspected or confirmed vasculitis should be treated following standard algorithms used in other cases of systemic vasculitis. Medications that penetrate the blood-brain barrier are always preferred. High-dose intravenous steroids and intravenous rituximab are the preferred therapeutic agents for acute cases of NMO, after which maintenance treatment with other immunosuppressants may be needed.[32,95]

Neuropathic pain can be treated with gabapentin, pregabalin, or duloxetine. Topical treatments, including lidocaine or capsaicin, are helpful and often overlooked treatments of neuropathic pain. Tricyclic antidepressants are also helpful but their use in patients with SS is somewhat problematic, as they can exacerbate sicca symptoms. Oral agents, such as baclofen and tizanidine, and botulinum toxin injections can be helpful in managing spasticity, which is often a residual symptom of myelopathy. Physical, occupational, and speech therapy are also very important in patients with corresponding deficits. Patients with mild cognitive dysfunction unrelated to CNS inflammatory disease sometimes respond to treatment of the underlying cause (e.g., sleep disturbance, depression) or cognitive remediation therapy.

Conclusions

CNS involvement is an uncommon extraglandular manifestation of SS. Manifestations span from asymptomatic white matter disease to vasculitic or demyelinating lesions of the brain or spinal cord. Optic neuritis and transverse myelitis secondary to SS, as well as overlapping demyelinating diseases, such as NMO and MS, can lead to debilitating residual deficits. There are no randomized, placebo-controlled, clinical trials in SS with CNS involvement. However, prompt recognition and treatment according to the current standards of care are needed in cases with acute or subacute onset, as well as with progressive neurologic deficits, as delay in treatment can lead to irreversible disability with a significant impact on patients' morbidity and quality of life.

References

1. Carvajal Alegria G, Guellec D, Mariette X, Gottenberg JE, Dernis E, Dubost JJ, Trouvin AP, Hachulla E, Larroche C, Le Guern V, Cornec D, Devauchelle-Pensec V, Saraux A. Epidemiology of neurological manifestations in Sjögren's syndrome: data from the French ASSESS Cohort. *RMD Open*. 2016;2(1):e000179.
2. Ramos-Casals M, Solans R, Rosas J, Camps MT, Gil A, Del Pino-Montes J, Calvo-Alen J, Jimenez-Alonso J, Mico ML, Beltran J, Belenguer R, Pallares L. Primary Sjögren syndrome in Spain: clinical and immunologic expression in 1010 patients. *Medicine*. 2008;87(4):210–219.
3. Alexander EL, Provost TT, Stevens MB, Alexander GE. Neurologic complications of primary Sjögren's syndrome. *Medicine*. 1982;61(4):247–257.
4. Alexander EL, Ranzenbach MR, Kumar AJ, Kozachuk WE, Rosenbaum AE, Patronas N, Harley JB, Reichlin M. Anti-Ro(SS-A) autoantibodies in central nervous system disease associated with Sjögren's syndrome (CNS-SS): clinical, neuroimaging, and angiographic correlates. *Neurology*. 1994;44(5):899–908.
5. Alexander EL, Arnett FC, Provost TT, Stevens MB. Sjögren's syndrome: association of anti-Ro(SS-A) antibodies with vasculitis, hematologic abnormalities, and serologic hyperreactivity. *Ann Intern Med*. 1983;98(2):155–159.
6. Bacman S, Perez Leiros C, Sterin-Borda L, Hubscher O, Arana R, Borda E. Autoantibodies against lacrimal gland M3 muscarinic acetylcholine receptors in patients with primary Sjögren's syndrome. *Investig Ophthalmol Vis Sci*. 1998;39(1):151–156.
7. Dawson LJ, Stanbury J, Venn N, Hasdimir B, Rogers SN, Smith PM. Antimuscarinic antibodies in primary Sjögren's syndrome reversibly inhibit the mechanism of fluid secretion by human submandibular salivary acinar cells. *Arthritis Rheum*. 2006;54(4): 1165–1173.

8. Nguyen KH, Brayer J, Cha S, Diggs S, Yasunari U, Hilal G, Peck AB, Humphreys-Beher MG. Evidence for antimuscarinic acetylcholine receptor antibody-mediated secretory dysfunction in nod mice. *Arthritis Rheum.* 2000;43(10):2297–2306.

9. Robinson CP, Brayer J, Yamachika S, Esch TR, Peck AB, Stewart CA, Peen E, Jonsson R, Humphreys-Beher MG. Transfer of human serum IgG to nonobese diabetic Igmu null mice reveals a role for autoantibodies in the loss of secretory function of exocrine tissues in Sjögren's syndrome. *Proc Natl Acad Sci USA.* 1998;95(13): 7538–7543.

10. Reina S, Sterin-Borda L, Orman B, Borda E. Autoantibodies against cerebral muscarinic cholinoceptors in Sjögren syndrome: functional and pathological implications. *J Neuroimmunol.* 2004;150(1–2):107–115.

11. Orman B, Sterin-Borda L, De Couto Pita A, Reina S, Borda E. Anti-brain cholinergic auto antibodies from primary Sjögren syndrome sera modify simultaneously cerebral nitric oxide and prostaglandin biosynthesis. *Int Immunopharmacol.* 2007;7(12): 1535–1543.

12. Dalmau J, Graus F. Antibody-mediated encephalitis. *N Engl J Med.* 2018;378(9): 840–851.

13. Tay SH, Fairhurst AM, Mak A. Clinical utility of circulating anti-N-methyl-d-aspartate receptor subunits NR2A/B antibody for the diagnosis of neuropsychiatric syndromes in systemic lupus erythematosus and Sjögren's syndrome: an updated meta-analysis. *Autoimmun Rev.* 2017;16(2):114–122.

14. Fox RI. Sjögren's syndrome. *Lancet.* 2005;366(9482):321–331.

15. Kapadia M, Sakic B. Autoimmune and inflammatory mechanisms of CNS damage. *Prog Neurobiol.* 2011;95(3):301–333.

16. Alexander EL, Provost TT, Sanders ME, Frank MM, Joiner KA. Serum complement activation in central nervous system disease in Sjögren's syndrome. *Am J Med.* 1988;85(4): 513–518.

17. Soliotis FC, Mavragani CP, Moutsopoulos HM. Central nervous system involvement in Sjögren's syndrome. *Ann Rheum Dis.* 2004;63(6):616–620.

18. Bakchine S, Duyckaerts C, Hassine L, Chaunu MP, Turell E, Wechsler B, Chain F. [Central and peripheral neurologic lesions in primary Gougerot-Sjögren syndrome. Clinicopathological study of a case]. *Rev Neurol.* 1991;147(5):368–375.

19. Megevand P, Chizzolini C, Chofflon M, Roux-Lombard P, Lalive PH, Picard F. Cerebrospinal fluid anti-SSA autoantibodies in primary Sjögren's syndrome with central nervous system involvement. *Eur Neurol.* 2007;57(3):166–171.

20. Alexander E, Provost TT. Sjögren's syndrome. Association of cutaneous vasculitis with central nervous system disease. *Arch Dermatol.* 1987;123(6):801–810.

21. Molina R, Provost TT, Alexander EL. Peripheral inflammatory vascular disease in Sjögren's syndrome. Association with nervous system complications. *Arthritis Rheum.* 1985;28(12):1341–1347.

22. Teixeira F, Moreira I, Silva AM, Vasconcelos C, Farinha F, Santos E. Neurological involvement in primary Sjögren syndrome. *Acta reumatologica portuguesa.* 2013; 38(1):29–36.

23. Morreale M, Marchione P, Giacomini P, Pontecorvo S, Marianetti M, Vento C, Tinelli E, Francia A. Neurological involvement in primary Sjögren syndrome: a focus on central nervous system. *PLoS One.* 2014;9(1):e84605.

24. Delalande S, de Seze J, Fauchais AL, Hachulla E, Stojkovic T, Ferriby D, Dubucquoi S, Pruvo JP, Vermersch P, Hatron PY. Neurologic manifestations in primary Sjögren syndrome: a study of 82 patients. *Medicine*. 2004;83(5):280–291.

25. Wong S, Pollock AN, Burnham JM, Sherry DD, Dlugos DJ. Acute cerebellar ataxia due to Sjögren syndrome. *Neurology*. 2004;62(12):2332–2333.

26. Yang H, Sun Y, Zhao L, Zhang X, Zhang F. Cerebellar involvement in patients with primary Sjögren's syndrome: diagnosis and treatment. *Clin Rheumatol*. 2018;37(5): 1207–1213.

27. Rafai MA, Boulaajaj FZ, Moutawakil F, Addali N, El Moutawakkil B, Fadel H, Hakim K, Bourezgui M, Sibai M, El Otmani H, Slassi I. Neurological manifestations revealing primitive Gougerot-Sjögren syndrome: 9 cases. *Jt Bone Spine : revue du rhumatisme*. 2009;76(2):139–145.

28. Zahlane S, Louhab N, El Mellakh M, Kissani N. Anterior horn syndrome: a rare manifestation of primary Sjögren's syndrome. Joint, bone, spine. *revue du rhumatisme*. 2016; 83(4):448–450.

29. Wingerchuk DM, Lennon VA, Lucchinetti CF, Pittock SJ, Weinshenker BG. The spectrum of neuromyelitis optica. *Lancet Neurol*. 2007;6(9):805–815.

30. Lennon VA, Wingerchuk DM, Kryzer TJ, Pittock SJ, Lucchinetti CF, Fujihara K, Nakashima I, Weinshenker BG. A serum autoantibody marker of neuromyelitis optica: distinction from multiple sclerosis. *Lancet*. 2004;364(9451):2106–2112.

31. Lennon VA, Kryzer TJ, Pittock SJ, Verkman AS, Hinson SR. IgG marker of optic-spinal multiple sclerosis binds to the aquaporin-4 water channel. *J Exp Med*. 2005;202(4): 473–477.

32. Stellmann JP, Krumbholz M, Friede T, Gahlen A, Borisow N, Fischer K, Hellwig K, Pache F, Ruprecht K, Havla J, Kumpfel T, Aktas O, Hartung HP, Ringelstein M, Geis C, Kleinschnitz C, Berthele A, Hemmer B, Angstwurm K, Young KL, Schuster S, Stangel M, Lauda F, Tumani H, Mayer C, Zeltner L, Ziemann U, Linker RA, Schwab M, Marziniak M, Then Bergh F, Hofstadt-van Oy U, Neuhaus O, Zettl U, Faiss J, Wildemann B, Paul F, Jarius S, Trebst C, Kleiter I. Immunotherapies in neuromyelitis optica spectrum disorder: efficacy and predictors of response. *J Neurol Neurosurg Psychiatry*. 2017;88(8):639–647.

33. Pittock SJ, Lucchinetti CF. Neuromyelitis optica and the evolving spectrum of autoimmune aquaporin-4 channelopathies: a decade later. *Ann N Y Acad Sci*. 2016;1366(1): 20–39.

34. Lee HJ, Chang SH, Kang EH, Lee YJ, Song YW, Ha YJ. A case of primary Sjögren's syndrome presenting as mass-like encephalitis, with progression to neuromyelitis optica spectrum disorder. *Archives of rheumatology*. 2017;32(4):353–357.

35. Ramos AB, Peters CW, Landry-Wegener B, Cannizzaro LA, Lovera J. A case of neuromyelitis optica spectrum disorder presenting with undiagnosed Sjögren's syndrome and a single, atypical tumefactive lesion: a clinical conundrum. *J Neurol Sci*. 2017;383: 216–218.

36. Wingerchuk DM, Banwell B, Bennett JL, Cabre P, Carroll W, Chitnis T, de Seze J, Fujihara K, Greenberg B, Jacob A, Jarius S, Lana-Peixoto M, Levy M, Simon JH, Tenembaum S, Traboulsee AL, Waters P, Wellik KE, Weinshenker BG. International consensus diagnostic criteria for neuromyelitis optica spectrum disorders. *Neurology*. 2015;85(2):177–189.

37. Wingerchuk DM, Hogancamp WF, O'Brien PC, Weinshenker BG. The clinical course of neuromyelitis optica (Devic's syndrome). *Neurology*. 1999;53(5):1107–1114.

38. Pittock SJ, Lennon VA, de Seze J, Vermersch P, Homburger HA, Wingerchuk DM, Lucchinetti CF, Zephir H, Moder K, Weinshenker BG. Neuromyelitis optica and non organ-specific autoimmunity. *Arch Neurol.* 2008;65(1):78–83.

39. Wandinger K-P, Stangel M, Witte T, Venables P, Charles P, Jarius S, Wildemann B, Probst C, Iking-Konert C, Schneider M. Autoantibodies against aquaporin-4 in patients with neuropsychiatric systemic lupus erythematosus and primary Sjögren's syndrome. *Arthritis Rheum.* 2010;62(4):1198–1200.

40. Bak E, Yang HK, Hwang JM. Optic neuropathy associated with primary Sjögren's syndrome: a case series. Optometry and vision science. *Official Publication of the American Academy of Optometry.* 2017;94(4):519–526.

41. McKeon A, Lennon VA, Lotze T, Tenenbaum S, Ness JM, Rensel M, Kuntz NL, Fryer JP, Homburger H, Hunter J, Weinshenker BG, Krecke K, Lucchinetti CF, Pittock SJ. CNS aquaporin-4 autoimmunity in children. *Neurology.* 2008;71(2):93–100.

42. Hummers LK, Krishnan C, Casciola-Rosen L, Rosen A, Morris S, Mahoney JA, Kerr DA, Wigley FM. Recurrent transverse myelitis associates with anti-Ro (SSA) autoantibodies. *Neurology.* 2004;62(1):147–149.

43. Chen C, Xiaobo S, Yuge W, Yaqing S, Ling F, Lisheng P, Zhengqi L, Wei Q. Multiple autoantibodies and neuromyelitis optica spectrum disorders. *Neuroimmunomodulation.* 2016;23(3):151–156.

44. Dellavance A, Alvarenga RR, Rodrigues SH, Kok F, de Souza AW, Andrade LE. Anti-aquaporin-4 antibodies in the context of assorted immune-mediated diseases. *Eur J Neurol.* 2012;19(2):248–252.

45. Tan EM, Feltkamp TE, Smolen JS, Butcher B, Dawkins R, Fritzler MJ, Gordon T, Hardin JA, Kalden JR, Lahita RG, Maini RN, McDougal JS, Rothfield NF, Smeenk RJ, Takasaki Y, Wiik A, Wilson MR, Koziol JA. Range of antinuclear antibodies in "healthy" individuals. *Arthritis Rheum.* 1997;40(9):1601–1611.

46. Wingerchuk DM, Weinshenker BG. Neuromyelitis optica: clinical predictors of a relapsing course and survival. *Neurology.* 2003;60(5):848–853.

47. Zhang B, Zhong Y, Wang Y, Dai Y, Qiu W, Zhang L, Li H, Lu Z. Neuromyelitis optica spectrum disorders without and with autoimmune diseases. *BMC Neurology.* 2014;14:162.

48. Gu LN, Zhang M, Zhu H, Liu JY. Higher frequency of brain abnormalities in neuromyelitis optica spectrum disorder patients without primary Sjögren's syndrome. *Neural regeneration research.* 2016;11(10):1633–1637.

49. Masuda H, Mori M, Uzawa A, Muto M, Uchida T, Kuwabara S. Serum antinuclear antibody may be associated with less severe disease activity in neuromyelitis optica. *Eur J Neurol.* 2016;23(2):276–281.

50. Jia N, Jing Y, Li QC, Liu L, Wang JW, Hu XM. Clinical features and prognostic analysis of neuromyelitisoptica spectrum disease with Sjögren syndrome. *Zhonghua Yi Xue Za Zhi.* 2017;97(11):827–832.

51. Zhong YH, Zhong ZG, Zhou Z, Ma ZY, Qiu MY, Peng FH, Zhang WX. Comparisons of presentations and outcomes of neuromyelitis optica patients with and without Sjögren's syndrome. *Neurol Sci : Official Journal of the Italian Neurological Society and of the Italian Society of Clinical Neurophysiology.* 2017;38(2):271–277.

52. Qiao L, Wang Q, Fei Y, Zhang W, Xu Y, Zhang Y, Zhao Y, Zeng X, Zhang F. The clinical characteristics of primary Sjögren's syndrome with neuromyelitis optica spectrum disorder in China: a STROBE-compliant article. *Medicine.* 2015;94(28):e1145.

53. Javed A, Balabanov R, Arnason BG, Kelly TJ, Sweiss NJ, Pytel P, Walsh R, Blair EA, Stemer A, Lazzaro M, Reder AT. Minor salivary gland inflammation in Devic's disease and longitudinally extensive myelitis. *Mult Scler*. 2008;14(6):809–814.

54. Yoshimura S, Nakamura H, Horai Y, Nakajima H, Shiraishi H, Hayashi T, Takahashi T, Kawakami A. Abnormal distribution of AQP5 in labial salivary glands is associated with poor saliva secretion in patients with Sjögren's syndrome including neuromyelitis optica complicated patients. *Mod Rheumatol*. 2016;26(3):384–390.

55. Tzartos JS, Stergiou C, Daoussis D, Zisimopoulou P, Andonopoulos AP, Zolota V, Tzartos SJ. Antibodies to aquaporins are frequent in patients with primary Sjögren's syndrome. *Rheumatol*. 2017;56(12):2114–2122.

56. Kothur K, Wienholt L, Brilot F, Dale RC. CSF cytokines/chemokines as biomarkers in neuroinflammatory CNS disorders: a systematic review. *Cytokine*. 2016;77: 227–237.

57. Wang H, Wang K, Zhong X, Qiu W, Dai Y, Wu A, Hu X. Cerebrospinal fluid BAFF and APRIL levels in neuromyelitis optica and multiple sclerosis patients during relapse. *J Clin Immunol*. 2012;32(5):1007–1011.

58. Cornec D, Costa S, Devauchelle-Pensec V, Jousse-Joulin S, Marcorelles P, Berthelot JM, Chiche L, Hachulla E, Hatron PY, Goeb V, Vittecoq O, Saraux A, Pers JO. Blood and salivary-gland BAFF-driven B-cell hyperactivity is associated to rituximab inefficacy in primary Sjögren's syndrome. *J Autoimmun*. 2016;67:102–110.

59. Deng F, Chen J, Zheng J, Chen Y, Huang R, Yin J, Gao X, Lin Q, Huang C, Gao Y, Yu X, Liu Z. Association of BAFF and IL-17A with subphenotypes of primary Sjögren's syndrome. *Int J Rheumat Dis*. 2016;19(7):715–720.

60. Lian Z, Liu J, Shi Z, Chen H, Zhang Q, Feng H, Du Q, Miao X, Zhou H. Association of TNFSF4 polymorphisms with neuromyelitis optica spectrum disorders in a Chinese population. *J Mol Neurosci*. 2017;63(3–4):396–402.

61. Reich DS, Lucchinetti CF, Calabresi PA. Multiple sclerosis. *N Engl J Med*. 2018;378(2): 169–180.

62. Thompson AJ, Banwell BL, Barkhof F, Carroll WM, Coetzee T, Comi G, Correale J, Fazekas F, Filippi M, Freedman MS, Fujihara K, Galetta SL, Hartung HP, Kappos L, Lublin FD, Marrie RA, Miller AE, Miller DH, Montalban X, Mowry EM, Sorensen PS, Tintore M, Traboulsee AL, Trojano M, Uitdehaag BMJ, Vukusic S, Waubant E, Weinshenker BG, Reingold SC, Cohen JA. Diagnosis of multiple sclerosis: 2017 revisions of the McDonald criteria. *Lancet Neurol*. 2018;17(2):162–173.

63. Alexander EL, Malinow K, Lejewski JE, Jerdan MS, Provost TT, Alexander GE. Primary Sjögren's syndrome with central nervous system disease mimicking multiple sclerosis. *Ann Intern Med*. 1986;104(3):323–330.

64. Miro J, Pena-Sagredo JL, Berciano J, Insua S, Leno C, Velarde R. Prevalence of primary Sjögren's syndrome in patients with multiple sclerosis. *Ann Neurol*. 1990;27(5): 582–584.

65. Sandberg-Wollheim M, Axell T, Hansen BU, Henricsson V, Ingesson E, Jacobsson L, Larsson A, Lieberkind K, Manthorpe R. Primary Sjögren's syndrome in patients with multiple sclerosis. *Neurology*. 1992;42(4):845–847.

66. Annunziata P, De Santi L, Di Rezze S, Millefiorini E, Capello E, Mancardi G, De Riz M, Scarpini E, Vecchio R, Patti F. Clinical features of Sjögren's syndrome in patients with multiple sclerosis. *Acta Neurol Scand*. 2011;124(2):109–114.

67. Noseworthy JH, Bass BH, Vandervoort MK, Ebers GC, Rice GP, Weinshenker BG, McLay CJ, Bell DA. The prevalence of primary Sjögren's syndrome in a multiple sclerosis population. *Ann Neurol.* 1989;25(1):95–98.

68. de Seze J, Devos D, Castelnovo G, Labauge P, Dubucquoi S, Stojkovic T, Ferriby D, Vermersch P. The prevalence of Sjögren syndrome in patients with primary progressive multiple sclerosis. *Neurology.* 2001;57(8):1359–1363.

69. de Andres C, Guillem A, Rodriguez-Mahou M, Lopez Longo FJ. Frequency and significance of anti-Ro (SS-A) antibodies in multiple sclerosis patients. *Acta Neurol Scand.* 2001;104(2):83–87.

70. Tsai KY, Tsai CP, Liao N. Sjögren's syndrome with central nervous system involvement presenting as multiple sclerosis with failure response to beta-interferon. *Eur Neurol.* 2001;45(1):59–60.

71. De Santi L, Costantini MC, Annunziata P. Long time interval between multiple sclerosis onset and occurrence of primary Sjögren's syndrome in a woman treated with interferon-beta. *Acta Neurol Scand.* 2005;112(3):194–196.

72. Flachenecker P, Reiners K, Krauser M, Wolf A, Toyka KV. Autonomic dysfunction in multiple sclerosis is related to disease activity and progression of disability. *Mult Scler.* 2001;7(5):327–334.

73. Alexander EL, Alexander GE. Aseptic meningoencephalitis in primary Sjögren's syndrome. *Neurology.* 1983;33(5):593–598.

74. Indart S, Hugon J, Guillausseau PJ, Gilbert A, Dumurgier J, Paquet C, Sene D. Impact of pain on cognitive functions in primary Sjögren syndrome with small fiber neuropathy: 10 cases and a literature review. *Medicine.* 2017;96(16):e6384.

75. Blanc F, Longato N, Jung B, Kleitz C, Di Bitonto L, Cretin B, Collongues N, Sordet C, Fleury M, Poindron V, Gottenberg JE, Anne O, Lipsker D, Martin T, Sibilia J, de Seze J. Cognitive dysfunction and dementia in primary Sjögren's syndrome. *ISRN Neurol.* 2013; 2013:501327.

76. Segal BM, Pogatchnik B, Holker E, Liu H, Sloan J, Rhodus N, Moser KL. Primary Sjögren's syndrome: cognitive symptoms, mood, and cognitive performance. *Acta Neurologica Scandinavica.* 2012;125(4):272–278.

77. Chen HH, Perng WT, Chiou JY, Wang YH, Huang JY, Wei JC. Risk of dementia among patients with Sjögren's syndrome: a nationwide population-based cohort study in Taiwan. *Semin Arthritis Rheum.* 2019;48(5):895–899.

78. Kulas JF, Naugle RI. Indications for neuropsychological assessment. *Clevel Clin J Med.* 2003;70(9):785–786, 8, 91-2.

79. Harboe E, Tjensvoll AB, Maroni S, Goransson LG, Greve OJ, Beyer MK, Herigstad A, Kvaloy JT, Omdal R. Neuropsychiatric syndromes in patients with systemic lupus erythematosus and primary Sjögren syndrome: a comparative population-based study. *Ann Rheum Dis.* 2009;68(10):1541–1546.

80. Malinow KL, Molina R, Gordon B, Selnes OA, Provost TT, Alexander EL. Neuropsychiatric dysfunction in primary Sjögren's syndrome. *Ann Intern Med.* 1985;103(3):344–350.

81. Massara A, Bonazza S, Castellino G, Caniatti L, Trotta F, Borrelli M, Feggi L, Govoni M. Central nervous system involvement in Sjögren's syndrome: unusual, but not unremarkable–clinical, serological characteristics and outcomes in a large cohort of Italian patients. *Rheumatology.* 2010;49(8):1540–1549.

82. Bourahoui A, De Seze J, Guttierez R, Onraed B, Hennache B, Ferriby D, Stojkovic T, Vermersch P. CSF isoelectrofocusing in a large cohort of MS and other neurological diseases. *Eur J Neurol.* 2004;11(8):525–529.

83. Coates T, Slavotinek JP, Rischmueller M, Schultz D, Anderson C, Dellamelva M, Sage MR, Gordon TP. Cerebral white matter lesions in primary Sjögren's syndrome: a controlled study. *J Rheumatol*. 1999;26(6):1301−1305.

84. Alexander EL, Beall SS, Gordon B, Selnes OA, Yannakakis GD, Patronas N, Provost TT, McFarland HF. Magnetic resonance imaging of cerebral lesions in patients with the Sjögren syndrome. *Ann Intern Med*. 1988;108(6):815−823.

85. Sarac H, Markeljevic J, Erdeljic V, Josipovic-Jelic Z, Hajnsek S, Klapan T, Batinica M, Barsic I, Sertic J, Dobrila Dintinjana R. Signal hyperintensities on brain magnetic resonance imaging in patients with primary Sjögren syndrome and frequent episodic tension-type headache: relation to platelet serotonin level and disease activity. *J Rheumatol*. 2013;40(8):1360−1366.

86. Harboe E, Beyer MK, Greve OJ, Goransson LG, Tjensvoll AB, Kvaloy JT, Omdal R. Cerebral white matter hyperintensities are not increased in patients with primary Sjögren's syndrome. *Eur J Neurol*. 2009;16(5):576−581.

87. Maggi P, Absinta M, Grammatico M, Vuolo L, Emmi G, Carlucci G, Spagni G, Barilaro A, Repice AM, Emmi L, Prisco D, Martinelli V, Scotti R, Sadeghi N, Perrotta G, Sati P, Dachy B, Reich DS, Filippi M, Massacesi L. Central vein sign differentiates Multiple Sclerosis from central nervous system inflammatory vasculopathies. *Ann Neurol*. 2018;83(2):283−294.

88. Limaye K, Samaniego EA, Adams Jr HP. Diagnosis and treatment of primary central nervous system Angiitis. *Curr Treat Options Neurol*. 2018;20(9):38.

89. Knopman DS, DeKosky ST, Cummings JL, Chui H, Corey-Bloom J, Relkin N, Small GW, Miller B, Stevens JC. Practice parameter: diagnosis of dementia (an evidence-based review). Report of the quality standards Subcommittee of the American academy of Neurology. *Neurology*. 2001;56(9):1143−1153.

90. Zerr I, Hermann P. Diagnostic challenges in rapidly progressive dementia. *Expert Rev Neurother*. 2018:1−12.

91. Lauvsnes MB, Beyer MK, Kvaloy JT, Greve OJ, Appenzeller S, Kvivik I, Harboe E, Tjensvoll AB, Goransson LG, Omdal R. Association of hippocampal atrophy with cerebrospinal fluid antibodies against the NR2 subtype of the N-methyl-D-aspartate receptor in patients with systemic lupus erythematosus and patients with primary Sjögren's syndrome. *Arthritis Rheumatol*. 2014;66(12):3387−3394.

92. Le Guern V, Belin C, Henegar C, Moroni C, Maillet D, Lacau C, Dumas JL, Vigneron N, Guillevin L. Cognitive function and 99mTc-ECD brain SPECT are significantly correlated in patients with primary Sjögren syndrome: a case-control study. *Ann Rheum Dis*. 2010;69(1):132−137.

93. Segal BM, Mueller BA, Zhu X, Prosser R, Pogatchnik B, Holker E, Carpenter AF, Lim KO. Disruption of brain white matter microstructure in primary Sjögren's syndrome: evidence from diffusion tensor imaging. *Rheumatol*. 2010;49(8):1530−1539.

94. Ramos-Casals M, Garcia-Hernandez FJ, de Ramon E, Callejas JL, Martinez-Berriotxoa A, Pallares L, Caminal-Montero L, Selva-O'Callaghan A, Oristrell J, Hidalgo C, Perez-Alvarez R, Mico ML, Medrano F, Gomez de la Torre R, Diaz-Lagares C, Camps M, Ortego N, Sanchez-Roman J. Off-label use of rituximab in 196 patients with severe, refractory systemic autoimmune diseases. *Clin Exp Rheumatol*. 2010;28(4):468−476.

95. Kim SH, Huh SY, Lee SJ, Joung A, Kim HJ. A 5-year follow-up of rituximab treatment in patients with neuromyelitis optica spectrum disorder. *JAMA neurology*. 2013;70(9):1110−1117.

Treatment of Sjögren's syndrome internal organ manifestations and constitutional symptoms

Rana Mongroo, MD[1], Bivin Varghese, MD[1], Steven Carsons, MD[2]

[1]*Fellow in Rheumatology, Division of Rheumatology, Allergy & Immunology, Department of Medicine, New York University Long Island School of Medicine, Mineola, NY, United States;* [2]*Professor of Medicine, Chief, Division of Rheumatology, Allergy & Immunology, Department of Medicine, New York University Long Island School of Medicine, Mineola, NY, United States*

Constitutional symptoms

A variety of constitutional symptoms may be seen in Sjögren's syndrome (SS) including fatigue, fever, and weight loss. Fever is estimated to occur in approximately 5% of primary SS patients.[1] Fever should prompt an investigation for infection, especially in patients treated with immunosuppressive medications. Fever may also be a sign of the development of a lymphoproliferative disorder in this high-risk population. Weight loss may also be a sign of the development of lymphoma or a consequence of gastrointestinal (GI) involvement (vide infra). Poor oral intake due to consequences of chronic xerostomia (Chapter 3) may also result in significant weight loss. Fatigue is one of the most common extraglandular symptoms in primary SS, occurring in up to 70%−80% of patients.[2] It is important to exclude alternate causes of fatigue before attributing fatigue to primary SS because some of these conditions are easily treated. Such conditions include anemia, thyroid disorders, and fibromyalgia (vide infra). Sleep disorders may affect up to 15% of primary SS patients[3] and are common causes of fatigue in the overall population. Snoring, obesity, and narcoleptic symptoms can be clues to the presence of obstructive sleep apnea and prompt a workup that includes polysomnography. Treatment guidelines for the management of fatigue have been published by the Clinical Practice Guidelines Committee of the Sjögren's Syndrome Foundation, Inc. (SSF).[4] The only treatment modality receiving a strong recommendation was education regarding self-care measures, which includes advice about exercise. Exercise has been demonstrated to reduce fatigue in systemic lupus erythematosus, rheumatoid arthritis (RA), multiple sclerosis, and, in one randomized controlled trial for SS.[5] A weak recommendation allowed for a trial of hydroxychloroquine in selected situations for the fatigue associated with SS.[4] Tumor necrosis factor (TNF) inhibitors were not recommended for use in the treatment of fatigue.[4]

Sjögren's Syndrome. https://doi.org/10.1016/B978-0-323-67534-5.00011-9

Rheumatologic manifestations

Inflammatory musculoskeletal pain

Articular involvement was described in Henrik Sjögren's original paper[6] and has been documented in 41%—53% of SS patients in other series.[1,7—14] Musculoskeletal symptoms (Chapter 6) may be the presenting manifestation of SS and can precede, follow, or occur together with typical sicca symptoms.[15—18] Major manifestations may include arthralgias, myalgias, or frank arthritis (Chapter 6). A nonerosive polyarthritis with small and large joint involvement that resembles RA has been described in 16%—35%.[3,19,20] Less commonly, asymmetric polyarthritis, oligoarthritis, or monoarthritis may occur.[10,16]

In some instances, overlap syndromes develop where patients meet criteria for both primary SS and RA.[17,21] Occasionally, patients develop RA or a rheumatoid-like arthritis after having primary SS alone for many years.[21] The use of rheumatoid factor (RF) to differentiate between SS-RA overlap and SS with inflammatory polyarthritis is limited by the high prevalence of RF found in SS (estimated to be 60% —70%) regardless of the presence or absence of joint involvement.[22] Anti-cyclic citrullinated peptide (anti-CCP) antibodies may be found in 7.5%—25% of patients with SS. However, most but not all studies suggest that anti-CCP positivity is associated with the development of synovitis and/or polyarthritis in SS.[17,19,23,24]

Management

It has been difficult to derive clear estimates of the efficacy of disease-modifying arthritis remittive drugs (DMARDs) and biological therapies for the articular manifestations of SS from existing clinical trial data. Table 11.1 depicts eleven oral and biologic DMARD trials in SS populations, along with the assessments and biomarkers used as the outcome measures for arthritis. In addition to routine biomarker measurements of erythrocyte sedimentation rate, C-reactive protein, and immunoglobulin levels, different trials have employed several different outcome measures to assess the effect of the trial medication on articular signs and symptoms as shown in Table 11.1, thus making comparisons difficult. Some trials did not assess the effect on musculoskeletal manifestations at all because the primary outcome measure of many SS trials consists of a core set of parameters comprising ocular and oral sicca, fatigue, and pain as measured by a visual analogue scale (VAS). The pain VAS is sometimes labeled as representing joint pain, but even so, it is often not specified as inflammatory arthritis or synovitis and might represent musculoskeletal pain from other concurrent entities such as osteoarthritis and fibromyalgia.

SS trials have begun to use the European League Against Rheumatism Sjögren's Syndrome Disease Activity Index (ESSDAI), a validated composite measure of systemic disease activity with 12 domains. The inclusion of an articular domain with different levels of severity depending on the number of swollen and tender joints should make comparison of musculoskeletal outcomes among trials easier in the future. Other issues regarding SS trial design include the magnitude of effect chosen to be necessary

Table 11.1 Recent oral and biologic DMARD trials in primary Sjögren's syndrome.

Study	Med	Pain VAS	Joint pain	Articular ESSDAI	SJC	TJC	Arthralgias	SDAI (RA)	Ig (any)	ESR	CRP	Design, References
JOQUER 2014	HCQ	Trend (0.06)	–		–	–	–	–	0.04	0.001	0.03	RCT[23]
ETA 2004	ETA	–	–		–	–	–	–	N (0.82)	0.004	–	RCT[122]
TRIPPS 2004	INF	N 0.46	–		N 0.75	N 0.97	–	–	0.001	N 0.97	N 0.96	RCT[123]
Meijer 2010	RTX	–	–		–	–	Trend (0.058)	–	<0.05	–	–	RCT[124]
St. Clair 2013	RTX	–	Trend 0.077		–	–	–	–	–	–	–	Open label[125]
Carubbi 2013	RTX	<0.01	–		–	–	–	.	N >0.05	–	–	Comparator[126]
TEARS 2014	RTX	N 0.29	–	N	–	–	–	–	<0.001	N 0.185	N 0.74	RCT[127]
Adler 2013	ABA	–	–	–	–	–	–	–	<0.005	–	–	Open label[120]
ROSE 2015	ABA	–	–	–	–	–	–	Y	<0.05	–	–	Open label; RA + SS[128]
ASAP 2014	ABA	–	–	Y	–	–	–	–	<0.05	–	–	Open label[129]
BELISS 2015	BAFF	N	–	Y	–	–	–	–	<0.0001	–	–	Open label[130]

CRP, C-reactive protein; DMARDs, disease-modifying antirheumatic drugs; HCQ, hydroxychloroquine; Ig, immunoglobulin; ESR, erythrocyte sedimentation rate; ETA, etanercept; INF, infliximab; RA, rheumatoid arthritis; RTX, rituximab; ABA, abatacept; BAFF, B cell–activating factor; ESSDAI, European League Against Rheumatism Sjögren's syndrome disease activity index; SJC, swollen joint count; TJC, tender joint count; SDAI, simplified disease activity index; RCT, randomized controlled trial; VAS, visual analogue scale; Y, yes; N, no.

to meet the outcome measure, dose of the medication, and duration of therapy.[25] Nonetheless, inspection of Table 11.1 reveals some signals that suggest that these therapies may be useful for the treatment of articular complaints in certain individuals with SS.

Three organizations have published guidelines for the management of primary SS.[4,26,27] In view of the issues with trial design mentioned earlier, guideline drafts were informed by expert opinion and extrapolation from use of the therapeutic agents for related autoimmune rheumatic diseases. The SSF clinical practice guidelines (CPG) for the treatment of inflammatory musculoskeletal pain associated with SS recommends first-line therapy with hydroxychloroquine.[4] Should hydroxychloroquine be ineffective, the CPG recommends either substitution or addition of low-dose weekly methotrexate. In the event methotrexate does not control symptoms, the CPG recommends addition of low-dose prednisone ($\leq$15 mg daily) for <1 month, with an option to taper over a longer period while switching to DMARDs/biologic drugs to attain disease control. Additional recommended options include sulfasalazine, leflunomide, and cyclosporine A. Azathioprine was recommended as an option for inflammatory musculoskeletal pain particularly in the context of other extraglandular manifestations (e.g., interstitial lung disease [ILD], vasculitis). Regarding the use of biologic drugs, the CPG did not recommend TNF-α inhibitors for sicca symptoms; however, the guidelines mention that TNF-α inhibitors can be used to treat severe polyarthritis unresponsive to DMARDs, especially in patients with overlapping features of RA. Rituximab was also recommended as an option to treat the extraglandular manifestations of SS, including inflammatory arthritis. The CPG determined that, at present, there was insufficient data to recommend the use of abatacept, tocilizumab, and belimumab but recommended further study of these agents.

Recommendations of the British Society for Rheumatology[26] were similar to the SSF CPG but emphasized the use of methotrexate as the first-line therapeutic agent for arthritis and did not recommend the use of leflunomide for the treatment of arthritis associated with SS. Guidelines developed by the Japanese Research Team for Autoimmune Diseases for the Research Program for Intractable Disease by the Ministry of Health Labor and Welfare[27] were similar for corticosteroids and rituximab; however, the guidelines addressed extraglandular manifestations as a group as opposed to specific manifestations. These recommendations also did not address the use of specific DMARDs.

Muscular involvement

SS can cause inflammatory myalgias that often respond to the same treatments as given for arthralgias and arthritis. Rarely, myalgias may also be caused by an inflammatory myositis. A review documented inflammatory myositis in 17 (1.3%) individuals among an Italian cohort of 1320 SS patients.[28] These subjects presented with weakness and either elevated creatine phosphokinase levels or an abnormal electromyographic result and muscle biopsies were abnormal in six, revealing polymyositis-like histology in five and a picture consistent with inclusion body myositis in one. Espitia-Thibault et al.[29] described a group of four patients with inflammatory myositis (among a cohort of 23 SS cases with muscle involvement) whose biopsy results demonstrated germinal center—like structures in addition to endomysial and perimysial inflammation. These lymphocyte clusters appeared as nodular infiltrates with follicular structures composed of central CD20$^+$ B cells surrounded by CD4$^+$ and CD8$^+$ T cells similar to those seen in labial salivary gland biopsies. Patients were successfully treated with corticosteroids and/or hydroxychloroquine and did well on follow-up, suggesting a good prognosis for this specific subtype of SS myopathy. Further studies are needed to confirm these findings. Inflammatory myositis in SS is typically treated with corticosteroids as the first-line therapy, followed by the initiation of other DMARDs such as methotrexate or azathioprine as steroid-sparing agents. For refractory cases biologic drugs such as intravenous rituximab, or intravenous immunoglobulin can also be used.

Fibromyalgia

Fibromyalgia syndrome (FMS) is a frequent comorbidity in SS and reported to occur in 15%—30% of cases.[30,31] FMS may contribute to arthralgias, myalgias, and fatigue in SS and must be addressed before instituting corticosteroids, DMARDs, and/or other immunosuppressive therapy for musculoskeletal symptoms. Patients should be counseled to practice good sleep hygiene (chapter 12) and encouraged to exercise. Stretching exercises and light aerobics as tolerated should be prescribed as the first-line therapy. Sicca symptoms that interfere with sleep should be treated more aggressively. Ocular ointments and gels can be applied to the eyes instead of artificial tears at bedtime for longer lasting relief. Secretagogues (e.g., pilocarpine, cevimeline) can be used to prevent nocturia related to excessive water drinking during the day. The last dose can be administered at bedtime to prevent awakening for nocturnal fluid ingestion. Other simple measures such as the use of an ultrasonic cool mist humidifier at night or coating the tongue and mucous membranes with lubricants such as vitamin E oil or moisturizing gels (e.g., Biotene Oral Balance®) at bedtime can also help alleviate nocturnal dryness.

A limitation of FMS pharmacotherapy in SS is the frequent anticholinergic side effects from standard tricyclic-type medications such as amitriptyline, nortriptyline, doxepin, and cyclobenzaprine, which can exacerbate ocular and oral dryness. Should medication be required, newer serotonin-norepinephrine reuptake inhibitors such as duloxetine, milnacipran, and pregabalin can be used, preferably, at the lowest possible doses. These agents are approved by the FDA for treatment of FMS and may also alleviate pain from other causes. Additional treatment options for FMS in SS are discussed in Chapter 12.

Respiratory manifestations

The prevalence of clinically significant pulmonary disease in SS ranges from 9.0% to 24%,[32] and other parts of the respiratory tract may also be involved. Pulmonary manifestations (Chapter 6) are associated with impairments in physical functioning and quality of life, when SS patients with respiratory symptoms are compared with those without lung involvement. It is important to note that pulmonary involvement in SS is associated with a fourfold increased risk of mortality after 10 years of disease.[33]

Upper respiratory tract and airway disease

Saliva serves as a buffer for refluxed gastric contents; its inadequacy can cause laryngeal reflux, which in turn leads to symptoms of globus sensation, excessive throat clearing, cough, and hoarseness. Lymphocytic inflammation and atrophy of the submucosal glands of the airways leads to dessication of the respiratory mucosa, changes in the viscosity of mucus, and compromised mucociliary clearance. These abnormalities may result in persistent dry cough, hoarseness, nasal dryness, crusting, epistaxis, and recurrent respiratory infections including bronchitis or sinusitis.[18,34,35] Other causes of a chronic cough in SS are discussed later. Symptoms may be relieved by therapeutic doses of secretagogues or antitussive agents such as guaifenesin with or without dextromethorphan. Laryngeal reflux is treated with dietary modifications, histamine receptor 2 (H_2) blockers and/or proton pump inhibitors. Treatment of bacterial infections may require extended courses of antibiotics. A variety of moisturizing nasal sprays and gels can also be used twice or thrice during the day and every night at bedtime to alleviate xeromycteria.

Interstitial lung disease

ILD is the most common pulmonary manifestation of SS and can precede the diagnosis and be the presenting manifestation of the disease or develop up to 10 years later in the course. Patients present with various features, most commonly dyspnea and cough, and, occasionally, also with sputum production, chest pain, and fever that mimics acute bacterial pneumonia. The severity of symptoms can range from asymptomatic disease to slowly progressive respiratory failure. Pulmonary function tests (PFTs) typically shows a restrictive pattern with low diffusing capacity; however, depending on the degree of concomitant airway disease, obstructive patterns may be observed. The different forms of ILD in SS are classified according to histologic and imaging features (Table 11.2) and include nonspecific interstitial pneumonitis (NSIP), usual interstitial pneumonitis (UIP), lymphocytic interstitial pneumonitis (LIP), and cryptogenic organizing pneumonia (COP). NSIP is most common followed by COP in most series.[36] LIP has been most closely associated with SS. UIP is the most challenging to treat and has the worst prognosis.[32,37,38]

Treatment of nonspecific interstitial pneumonitis

The prognosis of NSIP is generally good and depends on the degree of fibrosis at the time of diagnosis. In a case series by Katzenstein et al.,[39] no deaths occurred in the patients whose biopsy results showed pure inflammation without fibrosis, while the mortality rate was 11% for those patients with ILD with fibrosis. For patients who are asymptomatic and have normal or minimally abnormal PFT results, clinical and radiologic surveillance is recommended instead of active treatment. For patients who are symptomatic, with abnormal PFT results and/or radiographic progression of disease, initial treatment begins with high-dose corticosteroids (e.g., prednisone, 1 mg/kg/day of ideal body weight) followed by a steroid taper over 6 months.[38]

Table 11.2 Overview of interstitial lung disease in Sjögren's syndrome.

Subtypes	Histology	Radiographic findings	Location	Prognosis
Nonspecific interstitial pneumonitis	Interstitial inflammation, fibrosis, relative preservation of lung architecture	Patchy ground-glass opacities, intralobular reticulation, traction bronchiectasis	Bibasilar, symmetric	Good
Usual interstitial pneumonitis	Patchy lymphocytic inflammation, fibroblast foci, honeycombing, intermixed with normal lung	Reticular abnormalities, bronchiectasis, subpleural honeycombing	Bibasilar, peripheral, symmetric	Poor
Lymphocytic interstitial pneumonitis	Diffuse interstitial infiltration by lymphocytes and plasma cells, lymphoid follicles, germinal centers, follicular bronchiolitis	Ground-glass opacities, centrilobular/subpleural nodules, reticular opacities, septal thickening, bronchial and bronchiolar thickening, cysts	Bibasilar, symmetric	Fair
Cryptogenic organizing pneumonia	Small airway intraluminal inflammatory debris with fibroblasts/myofibroblasts, alveolar inflammation	Parenchymal consolidations with air bronchograms, ground-glass opacities, centrilobular nodules, tree-in-bud opacities	Peripheral	Fair

For patients in whom steroid treatment fails because of the lack of efficacy or side effects, other immunosuppressive agents (e.g., azathioprine) should be considered based on limited data. In a nonrandomized study of 11 patients treated with azathioprine for NSIP, there was a significant improvement in forced vital capacity at 6 months when compared with untreated patients.[40] Experience using mycophenolate mofetil (MMF) for ILD associated with connective tissue diseases (CTDs) suggests possible benefit for SS patients. In a series of 125 patients with CTDs, 5 of whom had SS, MMF was well tolerated and had a glucocorticoid-sparing effect.[41]

Rituximab may also have a potential role in the treatment of SS-associated ILD. In a French registry of 78 SS patients, 9 had SS-related pulmonary manifestations: 8 with ILD and 1 with bronchiolar involvement. Six of the eight patients with ILD responded to the first cycle of rituximab.[42] Additionally, in the latest treatment guidelines for SS, use of rituximab was mentioned as a moderate recommendation for the treatment of pulmonary disease.[43] For SS patients who have rapidly progressive initial disease, or progression despite treatment with glucocorticoids and a second-line immunosuppressive agent, use of intravenous or oral cyclophosphamide may be beneficial, based on limited data from case series and clinical experience in related CTDs.[44] Some data supports the use of cyclophosphamide with corticosteroids.[45] Data on the use of calcineurin inhibitors, which include cyclosporine and tacrolimus, for NSIP is very limited and should only be reserved for refractory disease.

Treatment of other Sjögren's syndrome interstitial lung disease

Among all the ILD subtypes associated with CTDs, UIP has the worst prognosis and this is true in SS as well.[38] There is no known treatment for UIP, but for patients with declining respiratory function, a treatment algorithm similar to that used for NSIP is suggested.

Patients with LIP generally respond well to initial corticosteroid therapy. There are also reports of rituximab improving more refractory cases of LIP.[46,47] Despite this steroid responsiveness, according to some studies, up to one-third may die within several years of diagnosis from progression of disease or infectious complications related to immunosuppressive therapy.[48]

Cryptogenic organizing pneumonia is a relatively uncommon clinicopathologic entity, and focal areas of OP can be seen in association with NSIP.[49] Corticosteroids are also the mainstay of therapy and response can be seen within several days to a few weeks. The optimum dose and length of treatment is not known and relapses are common.[50] Data for the use of immunosuppressive agents for OP is very limited.

Airway disease

Follicular bronchiolitis (FB) is one of the most common pulmonary manifestations of SS and often coexists with ILD. It is characterized by hyperplastic lymphoid follicles with reactive germinal centers along the bronchovascular bundles. The inflammatory infiltrate primarily affects the bronchioles and peribronchiolar interstitium and does not extend into the adjacent parenchyma. It is largely composed of mast cells, neutrophils, and lymphocytes (similar to that of asthma) and causes bronchial hyperreactivity, recurrent bronchitis, cough, and dyspnea.[48,51] Typical radiographic features include small 1–3 mm nodules, with a predominant centrilobular and peribronchial distribution. The prognosis of isolated FB is relatively good.[52] The best treatment strategy for FB in SS is unclear, but as it may be associated with NSIP, LIP, or organizing pneumonia, treatment is usually tailored toward the associated ILD.

Chronic obstructive pulmonary disease (COPD) has also been described in SS and may contribute to respiratory symptoms. In a Swedish cohort, 37% of SS patients met COPD criteria over 11 years of follow-up. In patients with SS, COPD was five times more prevalent among ever smokers and was also higher than expected in nonsmokers than in controls. These patients demonstrated evidence of both restrictive and obstructive disease on pulmonary function testing over time with significantly decreased vital capacity, total lung capacity, FEV_1 (forced expiratory volume in the first second of expiration), FEV_1/forced vital capacity, and DLCO (diffusing capacity of lung for carbon monoxide) and an increased residual volume.[53] Interestingly, respiratory symptoms often showed poor correlation with PFT results in SS patients with COPD.[54] Little has been written about the treatment of COPD in SS but, presumably, until more information becomes available, the treatment approach should be the same as in other groups with COPD.

Pulmonary lymphoma

Patients with SS have a higher risk of developing lymphoproliferative disorders, most commonly non-Hodgkin B-cell lymphoma (Chapter 8), than patients with other autoimmune disorders and the general population.[55] These lymphomas arise mainly in mucosal extranodal sites including the salivary and lacrimal glands, stomach, and lung. Primary pulmonary lymphomas are relatively infrequent, representing less than 1% of lung cancers[56] and less than 1% of malignant lymphomas.[57] These lymphomas may present with cough and dyspnea or be discovered as a coincidental finding on chest imaging.[58,59] A case series of 13 patients diagnosed with bronchus-associated lymphoid tissue (BALT) lymphoma found that two of those patients had underlying SS.[58] The prognosis of mucosa-associated lymphoid tissue (MALT) lymphomas is relatively good regardless of which organs are involved. In a study of 22 patients with MALT lymphoma, >80% survival at 5 years was reported.[60] Treatment of BALT in SS with intravenous rituximab may help other aspects of the disease as well.[4]

Pulmonary amyloidosis

The most common form of pulmonary amyloidosis is amyloid light chain (AL) amyloidosis (kappa or lambda), which is a recognized complication of SS. Nodular pulmonary amyloidosis is seen most often in SS and occurs almost exclusively in women. It can be an incidental finding on chest radiography (calcified or noncalcified nodules with or without cysts) but may cause dyspnea, cough, weakness, fatigue, or hemoptysis.[61,62] It is almost always localized. Surgical lung biopsy is usually required to establish the diagnosis and rule out lymphoma, especially in patients with expanding nodules or constitutional symptoms. The prognosis is very good and treatment is not always required. Symptomatic patients may get some benefit from corticosteroid use.[61,62] Systemic AL amyloidosis is very rarely described in association with SS, with only two cases reported in the literature.[63,64]

Pleural involvement

Pleural effusions rarely occur as a direct complication of SS and should always raise suspicion of an overlap syndrome with another underlying autoimmune disorder such as RA or systemic lupus erythematosus. In the literature, there are only 10 reports of pleural effusions (bilateral or unilateral) in association with SS in the absence of another cause.[65] In these cases, the pleural fluid analysis demonstrated an exudate with lymphocytic predominance, low complement levels, and elevated levels of SS-A/SS-B antibodies.[66] Pleurisy alone can be successfully managed with nonsteroidal antiinflammatory drugs at therapeutic doses, whereas effusions are treated with moderate doses of corticosteroids (e.g., prednisone, 20–30 mg/day) followed by a gradual taper.

Pulmonary arterial hypertension

There are less than 50 cases of SS-associated pulmonary arterial hypertension (PAH) described in the literature. Diagnosis of PAH requires right-heart catheterization, demonstrating elevated mean pulmonary artery pressures at rest or during exercise, in the setting of normal pulmonary capillary wedge pressure. Diagnosis is often delayed, as pulmonary symptoms are usually attributed to the underlying lung disease. Thus more severe disease is found at the time of diagnosis. Standard PAH therapy (endothelin receptor antagonists, phosphodiesterase type 5 inhibitors, or prostanoids) with or without immunosuppression can improve SS-associated PAH, although the best treatment strategy is still unclear.[67]

Management of gastrointestinal manifestations

SS may affect the entire GI tract including the mouth, esophagus, stomach, liver, pancreas, small intestine, and colon through a variety of mechanisms including lymphocytic infiltration of exocrine glands or GI mucosa, autonomic nerve dysfunction, or the development of an associated autoimmune disease that occurs with increased frequency in SS.

Mouth

Xerostomia is discussed in Chapter 3 and may cause numerous symptoms and complications including dysgeusia, dysphagia, dysphonia, tooth decay, and infections of the oral cavity.[68] All patients should be counseled to avoid medications with anticholinergic effects and to reduce the intake of highly acidic beverages, caffeine, alcohol, and nicotine.[69] The primary options for the treatment of dry mouth include topical agents and secretagogues.[70] Any type of mechanical and/or gustatory salivary stimulation will alleviate symptoms and can be achieved with the use of sugar-free gums, candies, and lozenges.[2] Products containing xylitol as the sweetener are preferred because of its possible anticaries effect.[71] Patients with no flow may benefit from the use of artificial saliva and oral lubricants.[2] Patients with persistent xerostomia and low salivary function despite the abovementioned options may benefit from muscarinic agonists such as pilocarpine or cevimeline that act as secretagogues.[72] Patients with SS are prone to candidiasis and oral preparations containing nystatin are the typical first-line agents.[73] Routine dental evaluation and follow-up every 6 months in addition to regular fluoride use is highly recommended.[74]

Esophagus

Dysphagia and gastroesophageal reflux disease (GERD) are the main esophageal symptoms of SS.[75] Poor dentition and hyposalivation impair preparation of the food bolus for the initial stages of deglutition. The lack of saliva may contribute to both dysphagia and reflux and should be treated with secretagogues as discussed earlier. GERD should be managed aggressively as previously outlined. Patients with persistent dysphagia despite this approach should be referred to a gastroenterologist for evaluation and management of abnormalities in motility or upper and/or lower esophageal sphincter pressures.[76,77]

Gastric involvement

Dyspepsia and gastritis are common GI manifestations of SS.[78] These features can be symptomatically addressed with H_2 blockers or proton pump inhibitors. There is conflicting evidence regarding an increased prevalence of *Helicobacter pylori* in SS, but histopathologic findings supporting *H. pylori* infection requires management with antibiotics and repeat endoscopic surveillance to assess resolution.[79] *H. pylori* treatment does not, however, reduce gastric lymphocytic infiltration, gastric atrophy, or dyspepsia in SS. Gastric MALT lymphoma may occur in SS but is rare. Hepatitis C infection in patients with hepatitis C virus (HCV)-induced sicca is strongly associated with gastric B-cell clonal expansion, which may rarely result in gastric MALT lymphoma. This needs to be assessed and addressed in at-risk patients.[80,81]

Chronic atrophic gastritis occurs with greater frequency in SS than in normal controls.[82] Treatment is directed at modification or elimination of environmental factors (e.g., *H. pylori*) that may cause or aggravate this condition and at prevention of complications, including iron and vitamin B_{12} deficiency.[83]

Gastropareseis is well documented in SS[84,85] and may cause nausea, abdominal discomfort, weight loss, early satiety, and postprandial bloating. Dietary modifications including smaller more frequent meals and ingestion of food that is low in fat and insoluble fiber may alleviate symptoms. Medical therapy includes the use of promotility agents (e.g., metoclopramide, domperidone, erythromycin) and antiemetics, with careful monitoring for side effects.

Liver

Abnormal liver function test results have been observed in up to 40% of SS patients. Common hepatic manifestations include primary biliary cholangitis (PBC), chronic active autoimmune hepatitis (AIH), drug toxicity (e.g., methotrexate), and nonalcoholic fatty liver disease associated with steroid therapy for SS.[86] SS may occur in up to one-third of patients with PBC [87,] and sicca symptoms may occur in PBC in the absence of SS.[88] Of the SS patients positive for antimitochondrial antibodies, 60% have an elevated alkaline phosphatase level, whereas 82% have histologic features of PBC.[89] Ursodeoxycholic acid has been approved for the treatment of PBC[90] and the prognosis is generally good.

AIH is a rare manifestation in patients with SS. The diagnosis is usually confirmed by liver biopsy, the presence of anti—smooth muscle antibodies, and the exclusion of other causes. The usual treatment regimen for AIH includes glucocorticoids and azathioprine.[91] Although AIH can progress to cirrhosis and even hepatocellular carcinoma, when properly treated, the 10-year survival rate is >90%. HCV infection can affect the salivary glands and cause xerostomia, which can mimic SS and can cause abnormal liver function test results. It must therefore be excluded in all patients being evaluated for SS.[92] HCV infection-sicca patients are more likely to have neurologic involvement, elevated transaminase levels, RF, and cryoglobulins and are less likely to have anti-SS-A/SS-B antibodies compared with SS patients without HCV infection.[93] Therapy for HCV infection may improve HCV infection—associated sicca symptoms.[94] Patients with hemochromatosis and subsequent iron overload may also develop sicca symptoms secondary to salivary gland damage. This may improve with iron chelation therapy.[95,96] Many of the treatments recommended for inflammatory musculoskeletal pain in SS are associated with an increased risk of hepatotoxicity and, therefore, require laboratory monitoring on a regular basis.[97]

Pancreas

Acute autoimmune pancreatitis causes abdominal pain and less commonly jaundice, is rarely observed in (<1%) SS,[98] and considered steroid responsive. Chronic pancreatitis has been described in ~2%[99] and flares are treated with enzyme replacement and bowel rest. Pancreatic exocrine insufficiency has been reported in a much larger group of SS patients (36%—63%) but is clinically silent in most cases, with steatorrhea being uncommon; prevalence varies according to the method of assessment of pancreatic exocrine function. Primary sclerosing cholangitis was reported to occur in association with chronic pancreatitis and SS in several cases dating back to the 1970s.[100] In retrospect, as many of these cases were men and had salivary gland swelling in addition to sicca symptoms, the majority of these patients most likely had IgG4-related systemic disease with Mikulicz syndrome rather than true SS.[101] Mikulicz syndrome is characterized by sicca symptoms associated with bilateral salivary and/or lacrimal swelling caused by infiltration of salivary glands by IgG4-positive plasma cells. IgG4-related systemic disease requires treatment with corticosteroids, rituximab, or oral immunosuppressive medications.[102]

Small and large intestines

Chronic diarrhea can occur in up to 9% of SS patients.[96] Celiac disease, confirmed by small bowel biopsy, was prevalent in 4.5%–14.7% of SS patients in two small studies, but not seen in larger studies. Gluten-free diets typically eliminate GI symptoms but do not improve sicca symptoms, except as reported in one study.[103–105] Diarrhea in SS may also occur as a side effect from regular use of secretagogues or lozenges containing xylitol or sorbitol to treat xerostomia, and will usually improve with a dosage reduction. Two studies reported an increased propensity for SS patients to develop irritable bowel syndrome (IBS) in the absence of celiac.[106,107] One report attributed symptoms of IBS to food hypersensitivities and observed that abdominal pain, bloating, diarrhea, and joint pain were eliminated with dietary restriction of foods to which hypersensitivity was demonstrated but recurred on rechallenge.[108] Cases of coexistent SS and Crohn disease or ulcerative colitis have also been reported in a handful of patients and must be considered in the evaluation and treatment of diarrhea in SS.[109,110] Rarely, vasculitis in SS may involve the gut and present as ischemic bowel with abdominal pain, acute or subacute diarrhea, and gross or occult blood in the stool, especially in the setting of type II cryoglobulinemia.[111] Treatment is discussed in Chapter 7.

In addition to the aforementioned problems, colonic involvement with chronic constipation has been reported in up to 23% of SS patients.[96] In addition to the usual measures, treatment with secretagogues (e.g., cevimeline) may also alleviate this problem.

Management of renal manifestations

As previously discussed (Chapter 6), clinically significant renal complications in SS primarily result from tubulointerstitial nephritis (TIN) and its sequelae or, less commonly, from membranoproliferative glomerulonephritis (MPGN) related to cryoglobulinemia. A prospective study in India[112] documented renal disease in 50% of SS patients ($n = 70$) diagnosed according to the 2002 American European Consensus Group criteria (Chapter 2) using the case definition outlined in Table 11.3.

Renal tubular dysfunction

TIN results from lymphocytic infiltration around epithelial structures in the kidneys and causes a variety of different defects in tubular function, including distal renal tubular acidosis (dRTA), nephrogenic diabetes insipidus (NDI), and proximal tubular dysfunction. dRTA is due to inadequate urinary H^+ secretion leading to possible metabolic acidosis and alkaline urine. A urine acidification test (UAT) should be performed in all SS patients who demonstrate a persistently alkaline urine and/or hyperchloremia with low serum bicarbonate. The UAT is performed by administration of ammonium chloride or furosemide and fludrocortisone.[113] dRTA also causes wasting of urinary K^+ leading to hypokalemia and possible paralysis and/or cardiac arrest. It may be complicated by nephrolithiasis or nephrocalcinosis leading to renal colic and possible

Table 11.3 Renal involvement in Sjögren's syndrome.

Complete dRTA
Incomplete dRTA (+ UAT without overt acidosis ± hypokalemia)
Renal colic/nephrolithiasis
Nephrocalcinosis/overt dRTA or + UAT
Fanconi syndrome
Creatinine clearance <60 mL/min
Proteinuria >500 mg/24 h
Active urinary sediment
Positive finding in renal biopsy
Tubulointerstitial nephritis
Glomerulonephritis
Both

dRTA, *Distal renal tubular acidosis;* UAT, *Urine acidification test.*
Modified from Ref. 108.

urosepsis.[114] Management of dRTA includes bicarbonate and potassium supplementation and monitoring for nephrolithiasis to avoid complications.

NDI is caused by dysfunction of the principal cells of the collecting duct and presents with polydipsia, polyuria, and nocturia. It is seen in approximately in 75% of patients with biopsy-proven TIN but only about 25% demonstrate symptoms. Specific management of NDI is generally not required in SS because patients' volume of water intake for xerostomia is usually sufficient to maintain normal serum sodium levels.[115] Rarely, excessive polydipsia from sicca leads to hyposthenuria and hyponatremia. This can be alleviated with the regular use of sugar-free gums, lozenges, and/or secretagogues.

Patients with presumed TIN in whom more conservative treatments fail and/or who demonstrate progressive loss of renal function should undergo a renal biopsy to confirm the diagnosis, estimate chronicity, and rule out other causes. Treatment with high-dose corticosteroids (e.g., prednisone, 0.5–1 mg/kg per day) followed by a taper over 3–6 months is generally beneficial in most cases.[112,116] If a steroid-sparing agent is required because of disease relapse or intolerable side effects, MMF[117] and azathioprine[118] have both been used with success. Registry data from France also reported benefit from B-cell depleting therapy with rituximab in treatment-refractory cases of TIN.[42]

Glomerulonephritis

MPGN from immune complex deposition by cryoglobulins and small vessel vasculitis[113] is uncommon in SS compared with TIN and, when present, it frequently coexists with TIN. Other glomerular lesions less commonly occur [116,] and treatment is based on renal biopsy findings. Most patients with glomerulonephritis related to cryoglobulinemia are treated with rituximab[42] and a tapering course of steroids; plasmapheresis may be reserved for rapidly progressive or life-threatening disease.[115] Other potentially useful treatments for MPGN include MMF, azathioprine, or cyclophosphamide.[116]

Other biologic drugs that are currently being evaluated for treatment of SS include belimumab (targets B cell–activating factor), secukinumab (targets Th17-related epithelial inflammation), and abatacept (interferes with T-cell signaling); these could also potentially be useful in the future for the treatment of renal manifestations.[119–121]

Conclusions

Musculoskeletal pain and constitutional symptoms, particularly fatigue, are common manifestations of SS. Clinical practice guidelines based on evidence and expert opinion have been published to aid clinicians in the management of these manifestations and have been summarized earlier. Organ-specific extraglandular manifestations including involvement of the lung, GI tract, and kidney occur less frequently but can result in significant morbidity. The relatively low prevalence of each manifestation (5%–20%) in cohorts of SS patients presents significant challenges in designing therapeutic trials that would yield high-quality evidence. Treatment recommendations based on extrapolation from other autoimmune conditions and the available literature are provided. Corticosteroids remain the mainstay of treatment of significant extraglandular disease. Oral DMARDs remain important as steroid-sparing agents. Although there is no established role for TNF-α blockade in SS management, some data suggests a role for B-cell depletion in selected situations.

References

1. Garcia-Carrasco M, Ramos-Casals M, Rosas J, Pallares L, Calvo-Alen J, Cervera R, Font J, Ingelmo M. Primary Sjögren syndrome: clinical and immunologic disease patterns in a cohort of 400 patients. *Medicine (Baltimore)*. 2002;81(4):270–280.
2. Vivino FB, Bunya VY, Massaro-Giordano G, Johr CR, Giattino SL, Schorpion A, Shafer B, Peck A, Sivils K, Rasmussen A, Chiorini JA, He J, Ambrus Jr JL. Sjögren's syndrome: an update on disease pathogenesis, clinical manifestations and treatment. *Clin Immunol*. 2019;203:81–121.
3. Flament T, Bigot A, Chaigne B, Henique H, Diot E, Marchand-Adam S. Pulmonary manifestations of Sjögren's syndrome. *Eur Respir Rev*. 2016;25(140):110–123.
4. Carsons SE, Vivino FB, Parke A, Carteron N, Sankar V, Brasington R, Brennan MT, Ehlers W, Fox R, Scofield H, Hammitt KM, Birnbaum J, Kassan S, Mandel S. Treatment guidelines for rheumatologic manifestations of Sjögren's syndrome: use of biologic agents, management of fatigue, and inflammatory musculoskeletal pain. *Arthritis Care Res*. 2017;69(4):517–527.
5. Strombeck BE, Theander E, Jacobsson LT. Effects of exercise on aerobic capacity and fatigue in women with primary Sjögren's syndrome. *Rheumatology*. 2007;46(5):868–871.

6. Sjögren H. Zur Kenntnis der keratoconjunctivitis sicca: Keratitis filiformis bei hypofunktion der tranendrusen. *Acta Opthalmologica.* 1933;11(Suppl. II):1−151.

7. Alamanos Y, Tsifetaki N, Voulgari PV, Venetsanopoulou AI, Siozos C, Drosos AA. Epidemiology of primary Sjögren's syndrome in North-west Greece, 1982−2003. *Rheumatology.* 2006;45(2):187−191.

8. Davidson BK, Kelly CA, Griffiths ID. Primary Sjögren's syndrome in the North East of England: a long-term follow-up study. *Rheumatology.* 1999;38(3):245−253.

9. Lin DF, Yan SM, Zhao Y, Zhang W, Li MT, Zeng XF, Zhang FC, Dong Y. Clinical and prognostic characteristics of 573 cases of primary Sjögren's syndrome. *Chin Med J.* 2010;123(22):3252−3257.

10. Ramos-Casals M, Brito-Zeron P, Seror R, Bootsma H, Bowman SJ, Dorner T, Gottenberg JE, Mariette X, Theander E, Bombardieri S, De Vita S, Mandl T, Ng WF, Kruize A, Tzioufas A, Vitali C, Force ESST. Characterization of systemic disease in primary Sjögren's syndrome: EULAR-SS Task Force recommendations for articular, cutaneous, pulmonary and renal involvements. *Rheumatology.* 2015;54(12):2230−2238.

11. Ramos-Casals M, Brito-Zeron P, Yague J, Akasbi M, Bautista R, Ruano M, Claver G, Gil V, Font J. Hypocomplementaemia as an immunological marker of morbidity and mortality in patients with primary Sjögren's syndrome. *Rheumatology.* 2005;44(1): 89−94.

12. Skopouli FN, Dafni U, Ioannidis JP, Moutsopoulos HM. Clinical evolution, and morbidity and mortality of primary Sjögren's syndrome. *Semin Arthritis Rheum.* 2000;29(5):296−304.

13. Theander E, Henriksson G, Ljungberg O, Mandl T, Manthorpe R, Jacobsson LT. Lymphoma and other malignancies in primary Sjögren's syndrome: a cohort study on cancer incidence and lymphoma predictors. *Ann Rheum Dis.* 2006;65(6):796−803.

14. Zhao Y DY, Guo XP, Tang FL. Clinical Analysis of primary Sjögren's syndrome. *Beijing Med J.* 1997;19:100−104.

15. Bloch KJ, Buchanan WW, Wohl MJ, Bunim JJ. Sjögren's syndrome. A clinical, pathological, and serological study of sixty-two cases. *Medicine (Baltimore).* 1965;71(6): 386−401. discussion 401-3.

16. Pease CT, Shattles W, Barrett NK, Maini RN. The arthropathy of Sjögren's syndrome. *Br J Rheumatol.* 1993;32(7):609−613.

17. Yang H, Bian S, Chen H, Wang L, Zhao L, Zhang X, Zhao Y, Zeng X, Zhang F. Clinical characteristics and risk factors for overlapping rheumatoid arthritis and Sjögren's syndrome. *Sci Rep.* 2018;8(1):6180.

18. Fauchais AL, Ouattara B, Gondran G, Lalloue F, Petit D, Ly K, Lambert M, Launay D, Loustaud-Ratti V, Bezanahari H, Liozon E, Hachulla E, Jauberteau MO, Vidal E, Hatron PY. Articular manifestations in primary Sjögren's syndrome: clinical significance and prognosis of 188 patients. *Rheumatol.* 2010;49(6):1164−1172.

19. Mirouse A, Seror R, Vicaut E, Mariette X, Dougados M, Fauchais AL, Deroux A, Dellal A, Costedoat-Chalumeau N, Denis G, Sellam J, Arlet JB, Lavigne C, Urbanski G, Fischer-Dumont D, Diallo A, Fain O, Mekinian A, Club Rhumatismes I, Snfmi. Arthritis in primary Sjögren's syndrome: characteristics, outcome and treatment from French multicenter retrospective study. *Autoimmun Rev.* 2019;18(1):9−14.

20. ter Borg EJ, Kelder JC. Polyarthritis in primary Sjögren's syndrome represents a distinct subset with less pronounced B cell proliferation a Dutch cohort with long-term follow-up. *Clin Rheumatol.* 2016;35(3):649−655.

21. Khan O, Carsons S. Occurrence of rheumatoid arthritis requiring oral and/or biological disease-modifying antirheumatic drug therapy following a diagnosis of primary Sjögren syndrome. *J Clin Rheumatol*. 2012;18(7):356−358.

22. Carsons S, Harris EK. In: Steven Carsons M, Harris EK, eds. *The new Sjögren's syndrome handbook*. New York: Oxford University Press; 1998.

23. Gottenberg JE, Ravaud P, Puechal X, Le Guern V, Sibilia J, Goeb V, Larroche C, Dubost JJ, Rist S, Saraux A, Devauchelle-Pensec V, Morel J, Hayem G, Hatron P, Perdriger A, Sene D, Zarnitsky C, Batouche D, Furlan V, Benessiano J, Perrodeau E, Seror R, Mariette X. Effects of hydroxychloroquine on symptomatic improvement in primary Sjögren syndrome: the JOQUER randomized clinical trial. *J Am Med Assoc*. 2014;312(3):249−258.

24. Kim SM, Park E, Lee JH, Lee SH, Kim HR. The clinical significance of anti-cyclic citrullinated peptide antibody in primary Sjögren syndrome. *Rheumatol Int*. 2012;32(12): 3963−3967.

25. Faustman DL, Vivino FB, Carsons SE. Treatment of primary Sjögren syndrome with rituximab. *Ann Intern Med*. 2014;161(5):376−377.

26. Price EJ, Rauz S, Tappuni AR, Sutcliffe N, Hackett KL, Barone F, Granata G, Ng WF, Fisher BA, Bombardieri M, Astorri E, Empson B, Larkin G, Crampton B, Bowman SJ, British Society for Rheumatology Standards G, Audit Working G. The British society for rheumatology guideline for the management of adults with primary Sjögren's syndrome. *Rheumatol*. 2017;56(10):1828.

27. Sumida T, Azuma N, Moriyama M, Takahashi H, Asashima H, Honda F, Abe S, Ono Y, Hirota T, Hirata S, Tanaka Y, Shimizu T, Nakamura H, Kawakami A, Sano H, Ogawa Y, Tsubota K, Ryo K, Saito I, Tanaka A, Nakamura S, Takamura E, Tanaka M, Suzuki K, Takeuchi T, Yamakawa N, Mimori T, Ohta A, Nishiyama S, Yoshihara T, Suzuki Y, Kawano M, Tomiita M, Tsuboi H. Clinical practice guideline for Sjögren's syndrome 2017. *Mod Rheumatol*. 2018;28(3):383−408.

28. Colafrancesco S, Priori R, Gattamelata A, Picarelli G, Minniti A, Brancatisano F, D'Amati G, Giordano C, Cerbelli B, Maset M, Quartuccio L, Bartoloni E, Carubbi F, Cipriani P, Baldini C, Luciano N, De Vita S, Gerli R, Giacomelli R, Bombardieri S, Valesini G. Myositis in primary Sjögren's syndrome: data from a multicentre cohort. *Clin Exp Rheumatol*. 2015;33(4):457−464.

29. Espitia-Thibault A, Masseau A, Neel A, Espitia O, Toquet C, Mussini JM, Hamidou M. Sjögren's syndrome-associated myositis with germinal centre-like structures. *Autoimmun Rev*. 2017;16(2):154−158.

30. Torrente-Segarra V, Corominas H, Sanchez-Piedra C, Fernandez-Castro M, Andreu JL, Martinez-Taboada VM, Olive A, Rosas J, Sanchez-Alonso F, S.S.G.o.t.S.S.o. Rheumatology. Fibromyalgia prevalence and associated factors in primary Sjögren's syndrome patients in a large cohort from the Spanish Society of Rheumatology registry (SJOGRENSER). *Clin Exp Rheumatol*. 2017. 35;105(3):28−34.

31. Choi BY, Oh HJ, Lee YJ, Song YW. Prevalence and clinical impact of fibromyalgia in patients with primary Sjögren's syndrome. *Clin Exp Rheumatol*. 2016;34(2 Suppl. 96). p. S9-13.

32. Kampolis CF, Fragkioudaki S, Mavragani CP, Zormpala A, Samakovli A, Moutsopoulos HM. Prevalence and spectrum of symptomatic pulmonary involvement in primary Sjögren's syndrome. *Clin Exp Rheumatol*. 2018;36(112(3)):94−101.

33. Palm O, Garen T, Berge Enger T, Jensen JL, Lund MB, Aalokken TM, Gran JT. Clinical pulmonary involvement in primary Sjögren's syndrome: prevalence, quality of life and

mortality–a retrospective study based on registry data. *Rheumatology.* 2013;52(1): 173−179.

34. Hatron PY, Tillie-Leblond I, Launay D, Hachulla E, Fauchais AL, Wallaert B. Pulmonary manifestations of Sjögren's syndrome. *Presse Med.* 2011;40(1 Pt 2). p. e49-64.

35. Butnor KJ, Khoor A. Collagen vascular diseases and disorders of connective tissue. In: Tomashefski Jr JF, ed. *Dail and hammar's pulmonary pathology.* New York: Springer; 2008:722−759.

36. Kreider M, Highland K. Pulmonary involvement in Sjögren syndrome. *Semin Respir Crit Care Med.* 2014;35(2):255−264.

37. Gao H, Zhang XW, He J, Zhang J, An Y, Sun Y, Jia RL, Li SG, Zhang LJ, Li ZG. Prevalence, risk factors, and prognosis of interstitial lung disease in a large cohort of Chinese primary Sjögren syndrome patients: a case-control study. *Medicine (Baltim).* 2018; 97(24):e11003.

38. Parambil JG, Myers JL, Lindell RM, Matteson EL, Ryu JH. Interstitial lung disease in primary Sjögren syndrome. *Chest.* 2006;130(5):1489−1495.

39. Katzenstein AL, Fiorelli RF. Nonspecific interstitial pneumonia/fibrosis. Histologic features and clinical significance. *Am J Surg Pathol.* 1994;18(2):136−147.

40. Deheinzelin D, Capelozzi VL, Kairalla RA, Barbas Filho JV, Saldiva PH, de Carvalho CR. Interstitial lung disease in primary Sjögren's syndrome. Clinical-pathological evaluation and response to treatment. *Am J Respir Crit Care Med.* 1996; 154(3 Pt 1):794−799.

41. Fischer A, Brown KK, Du Bois RM, Frankel SK, Cosgrove GP, Fernandez-Perez ER, Huie TJ, Krishnamoorthy M, Meehan RT, Olson AL, Solomon JJ, Swigris JJ. Mycophenolate mofetil improves lung function in connective tissue disease-associated interstitial lung disease. *J Rheumatol.* 2013;40(5):640−646.

42. Gottenberg JE, Cinquetti G, Larroche C, Combe B, Hachulla E, Meyer O, Pertuiset E, Kaplanski G, Chiche L, Berthelot JM, Gombert B, Goupille P, Marcelli C, Feuillet S, Leone J, Sibilia J, Zarnitsky C, Carli P, Rist S, Gaudin P, Salliot C, Piperno M, Deplas A, Breban M, Lequerre T, Richette P, Ghiringhelli C, Hamidou M, Ravaud P, Mariette X, Club Rhumatismes et I, the French Society of R. Efficacy of rituximab in systemic manifestations of primary Sjögren's syndrome: results in 78 patients of the AutoImmune and Rituximab registry. *Ann Rheum Dis.* 2013;72(6):1026−1031.

43. Vivino FB, Carsons SE, Foulks G, Daniels TE, Parke A, Brennan MT, Forstot SL, Scofield RH, Hammitt KM. New treatment guidelines for Sjögren's disease. *Rheum Dis Clin N Am.* 2016;42(3):531−551.

44. Wallace B, Vummidi D, Khanna D. Management of connective tissue diseases associated interstitial lung disease: a review of the published literature. *Curr Opin Rheumatol.* 2016;28(3):236−245.

45. Schnabel A, Reuter M, Gross WL. Intravenous pulse cyclophosphamide in the treatment of interstitial lung disease due to collagen vascular diseases. *Arthritis Rheum.* 1998;41(7):1215−1220.

46. Seror R, Sordet C, Guillevin L, Hachulla E, Masson C, Ittah M, Candon S, Le Guern V, Aouba A, Sibilia J, Gottenberg JE, Mariette X. Tolerance and efficacy of rituximab and changes in serum B cell biomarkers in patients with systemic complications of primary Sjögren's syndrome. *Ann Rheum Dis.* 2007;66(3):351−357.

47. Swartz MA, Vivino FB. Dramatic reversal of lymphocytic interstitial pneumonitis in Sjögren's syndrome with rituximab. *J Clin Rheumatol.* 2011;17(8):454.

48. Tian X, Yi ES, Ryu JH. Lymphocytic interstitial pneumonia and other benign lymphoid disorders. *Semin Respir Crit Care Med*. 2012;33(5):450−461.
49. Myers JL, Colby TV. Pathologic manifestations of bronchiolitis, constrictive bronchiolitis, cryptogenic organizing pneumonia, and diffuse panbronchiolitis. *Clin Chest Med*. 1993;14(4):611−622.
50. Bradley B, Branley HM, Egan JJ, Greaves MS, Hansell DM, Harrison NK, Hirani N, Hubbard R, Lake F, Millar AB, Wallace WA, Wells AU, Whyte MK, Wilsher ML, B.T.S.S.o.C.C. British Thoracic Society Interstitial Lung Disease Guideline Group, A. Thoracic Society of, S. New Zealand Thoracic, S. Irish Thoracic. Interstitial lung disease guideline: the British thoracic Society in collaboration with the thoracic Society of Australia and New Zealand and the Irish thoracic Society. *Thorax*. 2008;63(Suppl. 5). p. v1-58.
51. Mathieu A, Cauli A, Pala R, Satta L, Nurchis P, Loi GL, Garau P, Sanna G, Passiu G, Carta P, et al. Tracheo-bronchial mucociliary clearance in patients with primary and secondary Sjögren's syndrome. *Scand J Rheumatol*. 1995;24(5):300−304.
52. Bates CA, Ellison MC, Lynch DA, Cool CD, Brown KK, Routes JM. Granulomatous-lymphocytic lung disease shortens survival in common variable immunodeficiency. *J Allergy Clin Immunol*. 2004;114(2):415−421.
53. Mandl T, Diaz S, Ekberg O, Hesselstrand R, Piitulainen E, Wollmer P, Theander E. Frequent development of chronic obstructive pulmonary disease in primary SS–results of a longitudinal follow-up. *Rheumatol*. 2012;51(5):941−946.
54. Strevens Bolmgren V, Olsson P, Wollmer P, Hesselstrand R, Mandl T. Respiratory symptoms are poor predictors of concomitant chronic obstructive pulmonary disease in patients with primary Sjögren's syndrome. *Rheumatol Int*. 2017;37(5):813−818.
55. Alunno A, Leone MC, Giacomelli R, Gerli R, Carubbi F. Lymphoma and lymphomagenesis in primary Sjögren's syndrome. *Front Med*. 2018;5:102.
56. Miller DL, Allen MS. Rare pulmonary neoplasms. *Mayo Clin Proc*. 1993;68(5): 492−498.
57. Voulgarelis M, Dafni UG, Isenberg DA, Moutsopoulos HM. Malignant lymphoma in primary Sjögren's syndrome: a multicenter, retrospective, clinical study by the European Concerted Action on Sjögren's Syndrome. *Arthritis Rheum*. 1999;42(8): 1765−1772.
58. Imai H, Sunaga N, Kaira K, Kawashima O, Yanagitani N, Sato K, Tomizawa Y, Hisada T, Ishizuka T, Hirato J, Saito R, Nakajima T, Mori M. Clinicopathological features of patients with bronchial-associated lymphoid tissue lymphoma. *Intern Med*. 2009;48(5):301−306.
59. Yachoui R, Leon C, Sitwala K, Kreidy M. Pulmonary MALT lymphoma in patients with Sjögren's syndrome. *Clin Med Res*. 2017;15(1−2):6−12.
60. Thieblemont C, de la Fouchardiere A, Coiffier B. Nongastric mucosa-associated lymphoid tissue lymphomas. *Clin Lymphoma*. 2003;3(4):212−224.
61. Rajagopala S, Singh N, Gupta K, Gupta D. Pulmonary amyloidosis in Sjögren's syndrome: a case report and systematic review of the literature. *Respirology*. 2010;15(5): 860−866.
62. Kaur S, Salvatore M, Jacobi A, Gorevic P. Pulmonary amyloidosis associated with Sjögren's syndrome. *Appl Radiol*. 2015.
63. Perlat A, Decaux O, Gervais R, Rioux N, Grosbois B. Systemic light chain amyloidosis and Sjögren syndrome: an uncommon association. *Amyloid*. 2009;16(3):181−182.

64. Delevaux I, Andre M, Amoura Z, Kemeny JL, Piette JC, Aumaitre O. Concomitant diagnosis of primary Sjögren's syndrome and systemic AL amyloidosis. *Ann Rheum Dis*. 2001;60(7):694–695.

65. Hosoda C, Hosaka Y, Ryu K, Kinoshita A, Saito K, Kuwano K. Pleuritis associated with primary Sjögren syndrome. *Respirol Case Rep*. 2018;6(2):e00285.

66. Stojan G, Baer AN, Danoff SK. Pulmonary manifestations of Sjögren's syndrome. *Curr Allergy Asthma Rep*. 2013;13(4):354–360.

67. Launay D, Hachulla E, Hatron PY, Jais X, Simonneau G, Humbert M. Pulmonary arterial hypertension: a rare complication of primary Sjögren syndrome: report of 9 new cases and review of the literature. *Medicine (Baltim)*. 2007;86(5):299–315.

68. Doig JA, Whaley K, Dick WC, Nuki G, Williamson J, Buchanan WW. Otolaryngological aspects of Sjögren's syndrome. *Br Med J*. 1971;4(5785):460–463.

69. Silvestre-Donat FJ, Miralles-Jorda L, Martinez-Mihi V. Protocol for the clinical management of dry mouth. *Med Oral*. 2004;9(4):273–279.

70. Porter SR, Scully C, Hegarty AM. An update of the etiology and management of xerostomia. *Oral Surg Oral Med Oral Pathol Oral Radiol Endod*. 2004;97(1):28–46.

71. Maguire A, Rugg-Gunn AJ. Xylitol and caries prevention–is it a magic bullet? *Br Dent J*. 2003;194(8):429–436.

72. Papas AS, Sherrer YS, Charney M, Golden HE, Medsger Jr TA, Walsh BT, Trivedi M, Goldlust B, Gallagher SC. Successful treatment of dry mouth and dry eye symptoms in Sjögren's syndrome patients with oral pilocarpine: a randomized, placebo-controlled, dose-adjustment study. *J Clin Rheumatol*. 2004;10(4):169–177.

73. Yan Z, Young AL, Hua H, Xu Y. Multiple oral Candida infections in patients with Sjögren's syndrome – prevalence and clinical and drug susceptibility profiles. *J Rheumatol*. 2011;38(11):2428–2431.

74. Popov Y, Salomon-Escoto K. Gastrointestinal and hepatic disease in Sjögren syndrome. *Rheum Dis Clin N Am*. 2018;44(1):143–151.

75. Mandl T, Ekberg O, Wollmer P, Manthorpe R, Jacobsson LT. Dysphagia and dysmotility of the pharynx and oesophagus in patients with primary Sjögren's syndrome. *Scand J Rheumatol*. 2007;36(5):394–401.

76. Palma R, Freire A, Freitas J, Morbey A, Costa T, Saraiva F, Queiros F, Carvalhinhos A. Esophageal motility disorders in patients with Sjögren's syndrome. *Dig Dis Sci*. 1994;39(4):758–761.

77. Grande L, Lacima G, Ros E, Font J, Pera C. Esophageal motor function in primary Sjögren's syndrome. *Am J Gastroenterol*. 1993;88(3):378–381.

78. Collin P, Karvonen AL, Korpela M, Laippala P, Helin H. Gastritis classified in accordance with the Sydney system in patients with primary Sjögren's syndrome. *Scand J Gastroenterol*. 1997;32(2):108–111.

79. El Miedany YM, Baddour M, Ahmed I, Fahmy H. Sjögren's syndrome: concomitant *H. pylori* infection and possible correlation with clinical parameters. *Jt Bone Spine*. 2005;72(2):135–141.

80. Sorrentino D, Faller G, DeVita S, Avellini C, Labombarda A, Ferraccioli G, Kahlow-Toussaint S. *Helicobacter pylori* associated antigastric autoantibodies: role in Sjögren's syndrome gastritis. *Helicobacter*. 2004;9(1):46–53.

81. Schreuder MI, van den Brand M, Hebeda KM, Groenen P, van Krieken JH, Scheijen B. Novel developments in the pathogenesis and diagnosis of extranodal marginal zone lymphoma. *J Hematop*. 2017;10(3–4):91–107.

82. Pokorny G, Karacsony G, Lonovics J, Hudak J, Nemeth J, Varro V. Types of atrophic gastritis in patients with primary Sjögren's syndrome. *Ann Rheum Dis*. 1991;50(2): 97−100.

83. Minalyan A, Benhammou JN, Artashesyan A, Lewis MS, Pisegna JR. Autoimmune atrophic gastritis: current perspectives. *Clin Exp Gastroenterol*. 2017;10:19−27.

84. Hammar O, Ohlsson B, Wollmer P, Mandl T. Impaired gastric emptying in primary Sjögren's syndrome. *J Rheumatol*. 2010;37(11):2313−2318.

85. Imrich R, Alevizos I, Bebris L, Goldstein DS, Holmes CS, Illei GG, Nikolov NP. Predominant glandular cholinergic dysautonomia in patients with primary Sjögren's syndrome. *Arthritis Rheum*. 2015;67(5):1345−1352.

86. Pickartz T, Pickartz H, Lochs H, Ockenga J. Overlap syndrome of autoimmune pancreatitis and cholangitis associated with secondary Sjögren's syndrome. *Eur J Gastroenterol Hepatol*. 2004;16(12):1295−1299.

87. Wang L, Zhang FC, Chen H, Zhang X, Xu D, Li YZ, Wang Q, Gao LX, Yang YJ, Kong F, Wang K. Connective tissue diseases in primary biliary cirrhosis: a population-based cohort study. *World J Gastroenterol*. 2013;19(31):5131−5137.

88. Alarcon-Segovia D, Diaz-Jouanen E, Fishbein E. Features of Sjögren's syndrome in primary biliary cirrhosis. *Ann Intern Med*. 1973;79(1):31−36.

89. Skopouli FN, Barbatis C, Moutsopoulos HM. Liver involvement in primary Sjögren's syndrome. *Br J Rheumatol*. 1994;33(8):745−748.

90. Lindor KD, Gershwin ME, Poupon R, Kaplan M, Bergasa NV, Heathcote EJ, American Association for Study of Liver D. Primary biliary cirrhosis. *Hepatology*. 2009;50(1): 291−308.

91. Matsumoto T, Morizane T, Aoki Y, Yamasaki S, Nakajima M, Enomoto N, Kobayashi S, Hashimoto H. Autoimmune hepatitis in primary Sjögren's syndrome: pathological study of the livers and labial salivary glands in 17 patients with primary Sjögren's syndrome. *Pathol Int*. 2005;55(2):70−76.

92. Ferreiro MC, Prieto MH, Rodriguez SB, Vazquez RL, Iglesias AC, Dios PD. Whole stimulated salivary flow in patients with chronic hepatitis C virus infection. *J Oral Pathol Med*. 2002;31(2):117−120.

93. Jorgensen C, Legouffe MC, Perney P, Coste J, Tissot B, Segarra C, Bologna C, Bourrat L, Combe B, Blanc F, Sany J. Sicca syndrome associated with hepatitis C virus infection. *Arthritis Rheum*. 1996;39(7):1166−1171.

94. Prunoiu C, Georgescu EF, Georgescu M, Simionescu C. Sjögren's syndrome associated with chronic hepatitis C - the benefit of the antiviral treatment. *Rom J Morphol Embryol*. 2008;49(4):557−562.

95. Takeda Y, Ohya T. Sicca symptom in a patient with hemochromatosis: minor salivary gland biopsy for differential diagnosis. *Int J Oral Maxillofac Surg*. 1987;16(6): 745−748.

96. Ebert EC. Gastrointestinal and hepatic manifestations of Sjögren syndrome. *J Clin Gastroenterol*. 2012;46(1):25−30.

97. Singh JA, Saag KG, Bridges Jr SL, Akl EA, Bannuru RR, Sullivan MC, Vaysbrot E, McNaughton C, Osani M, Shmerling RH, Curtis JR, Furst DE, Parks D, Kavanaugh A, O'Dell J, King C, Leong A, Matteson EL, Schousboe JT, Drevlow B, Ginsberg S, Grober J, St Clair EW, Tindall E, Miller AS, McAlindon T, R. American College of. American college of Rheumatology guideline for the treatment of rheumatoid arthritis. *Arthritis Care Res*. 2015;68(1):1−25.

98. Chang CC, Chang YS, Wang SH, Lin SY, Chen YH, Chen JH. Primary Sjögren's syndrome and the risk of acute pancreatitis: a nationwide cohort study. *BMJ Open*. 2017; 7(8):e014807.

99. S R, P B-Z, C M, B K, N a-D, Ramos-Casals M. *Digestive involvement in primary Sjögren's syndrome*. vol. 13. 2017.

100. Montefusco PP, Geiss AC, Bronzo RL, Randall S, Kahn E, McKinley MJ. Sclerosing cholangitis, chronic pancreatitis, and Sjögren's syndrome: a syndrome complex. *Am J Surg*. 1984;147(6):822–826.

101. Brito-Zeron P, Ramos-Casals M, Bosch X, Stone JH. The clinical spectrum of IgG4-related disease. *Autoimmun Rev*. 2014;13(12):1203–1210.

102. Akiyama M, Takeuchi T. IgG4-Related disease: beyond glucocorticoids. *Drugs Aging*. 2018;35(4):275–287.

103. Alvarez-Celorio MD, Angeles-Angeles A, Kraus A. Primary Sjögren's syndrome and celiac disease: causal association or serendipity? *J Clin Rheumatol*. 2000;6(4): 194–197.

104. Iltanen S, Collin P, Korpela M, Holm K, Partanen J, Polvi A, Maki M. Celiac disease and markers of celiac disease latency in patients with primary Sjögren's syndrome. *Am J Gastroenterol*. 1999;94(4):1042–1046.

105. Maclaurin BP, Matthews N, Kilpatrick JkA. Coeliac disease associated with autoimmune thyroiditis, Sjögren's syndrome, and a lymphocytotoxic serum factor. *Aust N Z J Med*. 1972;2(4):405–411.

106. Liden M, Kristjansson G, Valtysdottir S, Venge P, Hallgren R. Cow's milk protein sensitivity assessed by the mucosal patch technique is related to irritable bowel syndrome in patients with primary Sjögren's syndrome. *Clin Exp Allergy*. 2008;38(6):929–935.

107. Szodoray P, Barta Z, Lakos G, Szakall S, Zeher M. Coeliac disease in Sjögren's syndrome–a study of 111 Hungarian patients. *Rheumatol Int*. 2004;24(5):278–282.

108. Kim-Lee C, Suresh L, Ambrus Jr JL. Gastrointestinal disease in Sjögren's syndrome: related to food hypersensitivities. *SpringerPlus*. 2015;4:766.

109. Gainey R, Rooney PJ, Alspaugh M. Sjögren's syndrome and Crohn's disease. *Clin Exp Rheumatol*. 1985;3(1):67–69.

110. Katsanos KH, Saougos V, Kosmidou M, Doukas M, Kamina S, Asproudis I, Tsianos EV. Sjögren's syndrome in a patient with ulcerative colitis and primary sclerosing cholangitis: case report and review of the literature. *J Crohns Colitis*. 2009; 3(3):200–203.

111. Doyle MK. Vasculitis associated with connective tissue disorders. *Curr Rheumatol Rep*. 2006;8(4):312–316.

112. Jain A, Srinivas BH, Emmanuel D, Jain VK, Parameshwaran S, Negi VS. Renal involvement in primary Sjögren's syndrome: a prospective cohort study. *Rheumatol Int*. 2018;38(12):2251–2262.

113. Goules AV, Tatouli IP, Moutsopoulos HM, Tzioufas AG. Clinically significant renal involvement in primary Sjögren's syndrome: clinical presentation and outcome. *Arthritis Rheum*. 2013;65(11):2945–2953.

114. Ren H, Wang WM, Chen XN, Zhang W, Pan XX, Wang XL, Lin Y, Zhang S, Chen N. Renal involvement and followup of 130 patients with primary Sjögren's syndrome. *J Rheumatol*. 2008;35(2):278–284.

115. Evans R, Zdebik A, Ciurtin C, Walsh SB. Renal involvement in primary Sjögren's syndrome. *Rheumatol*. 2015;54(9):1541–1548.

116. Francois H, Mariette X. Renal involvement in primary Sjögren syndrome. *Nat Rev Nephrol.* 2016;12(2):82−93.
117. Koratala A, Reeves WH, Segal MS. Tubulointerstitial nephritis in Sjögren syndrome treated with mycophenolate mofetil. *J Clin Rheumatol.* 2017;23(7):402−403.
118. Kaufman I, Schwartz D, Caspi D, Paran D. Sjögren's syndrome - not just Sicca: renal involvement in Sjögren's syndrome. *Scand J Rheumatol.* 2008;37(3):213−218.
119. Mariette X, Seror R, Quartuccio L, Baron G, Salvin S, Fabris M, Desmoulins F, Nocturne G, Ravaud P, De Vita S. Efficacy and safety of belimumab in primary Sjögren's syndrome: results of the BELISS open-label phase II study. *Ann Rheum Dis.* 2015; 74(3):526−531.
120. Adler S, Korner M, Forger F, Huscher D, Caversaccio MD, Villiger PM. Evaluation of histologic, serologic, and clinical changes in response to abatacept treatment of primary Sjögren's syndrome: a pilot study. *Arthritis Care Res.* 2013;65(11):1862−1868.
121. Alunno A, Carubbi F, Bistoni O, Caterbi S, Bartoloni E, Mirabelli G, Cannarile F, Cipriani P, Giacomelli R, Gerli R. T regulatory and T helper 17 cells in primary Sjögren's syndrome: facts and perspectives. *Mediat Inflamm.* 2015;2015:243723.
122. Sankar V, Brennan MT, Kok MR, Leakan RA, Smith JA, Manny J, Baum BJ, Pillemer SR. Etanercept in Sjögren's syndrome: a twelve-week randomized, double-blind, placebo-controlled pilot clinical trial. *Arthritis Rheum.* 2004;50(7):2240−2245.
123. Mariette X, Ravaud P, Steinfeld S, Baron G, Goetz J, Hachulla E, Combe B, Puechal X, Pennec Y, Sauvezie B, Perdriger A, Hayem G, Janin A, Sibilia J. Inefficacy of infliximab in primary Sjögren's syndrome: results of the randomized, controlled Trial of Remicade in Primary Sjögren's Syndrome (TRIPSS). *Arthritis Rheum.* 2004;50(4): 1270−1276.
124. Meijer JM, Meiners PM, Vissink A, Spijkervet FK, Abdulahad W, Kamminga N, Brouwer E, Kallenberg CG, Bootsma H. Effectiveness of rituximab treatment in primary Sjögren's syndrome: a randomized, double-blind, placebo-controlled trial. *Arthritis Rheum.* 2010;62(4):960−968.
125. St Clair EW, Levesque MC, Prak ET, Vivino FB, Alappatt CJ, Spychala ME, Wedgwood J, McNamara J, Moser Sivils KL, Fisher L, Cohen P, Autoimmunity Centers of E. Rituximab therapy for primary Sjögren's syndrome: an open-label clinical trial and mechanistic analysis. *Arthritis Rheum.* 2013;65(4):1097−1106.
126. Carubbi F, Cipriani P, Marrelli A, Benedetto P, Ruscitti P, Berardicurti O, Pantano I, Liakouli V, Alvaro S, Alunno A, Manzo A, Ciccia F, Gerli R, Triolo G, Giacomelli R. Efficacy and safety of rituximab treatment in early primary Sjögren's syndrome: a prospective, multi-center, follow-up study. *Arthritis Res Ther.* 2013; 15(5):R172.
127. Devauchelle-Pensec V, Mariette X, Jousse-Joulin S, Berthelot JM, Perdriger A, Puechal X, Le Guern V, Sibilia J, Gottenberg JE, Chiche L, Hachulla E, Hatron PY, Goeb V, Hayem G, Morel J, Zarnitsky C, Dubost JJ, Pers JO, Nowak E, Saraux A. Treatment of primary Sjögren syndrome with rituximab: a randomized trial. *Ann Intern Med.* 2014;160(4):233−242.
128. Tsuboi H, Matsumoto I, Hagiwara S, Hirota T, Takahashi H, Ebe H, Yokosawa M, Hagiya C, Asashima H, Takai C, Miki H, Umeda N, Kondo Y, Ogishima H, Suzuki T, Hirata S, Saito K, Tanaka Y, Horai Y, Nakamura H, Kawakami A, Sumida T. Efficacy and safety of abatacept for patients with Sjögren's syndrome associated with rheumatoid arthritis: rheumatoid arthritis with orencia trial toward Sjögren's

syndrome Endocrinopathy (ROSE) trial-an open-label, one-year, prospective study-Interim analysis of 32 patients for 24 weeks. *Mod Rheumatol.* 2015;25(2):187—193.

129. Meiners PM, Vissink A, Kroese FG, Spijkervet FK, Smitt-Kamminga NS, Abdulahad WH, Bulthuis-Kuiper J, Brouwer E, Arends S, Bootsma H. Abatacept treatment reduces disease activity in early primary Sjögren's syndrome (open-label proof of concept ASAP study). *Ann Rheum Dis.* 2014;73(7):1393—1396.

130. De Vita S, Quartuccio L, Seror R, Salvin S, Ravaud P, Fabris M, Nocturne G, Gandolfo S, Isola M, Mariette X. Efficacy and safety of belimumab given for 12 months in primary Sjögren's syndrome: the BELISS open-label phase II study. *Rheumatology.* 2015;54(12):2249—2256.

Integrative rheumatology: complementary and alternative medicine for the management of Sjögren's syndrome

Yiu Tak Leung, MD, PhD

Assistant Professor, Department of Internal Medicine, Division of Rheumatology, Thomas Jefferson University Hospital, Philadelphia, PA, United States

Introduction

Primary Sjögren's syndrome is a systemic autoimmune disease characterized by lymphocytic infiltration of exocrine glands, resulting in dry eyes and dry mouth in more than 95% of patients, as well as other sicca symptoms such as hoarseness, dry cough, constipation, dry skin, and vaginal dryness in women. The most common extraglandular features include generalized musculoskeletal pain and fatigue, as well as disturbed sleep, autonomic dysfunction, mood disturbances, cognitive and neuropsychiatric impairment, and an increased risk of lymphoma. These disease manifestations significantly reduce many patients' quality of life, impacting their daily activities and ability to work (Chapter 15). Conventional therapy principally focuses on pharmacologic interventions to target the adverse effects of keratoconjunctivitis sicca and xerostomia, often with less than optimal efficacy and side effects. The integration of nonpharmacologic treatments offers many further therapeutic options for a personalized treatment plan for individual patients.

Dietary modifications

Chronic inflammation is a hallmark of Sjögren's syndrome, along with other systemic autoimmune diseases. These chronic inflammatory diseases are set in a milieu of inflammatory immune cells and cytokines. These proinflammatory mediators are further promoted by the consumption of the "Western diet," which is typically exemplified by the habitual intake of high-fat, high-cholesterol, high-sugar, and high-salt processed foods. Additionally, many symptoms associated with xerostomia, such as dry mucous membranes, poor dentition, and reflux, may significantly restrict a patient's food intake, leading to poor nutrition and unintentional weight loss. Practical

Sjögren's Syndrome. https://doi.org/10.1016/B978-0-323-67534-5.00012-0

recommendations that may significantly improve patients' quality of life include ingesting foods that are moist, soft, and cut into small pieces to assist chewing and swallowing, as well as the use of sour foods to promote salivation and the avoidance of foods that aggravate gastroesophageal reflux symptoms. The effects of a liquid diet on salivary flow were evaluated in a small non–placebo-controlled study in which 23 patients with primary Sjögren's syndrome were placed on a liquid diet to avoid mastication in order to rest the glandular cells.[1] Both the salivary flow rate as measured by unstimulated whole salivary collection and the lacrimal flow rate as measured by Schirmer-I test were found to be significantly increased in the 23 patients who followed this regimen for 4 weeks.

Furthermore, food allergies and hypersensitivities may also be associated with Sjögren's syndrome. Patients with Sjögren's syndrome frequently have symptoms of irritable bowel syndrome and 14.7% were found to have celiac disease in one study.[2] Trials of elimination diets and gluten-free diets should be suggested for patients with symptoms of food allergy or intolerance.

A study investigating patients with primary ($n = 24$) and secondary ($n = 22$) Sjögren's syndrome found that nutrient intake is altered and there was a lower energy-adjusted consumption of unsupplemental vitamin C, polyunsaturated fat, linoleic acid (LA), omega-3 fatty acids, and specific other unsaturated fatty acids when compared with controls.[3] Research studies on therapeutic dietary interventions for Sjögren's syndrome are sparse and more data are needed to elucidate the association between dietary factors and disease; however, many patients consider dietary modifications as a primary, nonpharmacologic alternative therapy. An antiinflammatory diet is recommended by the Sjögren's Syndrome Foundation and the foundation encourages an abundant consumption of colorful vegetables and fruits, fiber, healthy fats, legumes, whole grains, tea, and spices such as garlic, ginger, and turmeric and a moderate intake of organic meat. Numerous studies have demonstrated an association between components of the antiinflammatory diet and a decrease in the levels of different serologic markers of inflammation (Table 12.1). Foods to be avoided include refined grains, sugars, trans fats, refined oils, and red meat, as well as processed food and artificial food additives such as preservatives, sweeteners, and emulsifiers.

Despite the paucity of clinical trials examining the impact of dietary modifications on Sjögren's syndrome, components of the anti-inflammatory diet, such as fatty acids, curcumin, and vitamins found in abundance in colorful vegetables and fruits, have been individually investigated as nutritional supplements, thereby providing additional support for the use of these therapeutic dietary measures in patients with Sjögren's syndrome. The studies on nutritional supplements are reviewed in the following sections.

Nutritional supplements

Vitamin A

Vitamin A is a critical micronutrient in the maintenance of ocular function and its deficiency can cause serious ocular pathologic conditions including blindness and

Table 12.1 Diet and inflammatory markers.

Study	Country	Food	Participants	Methods	Results
Jiang et al.[44]	China	Cruciferous vegetables	$n = 1005$ Female = 1005 Mean age = 58.1 years	Food frequency questionnaire	Decreased serum levels 12.66% for TNF-α (Ptrend = 0.01), 18.18% for IL-1β (Ptrend = 0.02), and 24.68% for IL-6 (Ptrend = 0.02) among women with highest intakes of cruciferous vegetables
Salehi-Abargouei et al.[45]	Multinational	Non-soy legumes	$n = 464$ in 8 studies included in meta-analysis	9 RCTs systematically reviewed Meta-analysis included 8 RCTs	Non-soy legumes consumption: a trend toward a significant effect on decreasing CRP and hs-CRP concentrations (mean difference = −0.21; 95% CI, −0.44 to 0.02; $P = .068$)
Jiao et al.[46]	Multinational	Dietary fiber or fiber-rich foods		Meta-analysis included 14 RCTs	Dietary fiber consumption: A slight but significant reduction of 0.37 mg/L (95% CI, −0.74, 0) in circulating CRP levels
Hajihashemi et al.[47]	Iran	Whole-grain foods	$n = 44$ Women = 44 Ages 8 −15 years	Randomized crossover clinical trial: 6 weeks, 4-week washout, 6 weeks	Whole-grain intake: Significant reduction of hs-CRP (−21.8 vs. +12.1%, $P = .03$)
Bassett et al.[48]	Multinational	Flaxseed flour: Rich source of the omega-3 fatty acid α-linolenic acid, dietary fiber, and phytoestrogen lignans		Review	Flaxseed intake reduces circulating levels of TC by 6%−11% and LDL cholesterol by 9%−18% in normolipemic humans and by 5% −17% for TC and 4%−10% for LDL cholesterol in hypercholesterolemic patients
Guasch-Ferre et al.[49]	Multinational	Walnuts	$n = 1059$ in 26 clinical trials	Random-effects meta-analyses of 26 clinical trials	Walnut-enriched diets: −6.99 mg/dL (95% CI: −9.39, −4.58 mg/dL; $P < .001$) for TC; −5.51 mg/dL (95% CI: −7.72, −3.29 mg/dL; $P < .001$) for LDL cholesterol; and −4.69 (95% CI: −8.93, −0.45; $P = .03$) for triglyceride levels.

CI, confidence interval; CRP, C-reactive protein; hs, high-sensitivity; IL, interleukin; LDL, low-density lipoprotein; RCTs, randomized controlled trials; TC, total cholesterol; TNF, tumor necrosis factor.

xerophthalmia.[4] With regard to xerophthalmia, severe vitamin A deficiency can result in loss of conjunctiva goblet cells, which are a source of mucin on the eye surface and in tears. In addition, localized vitamin A deficiency can develop on the ocular surface due to harsh environment, chronic inflammation, or use of contact lenses, leading to dryness.[5] Topical ophthalmic administration of vitamin A eye drops can help regenerate goblet cells and ameliorate sicca symptoms.

Several clinical investigations have been published studying the efficacy of topical vitamin A in xerophthalmia, but although the patients in the studies had sicca symptoms, they were not diagnosed with Sjögren's syndrome. Clinical improvement and regeneration of goblet cells were demonstrated in a study of six patients with keratoconjunctivitis sicca by using topical application of an ophthalmic ointment containing the vitamin A derivative all-*trans* retinoic acid.[6] Another study examining the repeated application of a retinol palmitate aqueous ophthalmic solution (1000 IU vitamin A per mL droplet) four times daily for 4 weeks found an increase in goblet cell concentrations ($1.3 \pm 2.6 \rightarrow 2.1 \pm 1.8$ cells/slides) in the conjunctival tissues of patients with xerophthalmia.[7] A study investigated the efficacy of vitamin A eye drops as compared to cyclosporine A 0.05% (Restasis®).[8] Patients with xerophthalmia ($n = 150$) were divided equally into three groups: (1) receiving twice daily cyclosporine A 0.05%, (2) receiving four times daily retinyl palmitate 0.05%, and (3) placebo controls; all patients received preservative-free artificial tears four times daily. Both vitamin A eye drops and topical cyclosporine A 0.05% treatments led to significant improvement in blurred vision, tear film breakup time, Schirmer-I test results, and goblet cell density as compared with the control group. There was no significant difference in any of these parameters between the vitamin A and the cyclosporine A group. A similar therapeutic trial for patients with Sjögren's syndrome is desirable to evaluate for the potential efficacy of topical administration of vitamin A in this patient population.

Vitamin C

Vitamin C supplementation may be considered for patients with Sjögren's syndrome. This recommendation is based on a study in which five healthy male volunteers were given a diet deprived of ascorbic acid for 3 months leading to scurvy. All five subjects developed one or more signs of Sjögren's syndrome, including keratoconjunctivitis sicca, xerostomia and salivary gland enlargement, dry skin, hair loss, and dental decay.[9] Salivary acinar cells also have a relatively high concentration of vitamin C, which may play an important role in saliva production.[10] Moreover, a clinical study showed that vitamin C supplementation may be therapeutic for xerophthalmia.[11] A clinical study in 60 patients with type 2 diabetes showed that supplementation of vitamin C, 1000 mg daily, in combination with vitamin E, 400 IU daily, for 10 days resulted in improvement in tear breakup time ($P < .001$), improvement in Schirmer-I test results ($P < .001$), and an increase in conjunctival goblet cell concentrations (50 cells/field before and 59 cells/field after supplementation [$P = .002$]). It is unclear if both vitamin C and vitamin E were effective therapeutic agents or whether the participants in the study were deficient in either nutrient. A larger, controlled therapeutic trial for Sjögren's syndrome patients is needed to clarify the clinical benefits of supplemental vitamins C and E in this disease.

Iron, vitamin B_{12}, and folic acid

Iron and vitamin deficiencies were found to be highly prevalent in patients with primary Sjögren's syndrome.[12] In one investigation, 43 patients were evaluated and 51% had iron deficiency, 25% had B_{12} deficiency, and 9% had folate deficiency. Another study examining 80 patients with primary Sjögren's syndrome discovered that the mean serum B_{12} level was 419 pg/mL, with 8.8% having deficient levels of less than 200 pg/mL and an additional 56% having less than 300 pg/mL of B_{12}.[13] Therefore this patient population should be tested for vitamin deficiencies and should receive supplements to optimize their nutritional status.

Vitamin D

Vitamin D deficiency has been shown to be associated with an increased risk of developing autoimmune diseases,[14] and low levels of vitamin D have been reported in systemic lupus erythematosus (SLE),[15] primary Sjögren's syndrome,[16] and inflammatory myopathies.[17] However, the association between vitamin D levels and Sjögren's syndrome remains unsettled, and a meta-analysis[18] of nine studies published between 1999 and 2018 found that four studies reported significantly lower vitamin D levels in patients with Sjögren's syndrome than in healthy controls, but five studies did not find significant differences in vitamin D levels. Although a series of common single-nucleotide polymorphisms in the vitamin D receptor gene have been linked to many diseases such as diabetes, cardiovascular disease, and cancer, no association was found between vitamin D receptor gene polymorphism and the prevalence or severity of Sjögren's syndrome.[19] In addition, there has not been any study done to evaluate the therapeutic effect of vitamin D supplementation in Sjögren's syndrome.

Coenzyme Q10

Coenzyme Q10 (CoQ10) was evaluated in a double-blinded study of 66 patients with xerostomia to examine the effects of CoQ10 on salivary secretion.[20] About 90% of these patients had a diagnosis of Sjögren's syndrome. The patients were given either 100 mg daily of CoQ10 or placebo for 1 month, and the treatment group was found to have significantly increased mean salivary secretion rate of 71% as well as an increased salivary CoQ10 content after treatment.

Polyunsaturated fatty acids

Humans evolved on a Paleolithic diet with a ratio of omega-6 fatty acids to omega-3 fatty acids of approximately 1:1 to 4:1.[21] Modern Western diets provide a much higher ratio of omega-6 fatty acids over omega-3 polyunsaturated fatty acids in the range of 11:1 to 25:1.

α-linoleic acid (LA) is a key omega-3 fatty acid that is converted into eicosapentaenoic acid (EPA) and docosahexaenoic acid (DHA), and the metabolism of EPA and DHA produces antiinflammatory cytokines and exerts suppressive effects on the pathogenesis of inflammatory diseases. Excessive amounts of the omega-6 fatty acid arachidonic acid (ARA) in modern diets leads to the overproduction of 2-series prostaglandins (PGs) and 4-series leukotrienes (LTs) with proinflammatory effects.[22] LA is converted into ARA, and γ-linoleic acid (GLA) is the first intermediate in the metabolic conversion of LA into ARA. Conversely, GLA is an essential omega-6 fatty acid with antiinflammatory effects. The elongation of GLA results in dihomogammalinolenic acid (DGLA), which is a precursor of 1-series PGs such as PGE_1. PGE_1 has a mostly inhibitory effect on inflammatory cells by increasing intracellular cyclic AMP levels and reducing the release of lysosomal enzymes, chemotaxis, and the adherence of leukocytes to blood vessels.[23] Furthermore, GLA competitively inhibits LT synthesis by blocking the transformation of ARA to LTs. Thus GLA and its precursor, LA, have antiinflammatory activity.

A cross-sectional study of 41 patients with primary Sjögren's syndrome showed that the levels of plasma and cell membrane essential fatty acids correlated with disease severity.[24] DHA levels inversely correlated with clinical disease status and levels of DGLA and EPA correlated inversely with the levels of rheumatoid factor and anti-SSA antibodies. Furthermore, levels of anti-SSA antibodies correlated with levels of proinflammatory ARA. These data further provide the basis for interventional studies with polyunsaturated fatty acids in Sjögren's syndrome.

Omega-6 fatty acids: linoleic acid and γ-linolenic acid

The GLA level was noted to be decreased in the serum and red cell membranes of patients with Sjögren's syndrome,[25] and the benefits of GLA supplementation, along with evening primrose oil, which contains both LA and GLA, have been examined in several clinical studies of Sjögren's syndrome. The results have been equivocal, with some trials showing clinical improvement and others with minimal benefits (Table 12.2). The conflicting findings from these studies may have been partly due to differing underlying fatty acid status of the patients, disease severity, and small sample sizes ranging between 17 and 40 patients. Large, well-conducted, randomized controlled trials (RCTs) are needed to conclusively determine the efficacy of LA and GLA supplementation in patients with Sjögren's syndrome.

Green tea catechins

Murine studies found that oral administration of green tea polyphenols decreased the serum total autoantibody levels and lymphocytic infiltration of submandibular glands.[26,27] Green tea polyphenols were also shown to have protective effects on human salivary acinar cells against tumor necrosis factor-α-induced cytotoxicity.[26] Epigallocatechin-3-gallate (EGCG) is a green tea polyphenol and the most abundant catechin in tea. In a murine model for human Sjögren's syndrome EGCG was

Table 12.2 Effects of linoleic acid and γ-linoleic acid on Sjögren's syndrome.

Study	Participants	Method	Dose	Results
Horrobin et al.[50]	$n = 17$ Patients with sicca syndrome (8) and Sjögren's syndrome (9)	2- to 6-week trial	3 g EPO, 150 mg pyridoxine, 3 g vitamin C in three divided doses daily	13 Patients reported subjective improvement or complete resolution of dry eye symptoms; 10 patients with increased tear production measured by Schirmer-I test.
Manthorpe et al.[51]	$n = 36$ Patients with primary Sjögren's syndrome	3-Week double-blind, placebo-controlled, randomized crossover trial	Efamol (EPO with 73% LA, 9% GLA) 1500 mg twice a day versus placebo for controls	Significantly improved Schirmer-I test scores ($P < .03$). No improvement in breakup time, van Bijsterveld score, cornea sensitivity, tear lysozyme levels, and nuclear chromatin levels in conjunctival epithelial cells.
Oxholm et al.[52]	$n = 28$ Patients with primary Sjögren's syndrome	8-Week double-blind, placebo-controlled, randomized crossover trial	Efamol (EPO with 73% LA, 9% GLA) 3 g daily versus placebo for controls	Schirmer-I test results, breakup time, and van Bijsterveld scores improved significantly during Efamol treatment when compared with pretrial values ($P < .05$) but not when compared with placebo values ($P < .2$). Dihomogammalinolenic acid concentrations increased both in plasma ($P < .001$) and in erythrocytes ($P < .001$) during treatment with Efamol.
Theander et al.[53]	$n = 19$ Patients with primary Sjögren's syndrome	6-Month double-blind placebo-controlled randomized trial	800 or 1600 mg/day of GLA (extracted from EPO) versus corn oil for controls	No statistically significant improvement in fatigue. No differences in VAS for eye and mouth dryness or muscle/joint pain. No significant changes in Schirmer-I test result, van Bijsterveld score, unstimulated whole sialometry, or use of artificial tears or analgesics.
Aragona et al.[54]	$n = 40$ Patients with primary Sjögren's syndrome	1-Month double-blind placebo-controlled randomized trial	112 mg LA and 15 mg GLA twice daily versus placebo for controls	Tear PGE$_1$ levels significantly increased in treatment group after 1 month of treatment (PGE$_1$ level: 44 ± 5.4 ng/mL increased to 58.3 ± 5.5 ng/mL; $P < .01$). Statistically significant reduction of symptom score in treatment group after 1 month of treatment ($P < .01$). Corneal fluorescein stain treatment group showed significant improvement ($P < .01$) after 1 month of treatment and the improvement persisted 15 days after suspension of treatment ($P < .02$).

EPO, evening primrose oil; GLA, γ-linoleic acid; LA, linoleic acid; PGE$_1$, prostaglandin E1; VAS, visual analogue scale.

demonstrated to have antiapoptotic, antiinflammatory, and autoantigen-inhibitory properties.[27] There was reduced salivary gland lymphocyte infiltration, as well as decreased apoptotic activity and reduced serum autoantibody levels.

A phase II clinical trial evaluating the clinical effects of tea catechins on xerostomia was conducted on 60 patients with xerostomia, including 10 patients with Sjögren's syndrome.[28] The 8-week double-blinded, placebo-controlled randomized study compared the effects of lozenges containing green tea catechins to placebo containing all-natural formulation ingredients and 500 mg xylitol but without the green tea extracts; the lozenges were taken every 4 h with a maximum of six per day. There were seven Sjögren's syndrome patients in the treatment group and three in the placebo group. After 8 weeks of treatment, the catechin treatment group had a statistically significant increase in unstimulated (3.8-fold) and stimulated (2.1–fold) (by chewing neutral wax) saliva output as compared with baseline. Saliva output did not change significantly in the xylitol placebo group. In just the Sjögren's syndrome treatment group, there was a significantly increased unstimulated saliva output by 11.5-fold, whereas the stimulated saliva output increased nonsignificantly by 58%. Overall, among the patients receiving active treatment, the patients with Sjögren's syndrome continued to have lower saliva output than those with xerostomia of other causes.

Curcumin

Curcumin is a polyphenol that is the most active ingredient in the spice turmeric. It is being studied extensively and has been found to interact with multiple targets and to have inhibitory properties on inflammatory cytokine production, tumorigenesis, metastasis, and platelet aggregation. In vitro studies demonstrated that heat-solubilized curcumin and turmeric significantly decreased the binding of Sjögren's syndrome autoantibody Ro60 by 43% and 70% to their respective cognate autoantigens.[29] The authors of the study suggested that the higher inhibition of binding by turmeric than by purified curcumin was due to some curcuminoid loss in the purification process. There was also inhibition of binding of autoantibody Ro273 to their cognate antigens in the sera of a mouse model of Sjögren's syndrome. A further in vivo investigation using SLE murine model MRL-lpr/lpr mice showed that heat-solubilized curcumin and turmeric significantly reduced cellular infiltration of the salivary glands.[30] There was also significantly decreased lymphoproliferation, proteinuria, tail lesions, and autoantibodies. Research trials evaluating curcumin and turmeric in patients with Sjögren's syndrome are needed to determine their clinical relevance and efficacy.

Ginger

Ginger has been used as a medicinal food in both traditional Chinese medicine and Ayurveda for thousands of years for its antiinflammatory and digestive aid properties. Ginger is also extensively used for its an antinausea and antivomiting effects, as well as for the management of dental pain and stimulation of saliva. A clinical trial investigating the effects of ginger on xerostomia was done on 20 patients with type 2 diabetes using an oral spray containing herbal extracts of ginger.[31]

Ginger spray significantly ($P < .001$) increased the amount of saliva rapidly that was significantly ($P < .0010$) different from the amount of saliva after treatment with placebo. Ginger is a safe, affordable, and effective treatment option to increase saliva production in the treatment of hyposalivation and xerostomia.

Acupuncture

Acupuncture is one of the most widely used forms of complementary and alternative medicine (CAM). Acupuncture has been used for symptomatic treatment of dry eyes and for treating xerostomia and hyposalivation; however, there is very little data on its use for these symptoms in the setting of primary or secondary Sjögren's syndrome. There are several RCTs evaluating the effects of acupuncture on dry eyes and dry mouth and they will be reviewed later.

Acupuncture is a treatment option for eye diseases, as it is believed to be able to regulate lacrimal gland function via modulation of the autonomic nervous system and the immune system. A systematic review, in 2011, examined six RCTs comparing acupuncture with conventional treatment using artificial tears for dry eyes.[32] Meta-analysis of the three RCTs in patients with xerophthalmia or Sjögren's syndrome found that acupuncture significantly improved tear breakup times, Schirmer-I test scores, symptomatic response rates, and fluorescent staining results more than artificial tears. In particular, the singular RCT on patients with Sjögren's syndrome involved 60 patients who were divided into two groups: the acupuncture group received 30-min acupuncture sessions daily for 30 days and the control group received artificial tears 6 times daily for 30 days.[33] The other three RCTs evaluated acupuncture plus artificial tears versus artificial tears alone, and two of the three trials showed no significant benefits from acupuncture. Although definite conclusions could not be drawn from these conflicting trial results, there was some evidence supporting the use of acupuncture for the treatment of dry eyes. Subsequently, a meta-analysis[34] evaluating the effectiveness of acupuncture for dry eye syndrome was published in 2015 and concluded that acupuncture therapy is more effective than artificial tears. The meta-analysis included seven RCTs, five of which were also included in the 2011 systematic review, as well as two newer RCTs from 2012. These studies evaluated a total of 198 patients treated with acupuncture, compared with 185 patients treated with artificial tears. Patients in the acupuncture group were found to have significantly longer tear breakup time ($P < .00,001$) as well as significantly higher Schirmer-I test scores than those in the artificial tears group ($P = .001$). Furthermore, the cornea fluorescent staining result of patients in the acupuncture group was significantly improved compared with that in the artificial tears group ($P < .0001$).

Acupuncture is also used therapeutically for xerostomia because of the hypothesis that acupuncture can stimulate the parasympathetic and sympathetic nervous systems by neuronal activation. Furthermore, acupuncture releases neuropeptides such as the vasodilator calcitonin gene–related peptide, which has antiinflammatory effects and can increase blood flow in the salivary gland. A systemic review studied the effects of acupuncture on xerostomia and hyposalivation in 10 RCTs.[35] Therapeutic acupuncture was compared to sham acupuncture in 5 of the 10 RCTs and to oral hygiene/usual care in 4 other RCTs and 1 RCT used oral care sessions for control. One of the trials evaluated 21 patients with Sjögren's syndrome receiving parotid, submandibular, and labial gland acupuncture for 10 weeks versus usual care as control.[36] Subjective posttreatment improvement as measured on a 10-point visual analogue scale for the degree of discomfort from mouth dryness, eye dryness, and mouth/tongue burning was reported but it was not statistically significant. There was a significant ($P \leq .05$) increase in paraffin-stimulated saliva secretion in patients treated with therapeutic acupuncture.

However, the RCTs were overall assessed to be not well designed, with low quality for all the main outcomes and high risks of bias. Therefore the results are inconclusive and further larger, better-designed trials are necessary.

A study protocol for a randomized, double-blinded, sham acupuncture controlled trial of acupuncture for alleviating the key symptoms of primary Sjögren's syndrome (dryness, pain, and fatigue) was initiated in 2017 and, if completed, would be the first such RCT studying the efficacy of acupuncture on Sjögren's syndrome patients.[37] Patients with primary Sjögren's syndrome ($n = 120$) will be recruited from a single center in China and randomly assigned to acupuncture or sham acupuncture groups for 8 weeks of needle intervention. The anticipated results of this study will hopefully be able to provide more definitive evidence as to whether acupuncture is an effective treatment option for Sjögren's syndrome.

Guided imagery

Clinical hypnotherapy and/or guided imagery is another CAM option to explore for the management of sicca symptoms. Guided imagery or guided self-hypnosis is a mind-body technique that uses words and music to evoke mental images that stimulate sensory perceptions. The following is an example of a mind-body therapy to increase the production of saliva, shared by Dr. Randy Horwitz at the University of Arizona Center for Integrative Medicine:

"I typically take a few moments in clinic to walk patients through the process of selecting a cold, ripe lemon from the fridge, slicing into it (smelling and feeling the fresh citrus spray in their face), and finally taking a big bite out of a segment. Most patients note the production of copious amounts of saliva, and are amazed at the results. This technique can be practiced regularly."

Clinical studies are needed to quantitatively measure the effects of guided imagery techniques on the symptoms of Sjögren's syndrome.

Psychodynamic group therapy

Forty-six female patients with rheumatoid arthritis or primary Sjögren's syndrome participated in a prospective, controlled study of psychodynamic, time-limited group therapy.[38] The qualitative outcome was evaluated according to the patients' perceptions of what was appreciated as being most helpful in the group. There was reported improvements in alexithymia (difficulty in identifying and describing emotions) scores 9 months after participating in psychodynamic group therapy. This is a psychosomatic approach to cope with psychosocial issues related to living with chronic diseases such as Sjögren's syndrome and it helps patients gain insight into managing their disease emotionally.

Cognitive behavior therapy

Cognitive behavior therapy (CBT) focuses on teaching skills for coping and to improve illness, such as changes in thoughts and behaviors. CBT has been shown to improve pain, fatigue, mood, coping skills and overall physical function.[39] Effective strategies include goal setting, relaxation training, meditation, communications skills training, and strategies for relapse prevention.

Sleep disorders

Sjögren's syndrome and many other autoimmune diseases are strongly associated with sleep disorders.[40] The two most common sleep disorders associated with rheumatologic conditions are insomnia and obstructive sleep apnea. Sleep disturbance reduces the pain threshold and contributes to cognitive difficulties (brain fogginess), irritability, fatigue, and reduced quality of life. This is highlighted by a study that showed that experimental disruption of slow wave (delta) sleep in healthy persons produces alpha-delta sleep and fibromyalgia-like symptoms of musculoskeletal pain, fatigue, and negative mood changes.[41]

An assessment of general "sleep hygiene" is important. Often, patients with chronic pain develop undesirable habits with regard to sleep that further worsen their sleep disorders.

Table 12.3 features behavior recommendations to improve sleep hygiene.

Nonpharmacologic therapies for management of fibromyalgia

Patients with Sjögren's syndrome often suffer from generalized chronic musculoskeletal pain and symptoms that overlap with those of fibromyalgia. The prevalence of fibromyalgia in primary Sjögren's syndrome was found to be 31% in one study.[42] In addition the prevalence of fibromyalgia in Sjögren's syndrome patients with moderate-to-severe depression was significantly higher than that of those with mild depression or without depression (odds ratio = 10.62, $P = .0009$).

Table 12.3 How to improve sleep hygiene.

Sleep Hygiene
Maintain regular bedtime hours
Avoid caffeine, nicotine, and alcohol for at least 6 hours before bedtime
Do not exercise for at least 4 hours before bedtime
Avoid naps during the day that last more than 20 minutes
Omit use of drugs that stimulate the central nervous system, such as diet supplements and decongestants
Minimize distractions such as excess noise and light
Do not watch TV or work on projects while in bed
Keep bedroom dark and at a comfortable temperature
Take relaxing measures to promote sleep such as reading or taking a warm bath
Develop bedtime rituals such as brushing teeth, setting the alarm, and reading a book
Consider taking melatonin, 0.3–3.0 mg, 45 minutes before sleep
Consider taking a combination of valerian/lemon balm 30–60 minutes before sleep

Pharmacologic therapy for fibromyalgia syndrome includes the use of many central nervous system agents, such as antidepressants, muscle relaxants, and anticonvulsants, that act to modulate the sensation and tolerance of pain. However, the use of these medications in clinical practice has shown that these treatments are often significantly limited by drug tolerance and poor efficacy. Nonmedicinal CAM therapies (Table 12.4) play an enormous and important role in the management of fibromyalgia syndrome and offer patients many safe and efficacious treatment options.[43]

Table 12.4 Nonpharmacologic therapies for fibromyalgia syndrome.[43]

Strong evidence for efficacy	Patient education: Group format using lectures, written materials, demonstrations; improvement sustained for 3–12 months
	Cardiovascular exercise: Efficacy not maintained if exercise stops
	Cognitive behavior therapy: Improvement often sustained for months
Moderate evidence for efficacy	Strength training
	Acupuncture
	Hypnotherapy, biofeedback, balneotherapy
Weak evidence for efficacy	Chiropractic and manual medicine
	Massage therapy
	Electrotherapy, ultrasound
No evidence for efficacy	Tender (trigger) point injections
	Flexibility exercises

Conclusions

An integrative management approach for Sjögren's syndrome and its associated comorbidities is most effective in delivering a personalized treatment plan for patients, which includes medications, integrative treatments, and self-management strategies. The continued burgeoning numbers of CAM clinical trials and studies will further provide support and evidence for the utilization of these therapies.

References

1. Peen E, Haga HJ, Haugen AJ, Kahrs GE, Haugen M. The effect of a liquid diet on salivary flow in primary Sjögren's syndrome. *Scand J Rheumatol*. 2008;37(3):236−237.
2. Iltanen S, Collin P, Korpela M, Holm K, Partanen J, Polvi A, Maki M. Celiac disease and markers of celiac disease latency in patients with primary Sjögren's syndrome. *Am J Gastroenterol*. 1999;94(4):1042−1046.
3. Cermak JM, Papas AS, Sullivan RM, Dana MR, Sullivan DA. Nutrient intake in women with primary and secondary Sjögren's syndrome. *Eur J Clin Nutr*. 2003;57(2):328−334.
4. Sommer A. Xerophthalmia and vitamin A status. *Prog Retin Eye Res*. 1998;17(1):9−31.
5. Sommer A. Effects of vitamin A deficiency on the ocular surface. *Ophthalmol*. 1983; 90(6):592−600.
6. Tseng SC, Maumenee AE, Stark WJ, Maumenee IH, Jensen AD, Green WR, Kenyon KR. Topical retinoid treatment for various dry-eye disorders. *Ophthalmol*. 1985;92(6):717−727.
7. Kobayashi TK, Tsubota K, Takamura E, Sawa M, Ohashi Y, Usui M. Effect of retinol palmitate as a treatment for dry eye: a cytological evaluation. *Ophthalmologica*. 1997; 211(6):358−361.
8. Kim EC, Choi JS, Joo CK. A comparison of vitamin a and cyclosporine a 0.05% eye drops for treatment of dry eye syndrome. *Am J Ophthalmol*. 2009;147(2), 206-213 e3.
9. Hood J, Burns CA, Hodges RE. Sjögren's syndrome in scurvy. *N Engl J Med*. 1970; 282(20):1120−1124.
10. Enwonwu CO. Ascorbate status and xerostomia. *Med Hypotheses*. 1992;39(1):53−57.
11. Peponis V, Bonovas S, Kapranou A, Peponi E, Filioussi K, Magkou C, Sitaras N. Conjunctival and tear film changes after vitamin C and E administration in non-insulin dependent diabetes mellitus. *Med Sci Monit*. 2004;10(5):CR213−C217.
12. Lundstrom IM, Lindstrom FD. Iron and vitamin deficiencies, endocrine and immune status in patients with primary Sjögren's syndrome. *Oral Dis*. 2001;7(3):144−149.
13. Andres E, Blickle F, Sordet C, Cohen-Solal J, Sibilia J, Sapin R. Primary Sjögren's syndrome and vitamin B12 deficiency: preliminary results in 80 patients. *Am J Med*. 2006; 119(6):e9−10.
14. Ramagopalan SV, Goldacre R, Disanto G, Giovannoni G, Goldacre MJ. Hospital admissions for vitamin D related conditions and subsequent immune-mediated disease: record-linkage studies. *BMC Med*. 2013;11:171.
15. Abou-Raya A, Abou-Raya S, Helmii M. The effect of vitamin D supplementation on inflammatory and hemostatic markers and disease activity in patients with systemic lupus

erythematosus: a randomized placebo-controlled trial. *J Rheumatol.* 2013;40(3): 265−272.

16. Erten S, Sahin A, Altunoglu A, Gemcioglu E, Koca C. Comparison of plasma vitamin D levels in patients with Sjögren's syndrome and healthy subjects. *Int J Rheum Dis.* 2015; 18(1):70−75.

17. Azali P, Barbasso Helmers S, Kockum I, Olsson T, Alfredsson L, Charles P, Piehl Aulin K, Lundberg I. Low serum levels of vitamin D in idiopathic inflammatory myopathies. *Ann Rheum Dis.* 2013;72(4):512−516.

18. Li L, Chen J, Jiang Y. The association between vitamin D level and Sjögren's syndrome: a meta-analysis. *Int J Rheum Dis.* 2019;22(3):532−533.

19. Zilahi E, Chen JQ, Papp G, Szanto A, Zeher M. Lack of association of vitamin D receptor gene polymorphisms/haplotypes in Sjögren's syndrome. *Clin Rheumatol.* 2015;34(2): 247−253.

20. Ryo K, Ito A, Takatori R, Tai Y, Arikawa K, Seido T, Yamada T, Fujii K, Yamamoto Y, Saito I. Effects of coenzyme Q10 on salivary secretion. *Clin Biochem.* 2011;44(8−9): 669−674.

21. Konner M, Eaton SB. Paleolithic nutrition: twenty-five years later. *Nutr Clin Pract.* 2010; 25(6):594−602.

22. Tortosa-Caparros E, Navas-Carrillo D, Marin F, Orenes-Pinero E. Anti-inflammatory effects of omega 3 and omega 6 polyunsaturated fatty acids in cardiovascular disease and metabolic syndrome. *Crit Rev Food Sci Nutr.* 2017;57(16):3421−3429.

23. Weissmann G, Smolen JE, Korchak H. Prostaglandins and inflammation: receptor/ cyclase coupling as an explanation of why PGEs and PGI2 inhibit functions of inflammatory cells. *Adv Prostaglandin Thromboxane Res.* 1980;8:1637−1653.

24. Oxholm P, Asmussen K, Wiik A, Horrobin DF. Essential fatty acid status in cell membranes and plasma of patients with primary Sjögren's syndrome. Correlations to clinical and immunologic variables using a new model for classification and assessment of disease manifestations. *Prostaglandins Leukot Essent Fatty Acids.* 1998;59(4):239−245.

25. Horrobin DF. Essential fatty acid metabolism in diseases of connective tissue with special reference to scleroderma and to Sjögren's syndrome. *Med Hypotheses.* 1984;14(3): 233−247.

26. Hsu SD, Dickinson DP, Qin H, Borke J, Ogbureke KU, Winger JN, Cambra AM, Bollag WB, Stoppler HJ, Sharawy MM, Schuster GS. Green tea polyphenols reduce autoimmune symptoms in a murine model for human Sjögren's syndrome and protect human salivary acinar cells from TNF-alpha-induced cytotoxicity. *Autoimmunity.* 2007;40(2):138−147.

27. Gillespie K, Kodani I, Dickinson DP, Ogbureke KU, Camba AM, Wu M, Looney S, Chu TC, Qin H, Bisch F, Sharawy M, Schuster GS, Hsu SD. Effects of oral consumption of the green tea polyphenol EGCG in a murine model for human Sjögren's syndrome, an autoimmune disease. *Life Sci.* 2008;83(17−18):581−588.

28. De Rossi SS, Thoppay J, Dickinson DP, Looney S, Stuart M, Ogbureke KU, HSU S. A phase II clinical trial of a natural formulation containing tea catechins for xerostomia. *Oral Surg Oral Med Oral Pathol Oral Radiol.* 2014;118(4):447−454 e3.

29. Kurien BT, D'Souza A, Scofield RH. Heat-solubilized curry spice curcumin inhibits antibody-antigen interaction in in vitro studies: a possible therapy to alleviate autoimmune disorders. *Mol Nutr Food Res.* 2010;54(8):1202−1209.

30. Kurien BT, Harris VM, Quadri SM, Coutinho-de Souza P, Cavett J, Moyer A, Ittig B, Metcalf A, Ramji H, Truong D, Kumar R, Koelsch KA, Centola M, Payne A,

Danda D, Scofield H. Significantly reduced lymphadenopathy, salivary gland infiltrates and proteinuria in MRL-lpr/lpr mice treated with ultrasoluble curcumin/turmeric: increased survival with curcumin treatment. *Lupus Sci Med.* 2015;2(1):e000114.

31. Mardani H, Ghannadi A, Rashnavadi B, Kamali R. The Effect of ginger herbal spray on reducing xerostomia in patients with type II diabetes. *Avicenna J Phytomed.* 2017;7(4): 308−316.

32. Lee MS, Shin BC, Choi TY, Ernst E. Acupuncture for treating dry eye: a systematic review. *Acta Ophthalmol.* 2011;89(2):101−106.

33. Pang YJ, Jia GQ, Feng JL. The effect of acupuncture on the tear production in patients with Sjögren's syndrome. *J Tradit Chin Opahthalmol.* 2003;13:18−20.

34. Yang L, Yang Z, Yu H, Song H. Acupuncture therapy is more effective than artificial tears for dry eye syndrome: evidence based on a meta-analysis. *Evid Based Complement Alternat Med.* 2015;2015:143858.

35. Assy Z, Brand HS. A systematic review of the effects of acupuncture on xerostomia and hyposalivation. *BMC Complement Altern Med.* 2018;18(1):57.

36. List T, Lundeberg T, Lundstrom I, Lindstrom F, Ravald N. The effect of acupuncture in the treatment of patients with primary Sjögren's syndrome. A controlled study. *Acta Odontol Scand.* 1998;56(2):95−99.

37. Jiang Q, Zhang H, Pang R, Chen J, Liu Z, Zhou X. Acupuncture for Primary Sjögren Syndrome (pSS) on symptomatic improvements: study protocol for a randomized controlled trial. *BMC Complement Altern Med.* 2017;17(1):61.

38. Poulsen A. Psychodynamic, time-limited group therapy in rheumatic disease–a controlled study with special reference to alexithymia. *Psychother Psychosom.* 1991; 56(1−2):12−23.

39. Bennett R, Nelson D. Cognitive behavioral therapy for fibromyalgia. *Nat Clin Pract Rheumatol.* 2006;2(8):416−424.

40. Abad VC, Sarinas PS, Guilleminault C. Sleep and rheumatologic disorders. *Sleep Med Rev.* 2008;12(3):211−228.

41. Moldofsky H, Scarisbrick P. Induction of neurasthenic musculoskeletal pain syndrome by selective sleep stage deprivation. *Psychosom Med.* 1976;38(1):35−44.

42. Choi BY, Oh HJ, Lee YJ, Song YW. Prevalence and clinical impact of fibromyalgia in patients with primary Sjögren's syndrome. *Clin Exp Rheumatol.* 2016;34(2 Suppl. 96): S9−S13.

43. Goldenberg DL, Burckhardt C, Crofford L. Management of fibromyalgia syndrome. *J Am Med Assoc.* 2004;292(19):2388−2395.

44. Jiang Y, Wu SH, Shu XO, Xiang YB, Ji BT, Milne GL, Cai Q, Zhang X, Gao YT, Zheng W, Yang G. Cruciferous vegetable intake is inversely correlated with circulating levels of proinflammatory markers in women. *J Acad Nutr Diet.* 2014;114(5):700−708 e2.

45. Salehi-Abargouei A, Saraf-Bank S, Bellissimo N, Azadbakht L. Effects of non-soy legume consumption on C-reactive protein: a systematic review and meta-analysis. *Nutrition.* 2015;31(5):631−639.

46. Jiao J, Xu JY, Zhang W, Han S, Qin LQ. Effect of dietary fiber on circulating C-reactive protein in overweight and obese adults: a meta-analysis of randomized controlled trials. *Int J Food Sci Nutr.* 2015;66(1):114−119.

47. Hajihashemi P, Azadbakht L, Hashemipor M, Kelishadi R, Esmaillzadeh A. Whole-grain intake favorably affects markers of systemic inflammation in obese children: a randomized controlled crossover clinical trial. *Mol Nutr Food Res.* 2014;58(6):1301−1308.

48. Bassett CM, Rodriguez-Leyva D, Pierce GN. Experimental and clinical research findings on the cardiovascular benefits of consuming flaxseed. *Appl Physiol Nutr Metabol.* 2009; 34(5):965—974.

49. Guasch-Ferre M, Li J, Hu FB, Salas-Salvado J, Tobias DK. Effects of walnut consumption on blood lipids and other cardiovascular risk factors: an updated meta-analysis and systematic review of controlled trials. *Am J Clin Nutr.* 2018;108(1):174—187.

50. Horrobin DF, Campbell A, McEwen CG. Treatment of the Sicca syndrome and Sjögren's syndrome with E.F.A., pyridoxine and vitamin C. *Prog Lipid Res.* 1981;20:253—254.

51. Manthorpe R, Hagen Petersen S, Prause JU. Primary Sjögren's syndrome treated with Efamol/Efavit. A double-blind cross-over investigation. *Rheumatol Int.* 1984;4(4): 165—167.

52. Oxholm P, Manthorpe R, Prause JU, Horrobin D. Patients with primary Sjögren's syndrome treated for two months with evening primrose oil. *Scand J Rheumatol.* 1986; 15(2):103—108.

53. Theander E, Horrobin DF, Jacobsson LT, Manthorpe R. Gammalinolenic acid treatment of fatigue associated with primary Sjögren's syndrome. *Scand J Rheumatol.* 2002;31(2): 72—79.

54. Aragona P, Bucolo C, Spinella R, Giuffrida S, Ferreri G. Systemic omega-6 essential fatty acid treatment and pge1 tear content in Sjögren's syndrome patients. *Investig Ophthalmol Vis Sci.* 2005;46(12):4474—4479.

Perioperative management of patients with Sjögren's syndrome

13

Michael D. George, MD, MSCE[1], Nora Sandorfi, MD[2]

[1]*Assistant Professor of Medicine, Division of Rheumatology, University of Pennsylvania Perelman School of Medicine, Philadelphia, PA, United States;* [2]*Associate of Medicine, Division of Rheumatology, University of Pennsylvania Perelman School of Medicine, Philadelphia, PA, United States*

Perioperative management specific to Sjögren's syndrome

Patients with Sjögren's syndrome require special perioperative care for their sicca symptoms and for the extraglandular manifestations of the disease. It is important to recognize that physical and emotional stress can contribute to disease flares, and this risk may be compounded if disease-modifying therapies have also been held before surgery. Patients should have special counseling and planning, which by itself can have a positive effect on handling emotional stress. Owing to the complexity of the condition, the patient's rheumatologist should always be actively involved once the patient is scheduled to undergo surgery.

Managing sicca preoperatively

Glandular manifestations of Sjögren's disease are the first to address before a surgical procedure. Topical formulations for oral and ocular dryness are appropriate and should be used perioperatively, although use of vitamin E oil should be held for 2 weeks before surgery because of its anticoagulant effect. Similarly, fish oils and plant seed oils should also be held before surgery. If the patient cannot take even small amounts of liquid for a prolonged time before surgery, at least frequent mouth rinsing should be allowed. Secretagogues should not be taken on the day of the surgery if the patient undergoes general anesthesia. Importantly, secretagogues and other over-the-counter drugs for dry eyes and mouth are typically nonformulary; patients should be advised to bring these products to the hospital and write out a schedule for perioperative administration.

Anesthetic gases and the use of general anesthesia causes dryness, and local anesthesia is preferred when this is an appropriate option. If general anesthesia is required, a humidifier should be added to the rebreathing system. Extra lubrication should be used when an endotracheal tube or nasal tubes are needed, as the dry mucosa can be friable. The patient's eyes should be taped shut with an ocular gel or ointment intraoperatively to prevent desiccation and corneal erosions.[1]

Managing extraglandular manifestations

It is very important to address the extraglandular manifestations of the patient's Sjögren's syndrome as well. As part of the preoperative evaluation, the management of specific organ involvement such as interstitial lung disease, pulmonary hypertension, and renal insufficiency is often addressed by specialists. In particular, patients with clinically significant interstitial lung disease or pulmonary hypertension should be evaluated by a pulmonologist or pulmonary hypertension specialist before surgery.

Other conditions such as Raynaud phenomenon, arthritis, and neuropathy are often overlooked and should be addressed by the primary rheumatologist. Raynaud disease is often treated with calcium channel blockers and low-dose aspirin. Unless otherwise instructed by the surgical team, both need to be discontinued preoperatively and other preventative measures should be utilized instead. It is important that the patient is properly covered to maintain core body temperature and to keep the hands and feet warm during surgery. Arthritic joints should be properly positioned. The neck, shoulders, and knees should not be overextended; if needed, soft support should be provided for proper positioning. Care should also be taken during transfer to and from the operating room table and the bed. Similar precautions should be applied for areas affected by peripheral neuropathy; if possible, constant and prolonged pressure should be avoided.

Postoperative care

Introduction of oral intake should be done carefully, accounting for potential swallowing problems of which many patients with Sjögren's syndrome may suffer. If possible, the patient should be postured in an upright position. In the recovery room, preservative-free eye drops and frequent small sips of liquid or ice chips should be offered hourly to the patient when awake. Saltines or dry crackers may not be appropriate for patients with sicca symptoms. More moist foods such as apple sauce are preferred.

If the patient remains intubated, humidified oxygen should be used, as intubated patients are at increased risk for the development of oral mucosal inflammation.[2] In addition, ventilator-associated pneumonia (VAP) is a common complication in intensive care unit (ICU) patients, occurring in 9%−78% of cases.[3] Early on (within the first 4 days), the common pathogens are *Staphylococcus aureus*, *Haemophilus influenzae*, and *Streptococcus pneumoniae*. In cases beyond 4 days, VAP is usually due to enterobacteriaceae, *Pseudomonas aeruginosa* and *S. aureus*. Oropharyngeal colonization can travel down the endotracheal tube and cause further infections.

Mouth and oral care are therefore extremely important, especially in patients who remain intubated. Chlorhexidine 0.12% mouthwash is recommended before the surgical procedure and even after surgery.[4] Lemon Glycerin swabs actually inhibit saliva production, and brushing with regular tap water is not recommended because it may contain bacteria. Using a soft suction sponge may be satisfactory to clean the surfaces in the oral cavity as long as the patient is intubated.

In addition to oral care, preservative-free artificial tears should be administered every 2–3 hours in the ICU to keep the eyes moisturized.

Risk of infection after surgery

Patients undergoing surgery are at risk of other postoperative infections. The specific infections and risks vary based on the procedure being performed. Cataract surgery, for example, carries a very low risk of local infection of approximately 0.1%.[5] In contrast, abdominal surgery carries greater surgical risk, with approximately 10% of patients experiencing infections (most commonly wound infections, pneumonia, urinary tract infections) after colectomy for diverticular disease or colon cancer.[6] Orthopedic surgery is particularly common, with rates of hip and knee replacement rising in the general population.[7,8] Risk of infection after hip or knee replacement is approximately 3%–5%, with urinary infections, pneumonia, and surgical site infections being the most common infection types.[9,10] Any surgery that includes implanted prosthetic material, such as joint replacement surgery, is of particular concern because of the potential for bacterial seeding of the prosthetic material. The risk of prosthetic joint infection after hip or knee replacement is approximately 0.5%–1%, especially in the first year after surgery[9–11]; these infections carry substantial morbidity.

Although the preoperative use of immunosuppressive medications may increase the risk of postoperative infection, it is important to remember that many other patient and surgical factors also influence the risk of infection after surgery. In orthopedic surgery, for example, comorbidities (especially diabetes), coagulopathy, male gender, body mass index, surgical technique and materials, and surgeon and hospital volume can all impact infection risk.[9,11–15] Patients with rheumatoid arthritis have also been shown to be at increased risk of postoperative infection after orthopedic surgery.[10,16,17] While many of these risk factors are not modifiable, patients should be encouraged to seek care at a high-volume center from a highly experienced surgeon who performs a high volume of the procedure whenever possible.

Management of immunosuppression

Understanding how to manage immunosuppression in the perioperative period requires understanding to what degree different therapies might contribute to the risk of infection, the potential benefits of holding therapy before surgery, and the risks of holding or stopping therapy, which vary from patient to patient. Additionally, the necessity and urgency of surgery is of importance in the decision-making process. Clearly, in patients requiring urgent or emergent surgery, there is limited ability to modify immunosuppression, at least in the preoperative period.

Much of the data about the contributions of immunosuppression to the risk of postoperative infection comes from studies of patients with rheumatoid arthritis who are undergoing orthopedic surgery because this scenario is particularly common.[18] There is little randomized controlled trial data available to address this issue. Therefore current recommendations on the management of perioperative immunosuppression are based on data of infection risk from nonsurgical studies and from observational studies of orthopedic surgery. In the following section, we will summarize data on the risks of individual immunosuppressive therapies, recognizing that this field continues to evolve.

Conventional disease-modifying antirheumatic drugs

Current recommendations from the American College of Rheumatology (ACR) and the American Association of Hip and Knee Surgeons are to continue the use of methotrexate, sulfasalazine, hydroxychloroquine, and leflunomide throughout the perioperative period without interruption[19] (Table 13.1). Several pieces of evidence support this recommendation.

In two small randomized trials, holding low-dose methotrexate administration in the preoperative period did not decrease the risk of postoperative infection.[20,21] In one of these studies, in fact, patients who stopped methotrexate use 14 days before surgery had a significantly greater risk of adverse outcomes and were also more likely to have a disease flare.[21] In another small randomized trial, stopping leflunomide intake preoperatively also failed to lower the risk of infection.[22]

Evidence from the nonsurgical setting is also reassuring. The risk of infection associated with methotrexate has been shown to be low.[23] Hydroxychloroquine and sulfasalazine are immunomodulatory rather than being immunosuppressive and have not been associated with an increase in infection risk.[24]

Medications such as azathioprine, mycophenolate, cyclosporine, and tacrolimus may occasionally be used for certain manifestations of Sjögren's syndrome, and there is limited data to guide the management of these medications. These treatments can impact T-cell function and cause leukopenia. They are associated with an increased risk of infection in the nonoperative setting and so could hypothetically increase the risk of postoperative infections. There is no direct evidence about the impact of stopping these therapies before surgery. Therefore in the individual patient, the hypothetical benefits of stopping therapy should be weighed against the risks of treatment interruption and possible disease flare. In support of this approach, current guidelines recommend continuing these therapies before elective surgery in patients with severe systemic lupus erythematosus (SLE) but holding these therapies for 1 week before elective surgery in patients with nonsevere SLE.[19] Similar

Table 13.1 Summary of the 2017 ACR medication management guidelines for patients undergoing elective hip or knee arthroplasty.

	ACR recommendations	Comments
Conventional DMARDs		
Hydroxychloroquine, sulfasalazine	Continue without interruption	Not associated with greater infection risk in nonsurgical studies
Methotrexate, leflunomide	Continue without interruption	Small randomized studies show no benefit from treatment interruption
Azathioprine, cyclosporine mycophenolate mofetil, tacrolimus	Stop 7 days before surgery in nonsevere SLE Continue without interruption in severe SLE	Weigh risks and benefits of holding depending on the indication for use in Sjögren's syndrome
Biologic/Targeted therapies		
TNF inhibitors (adalimumab, certolizumab, etanercept, golimumab, infliximab)	Stop for one dosing interval before surgery[a]	Greater infection risk in nonsurgical studies, but no benefit in holding infliximab in one observational study—weigh risks and benefits
Other biologic drugs (e.g., abatacept, rituximab, tocilizumab)	Stop for one dosing interval before surgery[a]	No direct studies of timing but infection risk is similar to that with TNF inhibitors in nonsurgical studies
Tofacitinib	Stop for 7 days before surgery	No direct studies of timing but risk is similar to that with biologic therapies
Glucocorticoids		
Prednisone, prednisolone, methylprednisolone, dexamethasone	Taper to <20 mg/day of prednisone or equivalent when possible	Risk of infection with glucocorticoids is greater than that with other therapies. Surgical studies suggest increased risk at dosages >10 −20 mg/day and possible risk at lower doses.

If a treatment is stopped before surgery the ACR guidelines recommend waiting at least 14 days after surgery to restart therapy, ensuring that the wound is healing well and there are no signs of local or systemic infection.
ACR, American College of Rheumatology; DMARDs, disease-modifying arthritis remittive drugs; SLE, systemic lupus erythematosus; TNF, tumor necrosis factor.
[a] At least one dosing interval has elapsed between the last medication administration and surgery.
Adapted from Ref. 19.

principles should apply to patients with Sjögren's syndrome. In patients with severe organ manifestations with a high risk of flare with medication interruptions, therapy should be continued, especially for low-risk procedures without prosthetic material. In patients with less severe disease manifestations or who are at low risk of flare with treatment interruptions, it is reasonable to briefly interrupt treatment in the perioperative setting, as long as this does not necessitate an increase in glucocorticoid use.

Biologic and targeted therapies

Tumor necrosis factor inhibitors (TNFis) are known to be associated with an increased risk of infection in the nonoperative setting, and TNFis carry a black box warning for serious infections.[25] However, many patients tolerate therapy with TNFis well, and the risk of serious infection in clinical trials is approximately 5% per year. Other biologic therapies seem to convey similar risk, although some studies have suggested that infection risk might be slightly lower with abatacept and etanercept than with other therapies [26,27].

Studies have shown that patients treated with a TNFi are at greater risk of infection after surgery,[28] but these patients also tend to have more severe disease. The direct contribution of TNFis to infection after surgery is not known. Additionally, it is not clear whether interrupting biologic treatment before surgery improves outcomes and, if so, what duration of interruption is required. A study of Medicare patients demonstrated that patients who stopped infliximab use before surgery had similar risk of postoperative infection to patients who received infliximab within 4 weeks of surgery.[29] A study from the Veterans Affairs administration also suggested that holding biologic therapy did not significantly reduce infection risk.[30]

Because of limited data, guidelines from the ACR were based on the known risk of biologic therapies from nonsurgical studies. These guidelines recommend holding biologic therapies for one dosing interval before hip and knee replacement.[19] This means that at least one dosing interval has elapsed between the last administration of the biologic drug and surgery and that on the day of surgery the biologic drug is overdue. For example, for a patient treated with infliximab every 8 weeks the last dose would be given 9 weeks (57–63 days) before surgery, for adalimumab dosed every 2 weeks the last dose would be administered 3 weeks (15–21 days) before surgery, for weekly etanercept administration the last dose would be given 2 weeks (8–14 days) before surgery, and for rituximab given every 6 months the last dose would be administered 7 months (181–210 days) before surgery.

Tofacitinib, a small-molecule Janus kinase inhibitor, has a short half-life but may have a longer immunosuppressive effect. It is known to increase the risk of infection with magnitude similar to that of TNFis.[31] Although again there is no direct data on stopping the therapy, recommendations from the ACR are to stop tofacitinib use 7 days before surgery.

Treatment with biologic therapies or tofacitinib can be resumed 14 days after surgery assuming that there are no complications, essentially providing time to ensure that the surgical site is healing well and that there are no signs of infection. These recommendations result in only short interruptions in treatment before surgery and they are reasonable for many patients. In patients with a severe disease at a high risk of flare, however, the hypothetical benefits of stopping therapy must be weighed against the risks of treatment interruption.

Glucocorticoids

Management of glucocorticoids in the perioperative period is particularly important. Chronic use of glucocorticoids, especially at higher doses, is associated with a greater risk of infection than conventional or biologic disease-modifying arthritis remittive drugs (DMARDs) in nonsurgical patients.[32] Studies have also consistently shown that glucocorticoids are associated with greater infection risk in patients undergoing surgery as well [29,33–35]. The risk of infection is greater at higher doses of glucocorticoids. Guidelines from the ACR recommend avoiding dosages above 20 mg per day of prednisone before hip and knee surgery.[19] This recommendation may be too liberal, however, because observational studies suggest a significantly increased risk of infection at dosages above 10 mg per day of prednisone and possibly even at lower doses.[36] The precise risk in the latter group on low-dose glucocorticoids remains unclear.

"Stress-dose steroids" are sometimes given in the perioperative period. It is unclear whether these doses, given for a very short period, contribute substantially to infection risk. It does seem, however, that stress-dose steroids may not be necessary in the majority of patients chronically treated with glucocorticoids. This practice is based largely on two cases from the 1950s: the deaths of young patients with rheumatoid arthritis in whom glucocorticoids were abruptly stopped before surgery.[37] The limited data available has not provided evidence that increasing the home glucocorticoid dose before surgery improves outcomes as long as the home glucocorticoid dose is continued on the day of surgery and in the postoperative period [37–40]. If hypotension that does not respond to routine measures does occur, glucocorticoids can always be given intraoperatively as an adjunctive therapy. Alternatively, in high-risk patients, a fasting cortisol level test or adrenocorticotrophic hormone stimulation test can be performed preoperatively to screen for adrenal insufficiency.

Key messages for immunosuppression

Based on the available data, it appears that conventional DMARDs such as hydroxychloroquine, sulfasalazine, methotrexate, and leflunomide do not contribute substantially to the risk of postoperative infection and can continue to be used throughout the perioperative period.

Medications such as mycophenolate, azathioprine, cyclosporine, tacrolimus, and biologic drugs may contribute to infection risk but it remains unclear whether stopping therapy substantially decreases infection risk. The decision on whether to stop these medications before surgery depends on the risk of the surgery versus the risk of stopping therapy. For patients undergoing high-risk surgery who lack severe organ manifestations, the risk of brief interruption in therapy is small; therefore, holding azathioprine or mycophenolate use for a week before surgery and holding biologic drug use for one dosing interval before surgery is reasonable. These medications can be restarted 2 weeks after surgery if the surgical site is healing well.

Glucocorticoids, however, especially at dosages above 10 mg per day, substantially increase the risk of infection. Patients requiring higher glucocorticoid doses should consider deferring any elective surgeries until the glucocorticoid dose can be lowered or stopped. In addition, if stopping other treatments is likely to lead to a disease flare and result in the need to increase glucocorticoid doses in a particular patient, it may be a better option to avoid interruptions of other therapies in some cases. The risk posed by glucocorticoids is likely greater than any small benefit achieved by interrupting other treatments.

Again, these recommendations apply only to patients undergoing elective surgery. In patients requiring more urgent or emergent surgery, it is not possible to change therapy before surgery, although biologic therapies should be held for at least 2 weeks after these surgeries have been completed to ensure that patients are healing well. Patients should, of course, be monitored for signs of postoperative infection, especially if they have been treated with chronic glucocorticoids.

Conclusions

Patients with Sjögren's syndrome should be carefully evaluated and counseled before surgery, with rheumatologists taking an active role in the planning process. This evaluation includes plans for the management of sicca symptoms before and after surgery, the extraglandular manifestations of the disease (with involvement by other specialists as appropriate), and recommendations for the management of immunosuppression in the perioperative period.

References

1. Petruzzi L, Vivino F. Sjögren's syndrome–implications for perioperative practice. *AORN J*. March 2003;77(3):612−621, 624; quiz 625, 627−8.
2. Sjögren P. Hospitalisation associated with a deterioration in oral health. *Evid Based Dent*. 2011;12(2):48.
3. Dennesen P, van der Ven A, Vlasveld M, Lokker L, Ramsay G, Kessels A, van den Keijbus P, van Nieuw Amerongen, Veerman E. Inadequate salivary flow and poor oral mucosal status in intubated intensive care unit patients. *Crit Care Med*. March 2003; 31(3):781−786.
4. Booker S, Murff S, Kitko L, Jablonski R. Mouth care to reduce ventilator-associated pneumonia. *Am J Nurs*. October 2013;113(10):24−30. quiz 31.

5. Creuzot-Garcher C, Mariet A, Benzenine E, Daien V, Korobelnik J, Bron A, Quantin C. Is combined cataract surgery associated with acute postoperative endophthalmitis? A nationwide study from 2005 to 2014. *Br J Ophthalmol*. June 20, 2018 [Epub ahead of print].

6. Van Arendonk K, Tymitz K, Gearhart S, Stem M, Lidor A. Outcomes and costs of elective surgery for diverticular disease: a comparison with other diseases requiring colectomy. *JAMA Surg*. April 2013;148(4):316–321.

7. Products - Data Briefs - Number 211 - August 2015 [Internet]. [cited 2018 Aug 16]. Available from: https://www.cdc.gov/nchs/products/databriefs/db210.htm.

8. Products - Data Briefs - Number 186 - February 2015 [Internet]. [cited 2018 Aug 16]. Available from: https://www.cdc.gov/nchs/data/databriefs/db186.htm.

9. Katz J, Barrett J, Mahomed N, Baron J, Wright R, Losina E. Association between hospital and surgeon procedure volume and the outcomes of total knee replacement. *J Bone Joint Surg Am*. September 2004;86-A(9), 1909–16.

10. Stundner O, Danninger T, Chiu Y, Sun X, Goodman S, Russell L, Figgie M, Mazumdar M, Memtsoudis S. Rheumatoid arthritis vs osteoarthritis in patients receiving total knee arthroplasty: perioperative outcomes. *J Arthroplast*. February 2014;29(2): 308–313.

11. Katz J, Losina E, Barrett J, Phillips C, Mahomed N, Lew R, Guadagnoli E, Harris W, Poss R, Baron J. Association between hospital and surgeon procedure volume and outcomes of total hip replacement in the United States Medicare population. *J Bone Joint Surg Am*. November 2001;83-A(11):1622–1629.

12. Bongartz T, Halligan C, Osmon D, Reinalda M, Bamlet W, Crowson C, Hanssen A, Matteson E. Incidence and risk factors of prosthetic joint infection after total hip or knee replacement in patients with rheumatoid arthritis. *Arthritis Rheum*. December 15, 2008;59(12):1713–1720.

13. Mahomed N, Barrett J, Katz J, Phillips C, Losina E, Lew R, Guadagnoli E, Harris W, Poss R, Baron J. Rates and outcomes of primary and revision total hip replacement in the United States medicare population. *J Bone Joint Surg Am*. January 2003;85-A(1): 27–32.

14. Bozic K, Lau E, Kurtz S, Ong K, Rubash H, Vail T, Berry D. Patient-related risk factors for periprosthetic joint infection and postoperative mortality following total hip arthroplasty in Medicare patients (American) [Internet] *J Bone Jt. Surg*; May 2, 2012 [cited 2015 Mar 6];94(9). Available from: http://jbjs.org/cgi/doi/10.2106/JBJS.K.00072.

15. Ravi B, Croxford R, Austin PC, Hollands S, Paterson JM, Bogoch E, et al. Increased surgeon experience with rheumatoid arthritis reduces the risk of complications following total joint arthroplasty: surgical experience performing TJA in RA is protective. *Arthritis & Rheumatology*. March 2014;66(3):488–496.

16. Ravi B, Escott B, Shah PS, Jenkinson R, Chahal J, Bogoch E, Kreder H, Hawker G. A systematic review and meta-analysis comparing complications following total joint arthroplasty for rheumatoid arthritis versus for osteoarthritis. *Arthritis Rheum*. December 2012;64(12):3839–3849.

17. Ravi B, Croxford R, Hollands S, Paterson J, Bogoch E, Kreder H, Hawker G. Increased risk of complications following total joint arthroplasty in patients with rheumatoid arthritis: increased risk of specific complications in TJA recipients with RA. *Arthritis & Rheumatology*. February 2014;66(2):254–263.

18. Shourt C, Crowson C, Gabriel S, Matteson E. Orthopedic surgery among patients with rheumatoid arthritis 1980–2007: a population-based study focused on surgery rates, sex, and mortality. *J Rheumatol*. March 1, 2012;39(3):481–485.

19. Goodman S, Springer B, Guyatt G, Abdel M, Dasa V, George M, Gewurz-Singer O, Giles J, Johnson B, Lee S, Mandl L, Mont M, Sculco P, Sporer S, Stryker L, Turgunbaev M, Brause B, Chen A, Gililland J, Goodman M, Hurley-Rosenblatt A, Kirou K, Losina E, MacKenzie R, Michaud K, Mikuls T, Russel L, Sah A, Miller A, Singh J. American College of Rheumatology/American association of hip and knee surgeons guideline for the perioperative management of antirheumatic medication in patients with rheumatic diseases undergoing elective total hip or total knee arthroplasty. *Arthritis Rheumatol.* 2017;69(8):1538–1551, 2017 Aug.

20. Sany J, Anaya J, Canovas F, Combe B, Jorgensen C, Saker S, Thaury M, Gavroy J. Influence of methotrexate on the frequency of postoperative infectious complications in patients with rheumatoid arthritis. *J Rheumatol.* July 1993;20(7):1129–1132.

21. Grennan D, Gray J, Loudon J, Fear S. Methotrexate and early postoperative complications in patients with rheumatoid arthritis undergoing elective orthopaedic surgery. *Ann Rheum Dis.* March 2001;60(3):214–217.

22. Tanaka N, Sakahashi H, Sato E, Hirose K, Ishima T, Ishii S. Examination of the risk of continuous leflunomide treatment on the incidence of infectious complications after joint arthroplasty in patients with rheumatoid arthritis. *J Clin Rheumatol.* April 2003;9(2):115–118.

23. Lopez-Olivo M, Siddhanamatha H, Shea B, Tugwell P, Wells G, Suarez-Almazor M. Methotrexate for treating rheumatoid arthritis. *Cochrane Database Syst Rev.* 2014;(6):CD000957.

24. Wolfe F, Caplan L, Michaud K. Treatment for rheumatoid arthritis and the risk of hospitalization for pneumonia: associations with prednisone, disease-modifying antirheumatic drugs, and anti-tumor necrosis factor therapy. *Arthritis Rheum.* February 2006;54(2):628–634.

25. Singh J, Cameron C, Noorbaloochi S, Cullis T, Tucker M, Christensen R, Ghogomu E, Coyle D, Clifford T, Tugwell P, Wells G. Risk of serious infection in biological treatment of patients with rheumatoid arthritis: a systematic review and meta-analysis. *Lancet.* July 18, 2015;386(9990):258–265.

26. Yun H, Xie F, Delzell E, Levitan E, Chen L, Lewis J, Saag K, Beukelman T, Winthrop K, Baddley J, Curtis J. Comparative risk of hospitalized infection associated with biologic agents in rheumatoid arthritis patients enrolled in medicare. *Arthritis Rheumatol.* January 2016;68(1):56–66.

27. Curtis J, Yang S, Patkar N, Chen L, Singh J, Cannon G, Mikuls T, Delzell E, Saag K, Safford M, DuVall S, Alexander K, Napalkov P, Winthrop K, Burton M, Kamauu A, Baddley J. Risk of hospitalized bacterial infections associated with biologic treatment among US veterans with rheumatoid arthritis. *Arthritis Care Res.* July 2014;66(7):990–997.

28. Goodman S, Menon I, Christos P, Smethurst R, Bykerk V. Management of perioperative tumour necrosis factor α inhibitors in rheumatoid arthritis patients undergoing arthroplasty: a systematic review and meta-analysis. *Rheumatology.* March 2016;55(3):573–582.

29. George M, Baker J, Hsu J, Wu Q, Xie F, Chen L, Yun H, Curtis J. Perioperative timing of infliximab and the risk of serious infection after elective hip and knee arthroplasty. *Arthritis Care Res.* December 2017;69(12):1845–1854.

30. Abou Zahr Z, Spiegelman A, Cantu M, Ng B. Perioperative use of anti-rheumatic agents does not increase early postoperative infection risks: a Veteran Affairs' administrative database study. *Rheumatol Int.* February 2015;35(2):265–272.

31. Cohen S, Radominski S, Gomez-Reino J, Wang L, Krishnaswami S, Wood S, Soma K, Nduaka C, Kowk K, Valdez H, Benda B, Riese R. Analysis of infections and all-cause mortality in phase II, phase III, and long-term extension studies of tofacitinib in patients with rheumatoid arthritis. *Arthritis Rheumatol*. November 2014;66(11):2924—2937.

32. Dixon W, Suissa S, Hudson M. The association between systemic glucocorticoid therapy and the risk of infection in patients with rheumatoid arthritis: systematic review and meta-analyses. *Arthritis Res Ther*. August 31, 2011;13(4):R139.

33. Michaud K, Fehringer E, Garvin K, O'Dell J, Mikuls T. Rheumatoid arthritis patients are not at increased risk for 30-day cardiovascular events, infections, or mortality after total joint arthroplasty. *Arthritis Res Ther*. 2013;15(6):R195.

34. Somayaji R, Barnabe C, Martin L. Risk factors for infection following total joint arthroplasty in rheumatoid arthritis. *Open Rheumatol J*. November 29, 2013;7:119—124.

35. Gilson M, Gossec L, Mariette X, Gherissi D, Guyot M, Berthelot J, Wendling D, Michelet C, Dellamonica P, Tubach F, Dougados M, Salmon D. Risk factors for total joint arthroplasty infection in patients receiving tumor necrosis factor α-blockers: a case-control study. *Arthritis Res Ther*. 2010;12(4):R145.

36. George M, Baker J, Winthrop K, Alemao E, Chen L, Connolly S, Hsu J, Simon T, Wu Q, Xie F, Curtis J. Risk of biologics and glucocorticoids in patients with rheumatoid arthritis undergoing arthroplasty: a cohort study. *Ann Intern Med*. May 2019 [Epub ahead of print].

37. Yong S, Marik P, Esposito M, Coulthard P. Supplemental perioperative steroids for surgical patients with adrenal insufficiency. *Cochrane Database Syst Rev*. October 2009;(4): CD005367.

38. Glowniak J, Loriaux D. A double-blind study of perioperative steroid requirements in secondary adrenal insufficiency. *Surgery*. February 1997;121(2):123—129.

39. Thomason J, Girdler N, Kendall-Taylor P, Wastell H, Weddel A, Seymour R. An investigation into the need for supplementary steroids in organ transplant patients undergoing gingival surgery. A double-blind, split-mouth, cross-over study. *J Clin Periodontol*. September 1999;26(9):577—582.

40. Zaghiyan K, Melmed G, Berel D, Ovsepyan G, Murrell Z, Fleshner P. A prospective, randomized, noninferiority trial of steroid dosing after major colorectal surgery. *Ann Surg*. January 2014;259(1):32—37.

Utility and safety of vaccines in Sjögren's syndrome

14

R. Hal Scofield, MD[1,2,3], Eliza F. Chakrabarty, MD, MPH[4,5]

[1]*Member, Arthritis & Clinical Immunology Program, Oklahoma Medical Research Foundation, Oklahoma City, OK, United States;* [2]*Professor, Department of Medicine, College of Medicine, University of Oklahoma Health Sciences Center, Oklahoma City, OK, United States;* [3]*Staff Physician, Associate Chief of Staff for Research, Medical Service, United States Department of Veterans Affairs Medical Center, Oklahoma City, OK, United States;* [4]*Arthritis & Clinical Immunology Program, Oklahoma Medical Research Foundation, Oklahoma City, OK, United States;* [5]*Department of Medicine, College of Medicine, University of Oklahoma Health Sciences Center, Oklahoma City, OK, United States*

Sjögren's syndrome is a chronic, autoimmune, rheumatic disease with both organ-specific and systemic manifestations.[1] The great majority (>90%) of patients are women and may experience onset at any age, especially, in the fifth and sixth decades.[1] The exocrine glands including the lacrimal and salivary glands are most commonly affected leading to the characteristic sicca symptoms. Treatment of these features is generally symptomatic because no effective disease-modifying therapy currently exists. About 25% of patients may also develop internal organ or extraglandular manifestations[2] that are associated with systemic autoimmunity.[3] Rheumatic manifestations and other mild disease features are commonly treated with hydroxychloroquine with variable results.[4–7] Hydroxychloroquine is an immunomodulating drug but not an immunosuppressive drug and is therefore not associated with an increased risk of infections. Patients with serious and/or life-threatening complications require stronger immunosuppressive drugs, including glucocorticoids and biologic drugs. Such therapy predisposes to infections and may alter the immune response to vaccines.

There is a paucity of data concerning response to vaccination in Sjögren's syndrome. This is especially true when Sjögren's syndrome is compared to related autoimmune diseases such as rheumatoid arthritis (RA) and systemic lupus erythematosus (SLE). For the latter, there are extensive data regarding vaccination against hepatitis B, influenza, herpes zoster, papillomavirus, and *Streptococcus pneumoniae*. Although Sjögren's syndrome and SLE are certainly related at both the clinical and immunologic levels, patients with SLE are much more likely to be treated with immunosuppressive drugs that might impair immune responses to vaccination. Given the similarities of these illnesses, we will review data concerning vaccination among patients with SLE insofar as these data relate to those patients

Sjögren's Syndrome. https://doi.org/10.1016/B978-0-323-67534-5.00014-4

with Sjögren's syndrome. We will review not only vaccination against infectious diseases in patients with Sjögren's syndrome but also the data concerning vaccination as a triggering event for the disease.

Vaccination: general considerations

History

Edward Jenner (1749–1823) coined the word vaccination to describe the procedure he developed in 1796 using material from cowpox lesions to prevent smallpox.[8] The singular nominative Latin word for cow is *vacca*, derived from the Proto-Indo-European *woḱeh₂*.[9] When the cowpox lesion fluid was inoculated into the arms of children in his village, it induced, what we now term, immunity to smallpox. The procedure rapidly spread throughout the world, including introduction to the New World by Benjamin Waterhouse in Boston[10] and Samuel Scofield in New York City.[11] Some would argue that Jenner's experiments can be considered the beginning of immunology, if not the beginning of modern experimental medicine.

Childhood vaccinations

A number of childhood vaccines are routinely given in most parts of the world. Among these are vaccines that have a several-generation history, including diphtheria, tetanus, pertussis, mumps, and measles. Other vaccines, such as pneumococcal, papillomavirus, *Haemophilus influenzae*, have only been added recently. Because of the usual age of onset of Sjögren's syndrome, most patients will have already undergone the traditional childhood vaccinations. However, there are recommendations for repeating some of these during adulthood (Table 14.1).[12]

Adult vaccinations

A number of vaccinations are recommended exclusively for adults (Table 14.1).[12] For example, vaccination against pneumococcal disease is a multistep process that begins at the age 65 years. Despite consistent recommendations that patients with autoimmune rheumatic disease should be vaccinated, vaccine administration to these patients remains low.[13–15] Although there may be occasional special considerations, adults with Sjögren's syndrome should be vaccinated as is currently recommended for the general population (Table 14.1). In particular, vaccination should

Table 14.1 US centers for disease Control and Prevention vaccination requirements for adults.

Vaccination[a]	Who should receive it?	When should it be given?
Seasonal influenza	All adults	Yearly
Tetanus, diphtheria, pertussis	All adults	Every 10 years, during every pregnancy
Zoster (shingles), recombinant	All adults	Age 50 years, two doses 2–6 months apart; even with past shingles
Pneumococcal	All adults	Age 65 years, both 23-valent and 13-valent sequentially
Chicken pox (varicella)	All adults without disease or vaccination as a child	Above the age 19 years
Papillomavirus	Adult women up to the age 26 years and adult men up to the age 21 years	Women <26 years of age and men <21 years of age

[a] Other vaccinations may be recommended depending on factors such as work-related disease exposure or travel, see Table 14.2.
Modified from Ref. 12

not be delayed or avoided among patients taking hydroxychloroquine or glucocorticoids. In fact, data (vide infra) suggest that vaccination while on these drugs might be preferred.[16] Vaccinations should be performed even when patients are taking immunosuppressive agents.[17]

Influenza vaccination

Seasonal, epidemic influenza is a serious illness that causes the death of many tens of thousands of people each year in the United States. The disease and the resulting deaths are largely preventable by vaccination.[18] However, there are only a few studies of influenza vaccination in Sjögren's syndrome patients. Milanovic and colleagues[19] studied 99 patients with inflammatory rheumatic disease, of whom 32 had Sjögren's syndrome, for over 4 years. A total of 35 subjects received a yearly influenza vaccination, while 12 others received at least one. The remaining 52 declined to receive influenza vaccination. The occurrence of both influenza and the subsequent post-viral lung infections was reduced in those receiving vaccination, with the 2010 vaccination lowering the risk of influenza by 87%. No vaccinated subject experienced a disease exacerbation following vaccination. The authors concluded that modern influenza vaccine was safe and effective in patients with rheumatic disease.[19] Another study examined the effects of H1N1 influenza vaccination in Sjögren's syndrome versus age- and sex-matched controls. Treatment-naive Sjögren's syndrome subjects developed higher titers of anti-H1N1 antibodies than controls. There were also increases in noninfluenza antibody titers, along with evidence of polyclonal B-cell hyperactivity. The B-cell hyperactivity found *in vivo* was not found among patients treated with hydroxychloroquine, while the changes found *in vitro* were abolished with exposure of the B cells to chloroquine.[16] Of note, this study examined the subjects at 1 and 3 weeks after vaccination; thus longer term consequences of B-cell hyperactivity or its effect on clinical illness (i.e., disease flares) was not assessed.

Influenza vaccination has been studied much more extensively among those with SLE, who are more likely than those with Sjögren's syndrome to be treated with immunosuppressive and antimalarial medications. Puges et al.[20] reviewed 17 studies of influenza vaccination in SLE cohorts and found that there was a reduced rate of seroconversion as well as seroprotection for influenza A but not influenza B. Another review concluded that seroprotection rates were lower among patients with SLE who were taking glucocorticoid or azathioprine but that there was not an excess of adverse events.[21] Thus the differences in the findings between subjects with Sjögren's syndrome and those with SLE is most likely related to the treatment of SLE.

None of these studies utilized the live attenuated influenza virus vaccine, which should be avoided in patients with Sjögren's syndrome, especially when taking immunosuppressive drugs, and in other patients with potentially immunocompromising conditions.

Pneumococcal vaccination

Pneumococcal infection remains an important and serious medical problem, despite the available effective antibiotics and vaccination, especially in older adults or those with chronic illness.[22–24] Mortality with invasive disease, defined as positive blood cultures, is from 20% to 35% in older adults.[22,23] Meanwhile, pneumococcal vaccination is safe and effective even in adults over the age 75 years and significantly reduces morbidity and mortality, up to 90% for the latter.[25] Most adults with invasive pneumococcal disease were candidates for vaccination and saw a physician within a year of contracting the disease, but did not receive vaccination.[26] Thus we recommend that Sjögren's syndrome patients receive pneumococcal vaccination following the same schedule as for healthy adults. At present, this means that immunization starts at the age 65 years. An argument has been made that because of the markedly increased incidence of pneumococcal infection, all patients with SLE regardless of age should receive pneumococcal vaccination as a protective measure.[27] One could make this same argument for Sjögren's syndrome, especially, before starting on immunosuppressive medications. However, the incidence of these infections is lower in Sjögren's syndrome than that in SLE.

Unfortunately, there are no studies of this vaccination among those with Sjögren's syndrome. On the other hand, those with SLE have been studied. According to some studies, treatment with immunosuppressive medications does not impair the immune response to 23-valent[28] or 13-valent[29] recombinant pneumococcal vaccine among patients with SLE. Others have shown poor response with <40% of patients with SLE on immunosuppressants demonstrating a fourfold rise in antibody response with the 23-valent vaccination.[30] Despite efficacy, in a study of 579 patients with SLE in Germany, a substantial fraction (37.5%) of the patients declined pneumococcal vaccination, while another 16.1% had been advised not to take it by their physician. Thus only about one-third of patients had been properly vaccinated against pneumococcal disease.[13] In contrast, another study found the most common reason patients with SLE failed to receive pneumococcal vaccination was that physicians failed to recommend it.[31] In a systematic review, Puges and colleagues[20] concluded that pneumococcal vaccination has no effect on lupus disease activity. A small ($n = 42$) but randomized, placebo-controlled trial of sequential pneumococcal vaccinations showed no exacerbation of the disease in the immunized compared with the placebo arm.[32]

Thus although data are unavailable about Sjögren's syndrome, the data extrapolated from SLE suggest that pneumococcal vaccination is safe and effective among patients with Sjögren's syndrome. A serious barrier to vaccine receipt is failure of physicians to recommend this vaccination. This is true in the general population as well as in those with SLE. Physicians should recommend pneumococcal vaccination to those with Sjögren's syndrome as part of their routine clinical care.

Zoster vaccination

Reactivation of herpes zoster as shingles grows more common with age, and this risk is exaggerated among patients with inflammatory rheumatic disease.[33,34] A nationwide, population-based study from Taiwan matched 4287 primary Sjögren's syndrome patients with more than 25,000 matched controls. The cumulative incidence among patients was 18.7 per 1000 subject-years, whereas the incidence among the controls was 8.55 per 1000 subjects-years. Compared with healthy controls, the risk of shingles was highest among Sjögren's syndrome patients taking both glucocorticoids and immunosuppressants (hazard ratio [HR] = 4.4), followed by immunosuppressants alone (HR = 3.24) and glucocorticoid alone (HR = 2.54). However, even those patients on no medication had a statistically increased risk of shingles (HR = 2.06). Hospitalizations related to both shingles and postherpetic neuralgia were increased in Sjögren's syndrome patients.[35] There are no studies on the response or efficacy of zoster vaccination in Sjögren's syndrome cohorts. A new zoster vaccine (Shingrix®, a recombinant vaccine) has become available, and the US Centers for Disease Control and Prevention recommends its use over the previously available live vaccine (Zostavax®) because of its increased efficacy as well as the absence of the theoretic risk of reactivation from the live attenuated Zostavax® vaccine. Although the live vaccine has been studied in SLE,[36] to the authors' knowledge, the new recombinant zoster vaccine has not been studied in autoimmune rheumatic illness. Nonetheless, based on the safety and efficacy data in healthy adults, we recommend that Sjögren's syndrome patients above the age 50 years should receive two doses of the recombinant vaccine at least 2 months but not more than 6 months apart (Table 14.1).

Papillomavirus vaccination

Vaccination against human papillomavirus, the causative agent of cervical cancer, is now recommended as a part of routine childhood vaccination. Without vaccination the greater majority of humans are infected by early adulthood. Most adults have not received this vaccine based on the timing of its introduction. Thus there are recommendations for adults who did not receive the vaccine in childhood from the Centers of Disease Control and Prevention as well as other organizations. Women who were not immunized as a child should receive the human papillomavirus vaccine if they are under the age 26 years, while men not immunized as a child should receive this vaccine if they are under the age 21 years. Certainly, diagnosis of Sjögren's syndrome under these ages is uncommon; thus the decision to vaccinate a Sjögren's syndrome patient will rarely be faced.

There has been only one study of human papillomavirus infection rates among Sjögren's syndrome patients. Cirpan et al. studied 33 women with Sjögren's syndrome and 67 without it who were referred for cervical cytology screening. There were no difference between the two groups in cervical cytology, colposcopic examination, or cervical human papillomavirus DNA testing.[37] To our knowledge, there is no study of the human papillomavirus vaccination in Sjögren's syndrome. This is not the case in SLE, in which both the vaccination and the infection have been well studied. In a study of 34 women with SLE, 100% had seroconversion and there were no SLE flares associated with human papillomavirus vaccination. Vaccine was received at 0, 2, and 6 months, with follow-up for 6 months after the last inoculation.[38] Other studies have had similar results.[39] In contrast to the data from the single study on Sjögren's syndrome patients, those with SLE have a higher incidence of human papillomavirus infection than matched controls,[40,41] although not all studies have found an increase.[41,42] This could be a result of increased infection rates following exposure or a reduced ability to clear the viral infection compared with healthy women. One study found a sevenfold increase in human papillomavirus infection in SLE even when risk factors were accounted for.[34] However, no increase in cervical cancer is found among patients with SLE.[41] These disparate results among those with SLE indicate that further studies are needed in those with Sjögren's syndrome.

Hepatitis B vaccination

There are no data concerning the efficacy or safety of hepatitis B vaccination in Sjögren's syndrome. There is, however, a single case report of the onset of Sjögren's syndrome occurring about 1 month after a second hepatitis B vaccination.[43] The patient had proximal interphalangeal joint arthritis, sicca symptoms, rheumatoid factor, positive result in minor salivary gland biopsy, and anti-Ro (or SSA). The last finding is of interest in that anti-Ro appears many years, if not decades, before the clinical onset of Sjögren's syndrome[44,45] or SLE.[46] Thus given these data and the lack of other case reports, we conclude that the hepatitis B vaccine in not a likely cause or trigger of Sjögren's syndrome. Sjögren's syndrome patients with

Table 14.2 Optional vaccinations for adults[a].

Vaccination	Who should receive it?	When should it be given?
Anthrax	Occupationally exposed[b]	Before exposure
Cholera	Travelers to at risk areas	Before travel
Japanese encephalitis	Long-term travelers to Asia; short-term travelers with high exposure risk	Before travel
Meningococcal	16- to 23-year—old persons	Prior at-risk social situation
Rabies	Those exposed Occupationally exposed[b]	After exposure Before exposure
Typhoid[c,e]	Travelers traveling to at-risk areas	Before travel
Yellow fever[d,e]	Travelers traveling to endemic areas	Before travel; required for entry into some countries

[a] *Recommendations are taken from the Advisory Committee on Immunization Practices.[12]*
[b] *Includes veterinarians and some agricultural workers. Other vaccinations may be recommended for microbiologists or other laboratory personnel at risk for exposure through work.*
[c] *The oral typhoid vaccine contains live attenuated virus.*
[d] *A live attenuated virus vaccination.*
[e] *Live attenuated virus vaccinations should be used with caution in immunocompromised persons.*

appropriate risks should receive hepatitis B vaccine if they were not vaccinated during routine childhood vaccination practices.

Other vaccines

Effective vaccines are available for numerous pathogens, including hepatitis A virus, *Neisseria meningitidis*, and *H. influenzae* type b. With appropriate risk factors for the diseases associated with these organisms, adult Sjögren's syndrome patients should receive vaccines for those diseases. Some of these other vaccines are live attenuated viruses that should be used with caution in immunocompromised patients and only after careful consideration of the risk-benefit ratio (Table 14.2).

Travel

There are a great many considerations with regard to vaccination for travel. These include endemic infections at any given destination, exposure to agricultural areas, exposure to specific environments such as caves, the length of stay, and the presence of chronic illness in the traveler. Diseases to consider are many and include but are not limited to yellow fever, rabies, cholera, Ebola, Japanese encephalitis, meningococcal disease, typhoid, and polio. Another consideration is travel to mass gatherings.[47,48] For instance, pneumococcal pneumonia may be a particular risk at an event such as the Hajj.[47,49,50] Meningococcal infection[51] and influenza[52,53] are also potentially at high prevalence at mass gatherings. We imagine that those with chronic medical conditions are at even higher risks when attending mass gatherings and, therefore, should receive vaccines before traveling to such events. Travel to some countries may require the yellow fever vaccination, which is a live attenuated virus. Persons taking immunosuppressive agents and traveling to countries for which yellow fever vaccination is recommended should consult a physician or clinic specializing in travel medicine.

Effect of immunosuppressive medications on vaccine effectiveness

There are data in both SLE and Sjögren's syndrome concerning the effect of medications, including immunosuppressive agents, on vaccination efficacy. However, these data are limited and include only a few specific vaccinations. The study of an H1N1 influenza vaccination among Sjögren's syndrome patients was discussed earlier. In this study, treatment-naive Sjögren's syndrome patients had a more robust response as evidenced by increased antibody titers.[16] Minimal additional data are available specific to Sjögren's syndrome. However, among patients with SLE receiving either the 23-valent or 13-valent pneumococcal vaccination, there was no effect of immunosuppressant medications on the response in most[28,29,54] but not all studies.[30] Thus we find it difficult to make definitive recommendations concerning vaccination efficacy while on immunosuppressive therapy. If such therapy is short term (for instance, glucocorticoids for skin vasculitis), then vaccination could be delayed until the course is completed. On the other hand, if immunosuppressive agents are given more long term, then the risk of infection is greater and patients should be vaccinated. Certainly, clinical decisions will need to be individualized.

The effect of rituximab, which can be used in Sjögren's syndrome for the treatment of severe manifestations,[4] on vaccination efficacy has been studied in other autoimmune diseases. In a study of RA treated with rituximab, RA treated with methotrexate, and matched healthy controls, there was no difference in the response to influenza vaccination between the controls and methotrexate-treated RA. However, the response to the vaccine was severely attenuated for 6–10 months after the last dose of rituximab.[55] Another RA study of patients on methotrexate randomized to rituximab or continued methotrexate alone showed an equal response to tetanus toxoid but there was a decreased response to both pneumococcal and keyhole limpet hemocyanin vaccinations among those in the rituximab group.[56] Thus these studies may indicate that a recall response, such as tetanus, is not impaired by rituximab, while vaccination with a new antigen is impaired. We and van Assen et al.[55] conclude that vaccines such as influenza should be given before rituximab therapy, if possible.

Vaccination as a potential trigger of disease

A number of infectious agents have been proposed as triggers of Sjögren's syndrome.[57] Of interest, chronic hepatitis C induces salivary gland pathology that is highly similar to that found in Sjögren's syndrome, and some with hepatitis C also have sicca symptoms.[58] Whether hepatitis C is a trigger for Sjögren's syndrome in a subset of patients remains controversial. Active chronic hepatitis C is an exclusion criteria in the newest research classification criteria,[59,60] as well as in the older, but still used, American-European Consensus Group criteria.[61] Of all the viruses touted to be involved in the pathogenesis of Sjögren's syndrome, Epstein-Barr virus (human herpesvirus 4) is best supported by the available evidence.[62–68] Newly published data indicate that Epstein-Barr nuclear antigen 2 colocalizes with transcription factor at SLE and Sjögren's syndrome genetic risk loci, which are predominately located in gene regulatory regions.[69] These data provide a molecular mechanism for gene-infection interaction that might lead to autoimmune disease. Notwithstanding the epidemiologic and mechanistic association of hepatitis C and Epstein-Barr virus with Sjögren's syndrome, there are no vaccinations to prevent these infections, and the infection itself can often be asymptomatic.

There remains a theoretic concern that by instigating an immune response, vaccination may be associated with a more generalized immune activation potentially leading to a flare of underlying autoimmune disease. In general, although there are case reports or case series of autoimmune disease after vaccination, there is no causal relationship established between any autoimmune disease and any vaccination.[70–72] There are studies that find a statistical association in meta-analysis[73] but other studies that find no risk associated with vaccination.[74] There are no epidemiologic data concerning risk of Sjögren's syndrome and vaccination, however.

A vaccine that has garnered attention as an environmental trigger for autoimmune disease is the human papillomavirus vaccine, although most of the data and theoretic considerations are about SLE, not Sjögren's syndrome. A report of six women with onset of SLE, along with another report of various inflammatory rheumatic diseases after human papillomavirus vaccination, brought into question whether this vaccine could trigger autoimmunity.[75,76] Shared protein sequence between human papillomavirus and lupus autoantigens has been proposed as a worrisome feature of human papillomavirus vaccine.[77,78] However, a study of hospitalizations and emergency visits for SLE in the United States found no increase in the years following the introduction of this vaccine in 2006.[79] A population-based study of more than 70,000 young women with at least 1 of 49 autoimmune diseases found no association of onset of a new autoimmune disease with human papillomavirus vaccination. This study included Sjögren's syndrome as one of the autoimmune diseases under study.[80] In another study, 50 Chinese patients with SLE receiving the vaccine and 50 patients not receiving the vaccine had a follow-up for 1 year after vaccination. It was found that there was no increase in anti–double-stranded DNA titer, no increase in disease activity, decrease in serum complement levels, orincrease in disease flares.[39] Thus although the epidemiologic group receiving the human papillomavirus vaccine—teenaged girls and young adult women—is at risk of SLE (but not Sjögren's syndrome), the population-based studies and the SLE cohort study are reassuring that this vaccine neither triggers nor exacerbates autoimmune disease.

Vaccines as treatment

There are a number of strategies by which vaccines might be used to treat inflammatory, autoimmune rheumatic illness. For example, a phase II trial showed that tumor necrosis factor (TNF) therapeutic vaccination produced anti-TNF antibodies and provided clinical benefit in patients with TNF antagonist—resistant RA.[81] Of course, anti-TNF therapy has not been effective in Sjögren's syndrome, and so similar trials in Sjögren's syndrome are not warranted. Other immunization strategies for treatment of autoimmune disease include cell-based therapies in which patients would receive autologous immune cells such as immature dendritic cells.[82] No therapeutic vaccines have been studied in human Sjögren's syndrome, but immunization of non-obese diabetic mice with complete Freund adjuvant resulted in restoration of salivary flow.[83]

Conclusions

Diseases preventable by efficacious vaccines remain common in the population. As there are no contraindications and high benefit from prevention of infections, Sjögren's syndrome patients should be vaccinated against such diseases as recommended for the general population. This is particularly important for patients on immunosuppressive agents. There is no evidence that vaccines will cause an exacerbation of the underlying autoimmune rheumatic disease. In certain situations, it may be advantageous to temporarily hold immunosuppressive therapy in order to optimize the vaccine effect.

References

1. Fox RI. Sjögren's syndrome. *Lancet*. 2005;366(9482):321–331.
2. Ter Borg EJ, Kelder JC. Is extra-glandular organ damage in primary Sjögren's syndrome related to the presence of systemic auto-antibodies and/or hypergammaglobulinemia? A long-term cohort study with 110 patients from The Netherlands. *Int J Rheumat Dis*. 2017; 20(7):875–881.
3. Fayyaz A, Kurien BT, Scofield RH. Autoantibodies in Sjögren's syndrome. *Rheum Dis Clin N Am*. 2016;42(3):419–434.

4. Carsons SE, Vivino FB, Parke A, Carteron N, Sankar V, Brasington R, Brennan MT, Ehlers W, Fox R, Scofield H, Hammitt KM, Birnbaum J, Kassan S, Mandel S. Treatment guidelines for rheumatologic manifestations of Sjögren's syndrome: use of biologic agents, management of fatigue, and inflammatory musculoskeletal pain. *Arthritis Care Res.* 2017;69(4):517–527.

5. Gottenberg JE, Ravaud P, Puéchal X, LeGuern V, Sibilia J, Goeb V, Larroche C, Dubost J, Rist S, Saraux A, Devauchelle-Pensec V, Morel J, Hayem G, Hatron P, Perdriger A, Sene D, Zarnitsky C, Batouche D, Furlan V, Benessiano J, Perrodeau E, Seror R, Mariette X. Effects of hydroxychloroquine on symptomatic improvement in primary Sjögren syndrome: the JOQUER randomized clinical trial. *J Am Med Assoc.* 2014; 312(3):249–258.

6. Kruize AA, Hene RJ, Kallenberg CG, van Bijsterveld OP, van der Heide A, Kater L, Bijlsma JW. Hydroxychloroquine treatment for primary Sjögren's syndrome: a two year double blind crossover trial. *Ann Rheum Dis.* 1993;52(5):360–364.

7. Yoon CH, Lee HJ, Lee EY, Lee EB, Lee WW, Kim MK, Wee WR. Effect of hydroxy-chloroquine treatment on dry eyes in subjects with primary Sjögren's syndrome: a double-blind randomized control study. *J Korean Med Sci.* 2016;31(7):1127–1135.

8. Rusnock AA. Historical context and the roots of Jenner's discovery. *Hum Vaccines Immunother.* 2016;12(8):2025–2028.

9. Mallory JPAD. *The oxford introduction to proto-Indo-European and the proto-Indo-European world (Oxford Linguistics).* New York: Oxford University Press; 2006.

10. Blake JB. Benjamin Waterhouse and the introduction of vaccination, 1957Blake JB, ed. *Rev Infect Dis.* 1987;9(5):1044–1052.

11. Scofield S. *A practical Treatise on Vaccina or Cowpock: Embellished with a Coloured Engraving, representing a View of the local affection in its different stages.* New York: Southwick and Pelsue; 1810.

12. Centers for Disease Control and Prevention. *Recommended adult immunization schedule for ages 19 years or older.* United States; 2019. https://www.cdc.gov/vaccines/schedules/hcp/imz/adult.html.

13. Chehab G, Richter JG, Brinks R, Fischer-Betz R, Winkler-Rohlfing B, Schneider M. Vaccination coverage in systemic lupus erythematosus-a cross-sectional analysis of the German long-term study (LuLa cohort). *Rheumatology.* 2018;57(8):1439–1447.

14. Krasselt M, Ivanov JP, Baerwald C, Seifert O. Low vaccination rates among patients with rheumatoid arthritis in a German outpatient clinic. *Rheumatol Int.* 2017;37(2):229–237.

15. Feuchtenberger M, Kleinert S, Schwab S, Roll P, Scharbatke EC, Ostermeier E, Voll RE, Schafer A, Hans-Peter T. Vaccination survey in patients with rheumatoid arthritis: a cross-sectional study. *Rheumatol Int.* 2012;32(6):1533–1539.

16. Brauner S, Folkersen L, Kvarnstrom M, Meisgen S, Petersen S, Franzen-Malmros M, Mofors J, Brokstad K, Klareskog L, Jonsson R, Westerberg L, Trollmo C, Malmstrom V, Ambrosi A, Kuchroo V, Nordmark G, Wahren-Herlenius M. H1N1 vacci-nation in Sjögren's syndrome triggers polyclonal B cell activation and promotes autoan-tibody production. *Ann Rheum Dis.* 2017;76(10):1755–1763.

17. Gluck T. Vaccinate your immunocompromised patients!. *Rheumatology.* 2006;45(1): 9–10.

18. Paules C, Subbarao K. *Influenza Lancet.* 2017;390(10095):697–708.

19. Milanovic M, Stojanovich L, Djokovic A, Kontic M, Gvozdenovic E. Influenza vaccina-tion in autoimmune rheumatic disease patients. *Tohoku J Exp Med.* 2013;229(1):29–34.

20. Puges M, Biscay P, Barnetche T, Truchetet ME, Richez C, Seneschal J, Gensous N, Lazaro E, Duffau P. Immunogenicity and impact on disease activity of influenza and pneumococcal vaccines in systemic lupus erythematosus: a systematic literature review and meta-analysis. *Rheumatol*. 2016;55(9):1664−1672.

21. Huang Y, Wang H, Wan L, Lu X, Tam WW. Is systemic lupus erythematosus associated with a declined immunogenicity and poor safety of influenza vaccination?: a systematic review and meta-analysis. *Medicine*. 2016;95(19):e3637.

22. Backhaus E, Berg S, Andersson R, Ockborn G, Malmstrom P, Dahl M, Nasic S, Trollfors B. Epidemiology of invasive pneumococcal infections: manifestations, incidence and case fatality rate correlated to age, gender and risk factors. *BMC Infect Dis*. 2016;16:367.

23. Marrie TJ, Tyrrell GJ, Majumdar SR, Eurich DT. Effect of age on the manifestations and outcomes of invasive pneumococcal disease in adults. *Am J Med*. 2018;131(1), 100.e1-.e7.

24. Zhang D, Petigara T, Yang X. Clinical and economic burden of pneumococcal disease in US adults aged 19−64 years with chronic or immunocompromising diseases: an observational database study. *BMC Infect Dis*. 2018;18(1):436.

25. Tsai YH, Hsieh MJ, Chang CJ, Wen YW, Hu HC, Chao YN, Huang YC, Yang CT, Huang CC. The 23-valent pneumococcal polysaccharide vaccine is effective in elderly adults over 75 years old–Taiwan's PPV vaccination program. *Vaccine*. 2015;33(25): 2897−2902.

26. Mieczkowski TA, Wilson SA. Adult pneumococcal vaccination: a review of physician and patient barriers. *Vaccine*. 2002;20(9−10):1383−1392.

27. Luijten RK, Cuppen BV, Bijlsma JW, Derksen RH. Serious infections in systemic lupus erythematosus with a focus on pneumococcal infections. *Lupus*. 2014;23(14): 1512−1516.

28. Nagel J, Saxne T, Geborek P, Bengtsson AA, Jacobsen S, Svaerke Joergensen C, Nilsson J, Skattum L, Jonsen A, Kapetanovic MC. Treatment with belimumab in systemic lupus erythematosus does not impair antibody response to 13-valent pneumococcal conjugate vaccine. *Lupus*. 2017;26(10):1072−1081.

29. Chatham W, Chadha A, Fettiplace J, Kleoudis C, Bass D, Roth D, Gordon D. A randomized, open-label study to investigate the effect of belimumab on pneumococcal vaccination in patients with active, autoantibody-positive systemic lupus erythematosus. *Lupus*. 2017;26(14):1483−1490.

30. Rezende RP, Ribeiro FM, Albuquerque EM, Gayer CR, Andrade LE, Klumb EM. Immunogenicity of pneumococcal polysaccharide vaccine in adult systemic lupus erythematosus patients undergoing immunosuppressive treatment. *Lupus*. 2016;25(11):1254−1259.

31. Lawson EF, Trupin L, Yelin EH, Yazdany J. Reasons for failure to receive pneumococcal and influenza vaccinations among immunosuppressed patients with systemic lupus erythematosus. *Semin Arthritis Rheum*. 2015;44(6):666−671.

32. Grabar S, Groh M, Bahuaud M, Le Guern V, Costedoat-Chalumeau N, Mathian A, Hanslik T, Guillevin L, Batteux F, Launay O, VACCILUP study group. Pneumococcal vaccination in patients with systemic lupus erythematosus: a multicenter placebo-controlled randomized double-blind study. *Vaccine*. 2017;35(37):4877−4885.

33. Chakravarty EF. Incidence and prevention of herpes zoster reactivation in patients with autoimmune diseases. *Rheum Dis Clin N Am*. 2017;43(1):111−121.

34. Chakravarty EF, Michaud K, Katz R, Wolfe F. Increased incidence of herpes zoster among patients with systemic lupus erythematosus. *Lupus*. 2013;22(3):238−244.

35. Chen JY, Wang LK, Feng PH, Chu CC, Cheng TJ, Weng SF, Wu SZ, Lu TH, Chang CY. Risk of shingles in adults with primary Sjögren's syndrome and treatments: a nationwide population-based cohort study. *PLoS One*. 2015;10(8):e0134930.

36. Guthridge JM, Cogman A, Merrill JT, Macwana S, Bean KM, Powe T, Roberts V, James JA, Chakravarty EF. Herpes zoster vaccination in SLE: a pilot study of immunogenicity. *J Rheumatol*. 2013;40(11):1875—1880.

37. Cirpan T, Guliyeva A, Onder G, Terek MC, Ozsaran A, Kabasakal Y, Zekioglu O, Yucebilgin S. Comparison of human papillomavirus testing and cervical cytology with colposcopic examination and biopsy in cervical cancer screening in a cohort of patients with Sjögren's syndrome. *Eur J Gynaecol Oncol*. 2007;28(4):302—306.

38. Dhar JP, Essenmacher L, Dhar R, Magee A, Ager J, Sokol RJ. The safety and immunogenicity of Quadrivalent HPV (qHPV) vaccine in systemic lupus erythematosus. *Vaccine*. 2017;35(20):2642—2646.

39. Mok CC, Ho LY, Fong LS, To CH. Immunogenicity and safety of a quadrivalent human papillomavirus vaccine in patients with systemic lupus erythematosus: a case-control study. *Ann Rheum Dis*. 2013;72(5):659—664.

40. Lyrio LD, Grassi MF, Santana IU, Olavarria VG, Gomes Ado N, CostaPinto L, Oliveira RC, Aquino RD, Santiago MB. Prevalence of cervical human papillomavirus infection in women with systemic lupus erythematosus. *Rheumatol Int*. 2013;33(2):335—340.

41. Santana IU, Gomes Ado N, Lyrio LD, Rios Grassi MF, Santiago MB. Systemic lupus erythematosus, human papillomavirus infection, cervical pre-malignant and malignant lesions: a systematic review. *Clin Rheumatol*. 2011;30(5):665—672.

42. Rojo-Contreras W, Olivas-Flores EM, Gamez-Nava JI, Montoya-Fuentes H, Trujillo-Hernandez B, Trujillo X, Suarez-Rincon AE, Baltazar-Rodriguez LM, Sanchez-Hernandez J, Ramirez-Flores M, Vazquez-Salcedo J, Rojo-Contreras J, Morales-Romero J, Gonzalez-Lopez L. Cervical human papillomavirus infection in Mexican women with systemic lupus erythematosus or rheumatoid arthritis. *Lupus*. 2012;21(4):365—372.

43. Toussirot E, Lohse A, Wendling D, Mougin C. Sjögren's syndrome occurring after hepatitis B vaccination. *Arthritis Rheum*. 2000;43(9):2139—2140.

44. Jonsson R, Theander E, Sjostrom B, Brokstad K, Henriksson G. Autoantibodies present before symptom onset in primary Sjögren syndrome. *J Am Med Assoc*. 2013;310(17):1854—1855.

45. Theander E, Jonsson R, Sjostrom B, Brokstad K, Olsson P, Henriksson G. Prediction of Sjögren's syndrome years before diagnosis and identification of patients with early onset and severe disease course by autoantibody profiling. *Arthritis Rheum*. 2015;67(9):2427—2436.

46. Arbuckle MR, McClain MT, Rubertone MV, Scofield RH, Dennis GJ, James JA, Harley JB. Development of autoantibodies before the clinical onset of systemic lupus erythematosus. *N Engl J Med*. 2003;349(16):1526—1533.

47. Al-Tawfiq JA, Memish ZA. Prevention of pneumococcal infections during mass gathering. *Hum Vaccines Immunother*. 2016;12(2):326—330.

48. Alqahtani AS, Alfelali M, Arbon P, Booy R, Rashid H. Burden of vaccine preventable diseases at large events. *Vaccine*. 2015;33(48):6552—6563.

49. Alqahtani AS, Tashani M, Ridda I, Gamil A, Booy R, Rashid H. Burden of clinical infections due to S. pneumoniae during Hajj: a systematic review. *Vaccine*. 2018;36(30):4440—4446.

50. Ridda I, King C, Rashid H. Pneumococcal infections at Hajj: current knowledge gaps. *Infect Disord − Drug Targets*. 2014;14(3):177−184.

51. Yezli S. The threat of meningococcal disease during the Hajj and Umrah mass gatherings: a comprehensive review. *Trav Med Infect Dis*. 2018;24:51−58.

52. Haworth E, Barasheed O, Memish ZA, Rashid H, Booy R. Prevention of influenza at Hajj: applications for mass gatherings. *J R Soc Med*. 2013;106(6):215−223.

53. Al-Tawfiq JA, Zumla A, Memish ZA. Respiratory tract infections during the annual Hajj: potential risks and mitigation strategies. *Curr Opin Pulm Med*. 2013;19(3):192−197.

54. Chatham WW, Wallace DJ, Stohl W, Latinis KM, Manzi S, McCune WJ, Tegzova D, McKay JD, Avila-Armengol HE, Utset TO, Zhong ZJ, Hough DR, Freimuth WW, Migone TS. Effect of belimumab on vaccine antigen antibodies to influenza, pneumococcal, and tetanus vaccines in patients with systemic lupus erythematosus in the BLISS-76 trial. *J Rheumatol*. 2012;39(8):1632−1640.

55. van Assen S, Holvast A, Benne CA, Posthumus MD, van Leeuwen MA, Voskuyl AE, Blom M, Risselada AP, deHaan A, Westra J, Kallenberg CG, Bijl M. Humoral responses after influenza vaccination are severely reduced in patients with rheumatoid arthritis treated with rituximab. *Arthritis Rheum*. 2010;62(1):75−81.

56. Bingham 3rd CO, Looney RJ, Deodhar A, Halsey N, Greenwald M, Codding C, et al. Immunization responses in rheumatoid arthritis patients treated with rituximab: results from a controlled clinical trial. *Arthritis Rheum*. 2010;62(1):64−74.

57. Igoe A, Scofield RH. Autoimmunity and infection in Sjögren's syndrome. *Curr Opin Rheumatol*. 2013;25(4):480−487.

58. Carrozzo M, Scally K. Oral manifestations of hepatitis C virus infection. *World J Gastroenterol*. 2014;20(24):7534−7543.

59. Shiboski S, Shiboski C, Criswell L, Baer A, Challacombe S, Lanfranchi h, Schiodt M, Umehara H, Vivino F, Zhao Y, Dong Y, Greenspan D, Heidenreich A, Helin P, Kirkham B, Kitagawa K, Larkin G, Li M, Lietman T, Lindegaard J, McNamara N, Sack K, Shirlaw P, Sugai S, Vollenweider C, Whitch WA, Zhang S, Zhang W, Greenspan J, Daniels T. American college of rheumatology classification criteria for Sjögren's syndrome, a data driven, expert consensus approach in the Sjögren's international collaborative clinical alliance cohort. *Arthritis Care Res*. 2012;64(4):475−487.

60. Shiboski CH, Shiboski SC, Seror R, Criswell LA, Labetoulle M, Lietman TM, Rasmussen A, Scofield H, Vitali C, Bowman S, Mariette X, The International Sjögren's Syndrome Criteria Working Group. 2016 American College of Rheumatology/European League against Rheumatism classification criteria for primary Sjögren's syndrome A consensus and data-driven methodology involving three international patient cohorts. *Ann Rheum Dis*. January 2017;76(1):9−16.

61. Vitali C, Bombardieri S, Jonsson R, Moutsopoulos HM, Alexander EL, Carsons SE, Daniels TE, Fox PC, Fox RI, Kassan SS, Pillemer SR, Talal N, Weisman MH. The European study group on classification criteria for Sjögren's syndrome. classification criteria for Sjögren's syndrome: a revised version of the european criteria proposed by the American-European consensus group. *Ann Rheum Dis*. 2002;61(6):554−558.

62. Horiuchi M, Yamano S, Inoue H, Ishii J, Nagata Y, Adachi H, Ono M, Renard JN, Mizuno F, Hayashi Y, Saito I. Possible involvement of IL-12 expression by Epstein-Barr virus in Sjögren syndrome. *J Clin Pathol*. 1999;52(11):833−837.

63. Mariette X, Gozlan J, Clerc D, Bisson M, Morinet F. Detection of Epstein-Barr virus DNA by in situ hybridization and polymerase chain reaction in salivary gland biopsy specimens from patients with Sjögren's syndrome. *Am J Med*. 1991;90(3):286−294.

64. Fox RI, Luppi M, Pisa P, Kang HI. Potential role of Epstein-Barr virus in Sjögren's syndrome and rheumatoid arthritis. *J Rheumatol Suppl.* 1992;32:18−24.

65. Fox RI, Luppi M, Kang HI, Pisa P. Reactivation of Epstein-Barr virus in Sjögren's syndrome. *Springer Semin Immunopathol.* 1991;13(2):217−231.

66. Nagata Y, Inoue H, Yamada K, Higashiyama H, Mishima K, Kizu Y, Takeda I, Mizuno F, Hayashi Y, Saito I. Activation of Epstein-Barr virus by saliva from Sjögren's syndrome patients. *Immunology.* 2004;111(2):223−229.

67. Nagata Y, Inoue H, Yamada K, Higashiyama H, Mishima K, Kizu Y, Takeda I, Mizuno F, Hayashi Y, Saito I. Aryl hydrocarbon receptor-mediated induction of EBV reactivation as a risk factor for Sjögren's syndrome. *J Immunol.* 2012;188(9):4654−4662.

68. Harley JB, Zoller EE. Editorial: what caused all these troubles, anyway? Epstein-Barr virus in Sjögren's syndrome reevaluated. *Arthritis Rheumatol.* 2014;66(9):2328−2330.

69. Harley JB, Chen X, Pujato M, Miller D, Maddox A, Forney C, Magnusen AF, Lynch A, Chetal K, Yukawa M, Barski A, Salomonis N, Kaufman K, Kottyan L, Weirauch MT. Transcription factors operate across disease loci, with EBNA2 implicated in autoimmunity. 2018;50(5):699−707.

70. Conti F, Rezai S, Valesini G. Vaccination and autoimmune rheumatic diseases. *Autoimmun Rev.* 2008;8(2):124−128.

71. Barbhaiya M, Costenbader KH. Environmental exposures and the development of systemic lupus erythematosus. *Curr Opin Rheumatol.* 2016;28(5):497−505.

72. Soriano A, Afeltra A, Shoenfeld Y. Immunization with vaccines and Sjögren's syndrome. *Expert Rev Clin Immunol.* 2014;10(4):429−435.

73. Wang B, Shao X, Wang D, Xu D, Zhang JA. Vaccinations and risk of systemic lupus erythematosus and rheumatoid arthritis: a systematic review and meta-analysis. *Autoimmun Rev.* 2017;16(7):756−765.

74. Grimaldi-Bensouda L, Le Guern V, Kone-Paut I, Aubrun E, Fain O, Ruel M, Machet L, Viallard JF, Magy-Bertrand N, Daugas E, Rossignol M, Abenhaim L, Costedoat-Chalumeau N, for the PGRx Lupus Study Group. The risk of systemic lupus erythematosus associated with vaccines: an international case-control study. *Arthritis Rheumatol.* 2014;66(6):1559−1567.

75. Gatto M, Agmon-Levin N, Soriano A, Manna R, Maoz-Segal R, Kivity S, Doria A, Shoenfeld Y. Human papillomavirus vaccine and systemic lupus erythematosus. *Clin Rheumatol.* 2013;32(9):1301−1307.

76. Anaya JM, Reyes B, Perdomo-Arciniegas AM, Camacho-Rodriguez B, Rojas-Villarraga A. Autoimmune/auto-inflammatory syndrome induced by adjuvants (ASIA) after quadrivalent human papillomavirus vaccination in Colombians: a call for personalised medicine. *Clin Exp Rheumatol.* 2015;33(4):545−548.

77. Segal Y, Dahan S, Calabro M, Kanduc D, Shoenfeld Y. HPV and systemic lupus erythematosus: a mosaic of potential crossreactions. *Immunol Res.* 2017;65(2):564−571.

78. Segal Y, Calabro M, Kanduc D, Shoenfeld Y. Human papilloma virus and lupus: the virus, the vaccine and the disease. *Curr Opin Rheumatol.* 2017;29(4):331−342.

79. Pellegrino P, Carnovale C, Perrone V, Salvati D, Gentili M, Antoniazzi S, Clementi E, Radice S. Human papillomavirus vaccine in patients with systemic lupus erythematosus. *Epidemiology.* 2014;25(1):155−156.

80. Gronlund O, Herweijer E, Sundstrom K, Arnheim-Dahlstrom L. Incidence of new-onset autoimmune disease in girls and women with pre-existing autoimmune disease after quadrivalent human papillomavirus vaccination: a cohort study. *J Intern Med.* 2016;280(6):618−626.

81. Durez P, Vandepapeliere P, Miranda P, Toncheva A, Berman A, Kehler T, Mociran E, Fautrel B, Mariette X, Dhellin O, Fanget B, Ouary S, Grouard-Vogel G, Boissier MC. Therapeutic vaccination with TNF-Kinoid in TNF antagonist-resistant rheumatoid arthritis: a phase II randomized, controlled clinical trial. *PLoS One*. 2014;9(12):e113465.

82. Sabado RL, Balan S, Bhardwaj N. Dendritic cell-based immunotherapy. *Cell Res*. 2017; 27(1):74—95.

83. Tran SD, Kodama S, Lodde BM, Szalayova I, Key S, Khalili S, Faustman D, Mezey E. Reversal of Sjögren's-like syndrome in non-obese diabetic mice. *Ann Rheum Dis*. 2007; 66(6):812—814.

The cost of Sjögren's syndrome and the value of patient resources and support in management

Katherine M. Hammitt, MA[1], Steven Taylor, MBA[2]

[1]*Vice President of Medical and Scientific Affairs, Sjögren's Foundation, Reston, VA, United States;*
[2]*CEO, Sjögren's Foundation, Reston, VA, United States*

Introduction

Being diagnosed with a medically complex and chronic, systemic illness such as Sjögren's syndrome can be highly stressful. Sometimes the best "medicine" can be talking with others who have the same disease to better understand firsthand the day-to-day physical struggles and the psychosocial ramifications that a Sjögren's syndrome diagnosis brings. In addition, learning about one's disease and its symptoms reduces stress and empowers patients to become better healthcare advocates. The Sjögren's Foundation (SF) provides this needed support as well as important resources that help patients cope and manage living with their disease. Hope for a better life in the future also springs from learning about and engaging in the many foundation initiatives to reduce the financial, psychosocial, and physical burdens of the disease and to increase public and healthcare professional awareness and knowledge. These activities are further complemented by ongoing SF initiatives to foster research on disease mechanisms and the development of novel therapies to lessen overall morbidity and improve patient quality of life.

Burden of illness

Sjögren's syndrome greatly diminishes quality of life and carries high financial costs. An SF national patient survey of 9252 members was executed by Harris Poll[1] in 2016. Among the 2962 responses received, 86% of patients responded that the disease presents an everyday challenge and 74% reported that Sjögren's syndrome adds a significant emotional burden. Over 7 in 10 Sjögren's syndrome patients (71%) agreed that Sjögren's syndrome interferes with daily activities, and almost 7 in 10 (67%) are struggling to cope with their disease.

In addition to suffering from a broad range of symptoms that can be severe and debilitating, the lack of predictability interferes with planning for everything from routine activities to special events. Living with Sjögren's syndrome comes with a

Sjögren's Syndrome. https://doi.org/10.1016/B978-0-323-67534-5.00015-6

high price to relationships (Fig. 15.1) and added burdens due to making necessary changes at home and work (Figs. 15.2 and 15.3).[1] The time and cost involved with one's healthcare decreases quality of life, with patients on average seeing 5 healthcare providers annually and using 8.8 treatments or medications to manage their illness [1.]

Two in three respondents in the survey reported that living with Sjögren's syndrome adds a significant financial burden to their lives.[1] Patients spent the most, on average, on dental care followed by prescription medications and healthcare appointments. The first study to determine costs came from the United Kingdom in 2007 and compared direct costs (those costs specific to medical management) in Sjögren's syndrome, rheumatoid arthritis (RA), and healthy controls.[2] Another study looking at indirect costs (including costs related to time lost from work, hired help, and transportation to appointments) was published in 2010.[3] While healthcare costs have accelerated even further as biologic therapies have become available, the healthcare costs cited in the two UK studies were already prohibitive. Costs associated with Sjögren's syndrome were about two-thirds that of RA and both were significantly higher than those in non-RA and non-Sjögren's syndrome controls (Table 15.1).

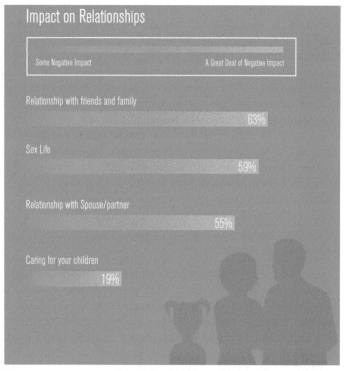

FIGURE 15.1

Effect of Sjögren's syndrome on interpersonal relationships.

Reproduced with permission from.[1]

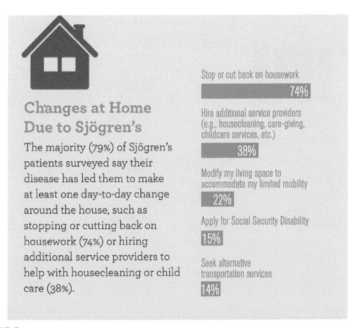

Changes at Home Due to Sjögren's

The majority (79%) of Sjögren's patients surveyed say their disease has led them to make at least one day-to-day change around the house, such as stopping or cutting back on housework (74%) or hiring additional service providers to help with housecleaning or child care (38%).

Stop or cut back on housework
74%

Hire additional service providers (e.g., housecleaning, care-giving, childcare services, etc.)
38%

Modify my living space to accommodate my limited mobility
22%

Apply for Social Security Disability
15%

Seek alternative transportation services
14%

FIGURE 15.2

Effect of Sjögren's syndrome on activities of daily living and employment.

Reproduced with permission from.[1]

Disability

Work disability is significant in Sjögren's syndrome, with the SF survey finding that 2 in 3 Sjögren's syndrome patients had to take days off work and 3 in 10 had to stop working, reduce hours, make a career change, or take a less demanding job due to Sjögren's syndrome. More than one in seven patients applied for the US Social Security disability due to their disease.[1] Mandl et al.[4] also found substantial disability among newly diagnosed patients with Sjögren's syndrome; 26% of patients had already experienced "work disability" (as defined by sick leave of more than 14 days in any 1-month period and/or receipt of a disability pension as gathered from the Swedish Social Insurance Agency) by the time of diagnosis. This percentage increased to 37% 12 months later and to 41% at 24 months after diagnosis.

Stress and Sjögren's syndrome

Stress undoubtedly ensues from the high burden of illness and cost of living with Sjögren's syndrome. Patients must deal with countless burdens including the awareness of being ill and the struggle to find and maintain support, to create and sustain good doctor-patient relationships, to deal with symptoms, and to learn to manage

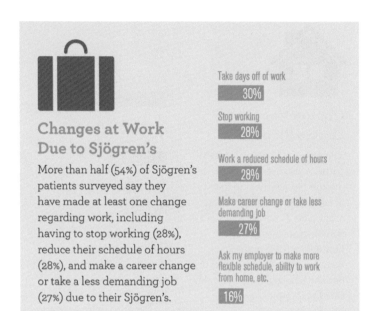

FIGURE 15.3

Effect of Sjögren's syndrome on work activities.

Reproduced with permission from.[1]

Table 15.1 Annual indirect and direct costs of SS, RA, and controls.

	Indirect costs		Direct costs	Total costs[a]
			Not including cost of biologic medications	
	Low range	**High range**		
Control group	£892 or US$1418	£3382 or US$5353	£949 or US$1499	£1841–£4331 or US$2909–$6843
SS patients	£7677 or US$12,150	£13,502 or US$21,369	£2188 or US$3457	£9865–£15,690 or US$15,587 –$24,790
RA patients	£10,444 or US$16,530	£17,070 or US$27,016	£2693 or US$4255	£13,137–£19,763 or US$20,756 –$31,226

RA, *rheumatoid arthritis*; SS, *Sjögren's syndrome*.
[a] *Costs based on studies published in 2006 (direct costs) and 2010 (indirect costs) with US dollars equivalent to British pound sterling for same period.*
Adapted from Refs. 2,3

one's disease on a day-to-day basis. Additionally, the frequent lack of understanding and support from friends, family, and/or colleagues further adds to the emotional burden of living with a chronic illness. The burden of illness also is clearly seen in the high rates of anxiety and depression found in Sjögren's syndrome. Anxiety is especially frequent, with a reported range of 33.8%—50% of Sjögren's syndrome patients (as rated by the Hospital Anxiety and Depression Scale), and depressive disorders occur at a rate ranging from 29.5% to 49%.[5-7]

Stress is also a natural part of everyone's lives and ranges from emotional stress from negative events to physical stresses, such as illness or traumatic accidents. In addition, a variety of positive emotional events may also cause stress, including moving into a new home, enduring home renovations, relocating to a new city, starting a new job or school, having a baby, and even exercise and travel when on vacation.

In Sjögren's syndrome, potential environmental stressors such as viruses, bacteria, and toxins may further exacerbate symptoms or contribute to disease pathogenesis. As discussed later, it is theorized that a genetic predisposition coupled with an environmental stressor and hormonal effects leads to the development of the disease. When the immune system becomes dysfunctional, this may perpetuate the cycle of chronic stress in the body.

The role of physical and emotional stressors in autoimmune reactivity is increasingly being recognized by investigators in psychoneuroimmunology and immunoendocrinology. One of the early investigators of the impact of emotional stress on the human body was Esther Sternberg, MD, who published the book "The Balance Within: The Science Connecting Health and Emotions" in 2001[5] while she was Director of the Integrative Neural Immune Program at the National Institutes of Health. She discussed, for the first time, the science behind stress and how it can influence the way specific hormones function and affect neural pathways and immune system function. Dr. Sternberg found that chronic stress and negative emotional situations can lead to increased inflammation and exacerbation of autoimmune disease. Hormones, produced through the stress response, and neurotransmitters can affect the ramping up or tampering down of the immune system. For example, the antiinflammatory effects of glucocorticoids, produced by the adrenal glands, may be altered in stressful situations. Cortisol, especially, affects the immune system's response by acting upon cytokines. Too much cortisol leads to immune dysfunction and subsequent greater vulnerability to infection, whereas too little cortisol leads to immune dysfunction through increased production of proinflammatory cytokines and downstream events resulting in a cycle of dysregulation. The delicate interplay among the nervous, endocrine/hormonal/adrenal, and immune systems is critical for the proper function of the immune system.[8,9]

Others followed this line of investigation, including O'Donovan et al.[10] who published a study in 2015 demonstrating an increased incidence of autoimmune disease among veterans of the Iraq and Afghanistan conflicts who suffered from posttraumatic stress disorder (PTSD). PTSD was correlated with endocrine and immune abnormalities associated with autoimmune disease development. The authors attributed this phenomenon to reduced immunomodulatory glucocorticoid activity (caused by reduced levels of glucocorticoids leading to decreased signaling through antiinflammatory glucocorticoid receptor transcriptional control pathways), increased inflammation, altered gene expression in immune cells, reduced methylation of immune-regulated genes, and accelerated immune cell aging. More studies focusing on the mechanisms by which stress affects the immune system[11–13] have demonstrated how physical and/or emotional stress can impact the immune system directly or indirectly via the hypothalamic-pituitary-adrenal axis and/or the autonomic nervous system (ANS) and can trigger increased cytokine production and subsequent inflammation.

No studies were done specifically in Sjögren's syndrome until a 2009 publication from the Sjögren's syndrome group in Greece reported that high levels of stress brought on by a major negative event often preceded the diagnosis of Sjögren's syndrome.[14] In a subsequent publication, Skopouli and Katsiougiannis[15] not only examined the impact stress might have on developing and/or perpetuating Sjögren's syndrome but also studied the specific effects of stress on salivary gland epithelial cells and ANS function. The investigators postulated that alteration of normal ANS function in a chronically stressed state may trigger apoptosis of salivary gland epithelial cells and an autoimmune response.

Of importance to note, these studies do not blame the patients for somehow causing or exacerbating their own illness and its progression. However, this scientific work does provide evidence to support the strategy that once diagnosed, patients with chronic illnesses such as Sjögren's syndrome can potentially improve their physical and emotional health by finding ways to reduce stress and enlarge their community of support.

Support and availability of resources linked to better health

Since the 1970s, numerous studies have linked improved physical and emotional health with access to social support networks and appropriate resources for information. Seminal work from the late 1970s and early 1980s empirically demonstrated a relationship between lack of social connectedness and increased mortality. Social scientists stratified the concept of social support into four modalities:[16,17]

- Emotional (having others acknowledge and validate a person's struggles)
- Instrumental (providing direct assistance with everyday needs)
- Appraisal (finding a means to obtain constructive feedback and help with decision-making from others)
- Informational (having access to informational materials and services)

O. Carl Simonton, MD, pioneered what became to be known as the field of psycho-oncology in the 1970s when he established a cancer center that promoted the positive impact of emotional support on survival.[18] His work was not initially accepted by the American Cancer Society, and the first independent evidence to verify the benefits of this approach was not published until 1989. At that time, investigators at the Stanford University and the University of California at Berkeley reported that women with advanced breast cancer who engaged in professional, supportive counseling and/or support groups lived twice as long as those who did not.[19] A study looking at cancer patients demonstrated that those reporting higher levels of social support had lower levels of markers of inflammation, including lower levels of C-reactive protein, interleukin 6, and tumor necrosis factor α, as well as, ultimately, lower mortality rates.[20]

Specific examples demonstrating how the lack of social support can lead to the development or exacerbation of physical health issues also have focused on cardiovascular events. One study reported that monkeys housed alone compared with others housed in small groups developed more atherosclerosis.[21] Another study found that subjects who were told that support was available before engaging in public speaking had lower systolic and diastolic blood pressures than those who were not offered support.[22] Another study showed a direct link between involvement with multiple social venues and a decreased susceptibility to the common cold.[23] Uchino[24] illustrated the physiologic mechanisms that link social support to positive changes in cardiovascular, neuroendocrine, and immune function. Other investigators have also reported that patients with cancer, diabetes, heart disease, and hypertension and those who have had a stroke all fared better when they had social support systems, and the greater the social support, the higher the resulting physical and emotional well-being.[25]

Berkman et al.[26] add that social connectedness increases self-efficacy or the desire to follow specific behaviors (such as exercise, rest, and diet) that can positively impact health and functional outcomes. When people join a social community that promotes healthy actions, they are more likely to adapt those healthy actions. Interestingly, the authors also state that if a person has social connections that are not supportive and positive, health can worsen. In this case, support from outside the family or those who are not supportive becomes even more critical.

The Sjögren's Foundation: creating a community of support

The SF in Reston, VA, is a national patient heath agency and support organization that was founded in 1983 by a patient searching for answers and looking for a way to fight back against her disease. It is the only voluntary, nonprofit, 501(c)(3) organization in the United States to focus exclusively on Sjögren's syndrome and has gradually expanded over the years to include several thousand friends and members worldwide. The SF members and staff actively strive to fulfill its vision statement, "To "create a community where patients, healthcare professionals and researchers come together to conquer the complexities of Sjögren's." The SF has been recognized annually since 2005 for meeting the National Health Council Standards of Excellence and has also received the Independent Charities of America Seal of Excellence.

Today, the foundation provides a community for Sjögren's syndrome patients with multiple modalities for social connectiveness (emotional support), for accessing information (informational support): planning care strategies (appraisal support), and for ensuring a better world in which access to therapies and knowledgeable clinicians is available (instrumental support). To accomplish these goals, the SF closely adheres to its core missions

- to support Sjögren's syndrome patients and their loved ones through education, resources, and services;
- to provide credible resources and education to healthcare professionals;
- to serve as the voice for all Sjögren's syndrome patients through advocacy and awareness initiatives;
- to lead, encourage, and fund innovative research projects to better understand, diagnose, and treat Sjögren's syndrome.

Some examples are provided in the following.

Support and communication

As discussed, evidence suggests that being part of a social community helps alleviate symptoms and improve overall health. The SF offers a variety of means for support, including 65 local support groups in the United States, 100 patient-volunteers who take calls from other patients, and the ability to expand patient connections with 30 additional groups worldwide through the International Sjögren's Network. Patients also engage in discussions with one another via Facebook, the *Smart Patients* online forum, and the SSF blog on *Conquering Sjögren's*. In addition, the SF holds an annual National Patient Conference that brings more than 450 patients together and provides a wonderful opportunity for patients to interact while also hearing the latest information on the disease from noted healthcare professionals. The SF also sponsors a series of "walkabouts" throughout the year in different parts of the country in order to bring people together in an effort to raise the much needed funds for research.

Patient education

The SF provides a wealth of Web-based and other written materials on Sjögren's syndrome, including information on diagnosis, symptoms, risk factors for potential complications, and management and treatment. All materials are vetted by the SF Medical and Scientific Advisory Board, which is composed of leading clinicians and researchers representing all related disciplines. Having easy access to reliable and credible information helps patients reduce stress by better understanding their disease and learning about best clinical practices. Informational resources are readily available from the SF via

- the SF website at www.sjögrens.org;
- The Sjögren's Book, a publication for patients published by Oxford University Press;[27]

- brochures, patient education sheets, other Sjögren's syndrome—related books, and CDs;
- *The Moisture Seekers* patient newsletter, published nine times a year;
- the SF Clinical Practice Guidelines for management and treatment of Sjögren's syndrome, an ongoing initiative that has resulted in 4 publications to date[28–31] and will eventually cover 16 rheumatology/systemic areas and all aspects of oral and ocular management;
- Web-based links to social media, including Facebook, the online forum *Smart Patients*, Twitter, Instagram, Pinterest, LinkedIn, and YouTube.

The SF brings much needed hope to patients and their families through its many initiatives to improve quality of life. Two of the most important areas that will profoundly impact patients' lives in the coming years are the development of Clinical Practice Guidelines and the formation of the SF Clinical Trials Consortium.

Engaging the professional community

The SF Clinical Practice Guidelines for the oral, ocular, and systemic management of the disease represent an ambitious undertaking involving a rigorous and transparent methodology and including a Delphi consensus process utilizing Consensus Expert Panels. Phase 1 has already involved 172 expert clinician-volunteers and other stakeholders, generated 56 recommendations on the management of Sjögren's syndrome, and resulted in 6 posters at professional meetings and 4 publications in the medical literature. Phase 2 of the Clinical Practice Guidelines will involve many additional specialists outside rheumatology and oral and ocular medicine who also see Sjögren's syndrome patients, including specialists in pulmonology, neurology, neuro-ophthalmology, neuropsychology, psychiatry, oncology, and sleep medicine.

The SF Clinical Trials Consortium comprises an international effort to advance the development of new therapies for Sjögren's syndrome. Its goals are to support and promote objectives that facilitate the design and implementation of clinical trials, to increase industry partnerships, and to engage in dialogue with government agencies that oversee therapy approval. As such, the consortium started by initiating meetings with the US Food and Drug Administration to define parameters for medication approval. The SF has also now developed an online educational tool called STEP (Sjögren's Training and Educational Platform), which provides training by international experts for using ESSDAI (European League Against Rheumatism Sjögren's Syndrome Disease Activity Index)[32] in clinical trials. STEP also will provide training on the execution and interpretation of various outcome measures and testing used in Sjögren's syndrome research. The consortium is also working to develop better endpoints and novel biomarkers for use in clinical trials and/or other aspects of care.

The SF also increases professional awareness and education through its complimentary newsletter for healthcare professionals, the *Sjögren's Quarterly*, as well as through the Clinical Practice Guidelines and all the SF multimedia communication venues mentioned earlier. The foundation regularly recruits patient-volunteers to act as Awareness Ambassadors to help educate and support their local community of medical providers by providing them with complimentary up-to-date patient materials on various aspects of the disease as well as information on various SF activities. This practice not only increases the awareness of Sjögren's syndrome and its morbidities among professionals but also offers patients a means of empowerment and an important role in shaping how professionals view this serious disorder.

Finally, with new discoveries comes new hope for improving patients' lives. To that end the SF annually awards thousands of dollars of research grants and supports other research programs to keep investigators focused on finding answers that will improve our knowledge of Sjögren's syndrome and, subsequently, lead to advances in treatment. Additionally, SF representatives regularly advocate on Capitol Hill to increase federal research funding for Sjögren's syndrome. The foundation has also added a strong voice to the various medical and patient coalitions that support legislation to increase patient access to more therapies and at a more reasonable cost, including both prescription drugs and over-the-counter products.

Conclusions

In summary, healthcare providers should refer their patients to the SF as part of their overall management plan. Sjögren's syndrome patients can add their voices to thousands of others to create a formidable force for advocacy to change the way their disease is perceived, managed, and treated. This alone provides an important empowerment tool for every individual. Most of all, joining the SF brings patients into a community that provides validation for the many difficulties they face and vital social support that can improve their health both physically and emotionally. As two Sjögren's syndrome patients, Corrie and Stacey, stated in the online SF forum *Smart Patients*, "Our paths may not be identical, but you will never walk alone. We are stronger and smarter together." Patients may contact the SF by calling 1-800-475-673 or visiting www.sjögrens.org.

References

1. Sjögren's Syndrome Foundation. Burden of illness high in Sjögren's — SSF national patient survey results are in. *Sjögren's Quarterly*. 2017;12(2):6—9, 1.
2. Callaghan R, Prabu A, Allan RB, Clarke AE, Sutcliffe N, Pierre YS, Gordon C, Bowman SJ. Direct healthcare costs and predictors of costs in patients with primary Sjögren's syndrome. *Rheumatol*. January 2007;46(1):105—111.
3. Bowman SJ, St Pierre Y, Sutcliffe N, Isenberg DA, Goldblatt F, Price E, Hamburger J, Richards A, Rauz S, Regan M, Rigby S, Jones A, Mulherin D, Clarke AE. Estimating indirect costs in primary Sjögren's syndrome. *J Rheumatol*. May 2010;37(5):1010—1015.
4. Mandl TJ, Jørgensen TS, Skougaard M, Olsson P, Kristensen LE. Work disability in newly diagnosed patients with primary Sjögren syndrome. *J Rheumatol*. February 2017;44(2):209—215.

5. Lisitsyna TA, Veltishchev DY, Seravina OF, Kovalevskaya OB, Starovoytova MN, Desinova OV, Abramkin AA, Ovcharov PS, Vasil'ev VI, Alekberova ZS, Krasnov VN, Nasonov EL. Comparative analysis of anxiety-depressive spectrum disorders in patients with rheumatic diseases. *Ter Arkhiv*. May 11, 2018;90(5):30−37.

6. Omma A, Tecer D, Kucuksahin O, Sandikci SC, Yildiz F, Erten S. Do the European League against Rheumatism (EULAR) Sjögren's syndrome outcome measures correlate with impaired quality of life, fatigue, anxiety and depression in primary Sjögren's syndrome? *Arch Med Sci*. June 2018;14(4):830−837.

7. Cui Y, Xia L, Li L, Zhao Q, Chen S, Gu Z. Anxiety and depression in primary Sjögren's syndrome: a cross-sectional study. *BMC Psychiatry*. May 16, 2018;18(1):131.

8. Sternberg EM. *The balance within: the science connecting health and Emotions*. New York: WH Freeman and Co.; 2001.

9. Silverman MN, Sternberg EM. Glucocorticoid regulation of inflammation and its functional correlates: from HPA axis to glucocorticoid receptor dysfunction. *Ann N Y Acad Sci*. July 2012;1261:55−63.

10. O'Donovan A, Cohen BE, Seal KH, Bertenthal D, Margaretten M, Nishimi K, Neylan TC. Elevated risk for autoimmune disorders in Iraq and Afghanistan veterans with posttraumatic stress disorder. *Biol Psychiatry*. February 15, 2015;77(4): 365−374.

11. Jara LJ, Navaro C, Medina G, Vera-Lastra O, Blanco F. Immune-neuroendocrine interactions and autoimmune diseases. *Clin Dev Immunol*. 2006;13:109−123.

12. Dhabhar FS. Enhancing versus suppressive effects of stress on immune function: implications for immunoprotection and immunopathology. *Neuroimmunomodulation*. 2009; 16:300−317.

13. Elenkov IJ, Chrousos GP. Stress hormones, proinflammatory and anti-inflammatory cytokines, and autoimmunity. *Ann N Y Acad Sci*. 2002;966:290−303.

14. Karaiskos D, Mavragani CP, Makaroni S, Zinzaras E, Vougarelis M, Rabavilas A, Moutsopoulos HM. Stress, coping strategies and social support in patients with primary Sjögren's syndrome prior to disease onset: a retrospective case-control study. *Ann Rheum Dis*. January 2009;68(1):40−46.

15. Skopouli FN, Katsiougiannis S. How stress contributes to autoimmunity-lessons from Sjögren's syndrome. *FEBS Lett*. January 2018;592(1):5−14.

16. House JS, Landis KR, Umberson D. Social relationships and health. *Science*. July 29, 1988;241(4865):540−545.

17. House J, Robbins C, Metzner H. The association of social relationships and activities with mortality: prospective evidence from the Tecumseh Community Health Study. *Am J Epidemiol*. July 1982;116(1):123−140.

18. Simonton OC, Creighton J, Simonton SM. *Getting well Again*. New York: Bantam Books; 1980. First published by JP Tercher 1978.

19. Spiegel D, Bloom JR, Kraemer HC, Gottheil E. Effect of psychosocial treatment on survival of patients with metastatic breast cancer. *Lancet*. October 14, 1989;2(8668): 888−891.

20. Boen CE, Barrow DA, Bensen JT, Farnan L, Gerstel A, Hendrix LH, Yang YC. Social relationships, inflammation, and cancer survival. *Cancer Epidemiol Biomark Prev*. May 2018;27(5):541−549.

21. Shively C, Clarkson T, Kaplan J. Social deprivation and coronary artery atherosclerosis in female cynomolgus monkey. *Atherosclerosis*. May 1989;77(1):69−76.

22. Kamark T, Mannuck S, Jennings J. Social support reduces cardiovascular reactivity to psychological challenge: a laboratory model. *Psychosom Med.* 1990 Jan-Feb;52(1): 42−58.

23. Cohen S, Doyle WJ, Skoner DP, Raben BS, Gwaltney Jr JM. Social ties and susceptibility to the common cold. *J Am Med Assoc.* June 25, 1997;277(24):1940−1944.

24. Uchino BN. Social Support and health: a review of physiological processes potentially underlying links to disease outcomes. *J Behav Med.* August 2006;29(4):377−387.

25. Heinze JE, Kruger DJ, Reischl TM, Cupal S, Zimmerman MA. Relationships among disease, social support, and perceived health: a lifespan approach. *Am J Community Psychol.* December 2015;56(3−4):268−279.

26. Berkman LF, Glass T, Brissette I, Seeman TE. From social integration to health: Durkheim in the new millennium. *Soc Sci Med.* September 2000;51(6):843−857.

27. Wallace D, Carsons S, Alexander E, Vivino F, Morland Hammitt K, Taylor S. In: Assoc, ed. *The Sjögren's book.* NY, NY: Oxford University Press; 2012.

28. Vivino FB, Carsons SE, Foulks G, Daniels TE, Parke A, Brennan MT, Forstot SL, Scofield RH, Hammitt KM. New treatment guidelines for Sjögren's disease. *Rheum Dis Clin N Am.* August 2016;42(3):531−551.

29. Carsons SE, Vivino FB, Parke A, Carteron N, Sankar V, Brasington R, Brennan MT, Ehlers W, Fox R, Scofield H, Hammitt KM, Birnbaum J, Kassan S, Mandel S. Treatment guidelines for rheumatologic manifestations of Sjögren's: use of biologics, management of fatigue & inflammatory musculoskeletal pain. *Arthritis Care Res.* April 2017;69(4): 517−527.

30. Zero DT, Brennan MT, Daniels TE, Papas A, Steward C, Pinto A, Al-Hashimi I, Navazesh M, Rhodus N, Sciubba J, Singh M, Wu A, Frantsve-Hawley J, Tracy S, Fox PC, Lawrence-Ford T, Cohen S, Vivino F, Hammitt KM. Clinical practice guidelines for oral management in Sjögren's disease: dental caries prevention. *J Am Dent Assoc.* April 2016;147(4):295−305.

31. Foulks GN, Forstot SL, Donshik PC, Forstot JZ, Goldstein MH, Lemp MA, Nelson JD, Nichols KK, Pflugfelder SC, Tanzer JM, Asbell P, Hammitt K, Jacobs DS. Clinical guidelines for management of dry eye associated with Sjögren disease. *Ocul Surf.* April 2015;13(2):118−132.

32. Seror R, Ravaud P, Bowman SJ, Baron G, Tzioufas A, Theander E, Gottenberg JE, Bootsma H, Mariette X, Vitali C, EULAR Sjögren's Task Force. EULAR Sjögren's syndrome disease activity index: development of a consensus systemic disease activity index for primary Sjögren's syndrome. *Ann Rheum Dis.* June 2010;69(6):1103−1109.

Index

Printed and bound by CPI Group (UK) Ltd, Croydon, CR0 4YY

03/10/2024

01040349-0003